T0260427

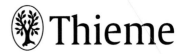

Emergency Imaging

A Practical Guide

Alexander B. Baxter, MD
Assistant Professor
Department of Radiology
New York University School of Medicine
New York, New York

with research and contributions by
Trudi Cloyd, MD
New York University Medical Center
New York, New York

1727 illustrations

Thieme
New York • Stuttgart • Delhi • Rio de Janeiro

Executive Editor: William Lamsback
Director, Editorial Services: Mary Jo Casey
Managing Editor: J. Owen Zurhellen IV
Production Editor: Kenneth L. Chumbley
International Production Director: Andreas Schabert
Vice President, Editorial and E-Product
  Development: Vera Spillner
International Marketing Director: Fiona Henderson
International Sales Director: Louisa Turrell
Director of Sales, North America: Mike Roseman
Senior Vice President and Chief Operating Officer:
  Sarah Vanderbilt
President: Brian D. Scanlan

Library of Congress Cataloging-in-Publication Data

Baxter, Alexander B., author.
Emergency imaging : a practical guide / Alexander
B. Baxter.
  p. ; cm.
  ISBN 978-1-60406-742-2 (alk. paper)
I. Title.
[DNLM: 1. Diagnostic Imaging. 2. Emergency
Medicine—methods. WN 180]
RC78.7.D53
616.07′54—dc23
                                    2015010462

© 2016 Thieme Medical Publishers, Inc.
Thieme Publishers New York
333 Seventh Avenue, New York, NY 10001 USA
+1 800 782 3488, customerservice@thieme.com

Thieme Publishers Stuttgart
Rüdigerstrasse 14, 70469 Stuttgart, Germany
+49 [0]711 8931 421, customerservice@thieme.de

Thieme Publishers Delhi
A-12, Second Floor, Sector-2, Noida-201301
Uttar Pradesh, India
+91 120 45 566 00, customerservice@thieme.in

Thieme Publishers Rio de Janeiro,
Thieme Publicações Ltda.
Argentina Building 16th floor, Ala A,
228 Praia do Botafogo
Rio de Janeiro 22250-040 Brazil
+55 21 3736-3631

Cover design: Thieme Publishing Group
Typesetting by Prairie Papers

Printed in the United States of
America by Sheridan Books, Inc.   5 4 3 2 1

ISBN 978-1-60406-742-2

Also available as an e-book:
eISBN 978-1-60406-743-9

Important note: Medicine is an ever-changing science undergoing continual development. Research and clinical experience are continually expanding our knowledge, in particular our knowledge of proper treatment and drug therapy. Insofar as this book mentions any dosage or application, readers may rest assured that the authors, editors, and publishers have made every effort to ensure that such references are in accordance with the state of knowledge at the time of production of the book.

Nevertheless, this does not involve, imply, or express any guarantee or responsibility on the part of the publishers in respect to any dosage instructions and forms of applications stated in the book. Every user is requested to examine carefully the manufacturers' leaflets accompanying each drug and to check, if necessary in consultation with a physician or specialist, whether the dosage schedules mentioned therein or the contraindications stated by the manufacturers differ from the state- ments made in the present book. Such examination is particularly important with drugs that are either rarely used or have been newly released on the market. Every dosage schedule or every form of application used is entirely at the user's own risk and responsibility. The authors and publishers request every user to report to the publishers any discrepancies or inaccuracies noticed. If errors in this work are found after publication, errata will be posted at www.thieme.com on the product description page.

Some of the product names, patents, and registered designs referred to in this book are in fact registered trademarks or proprietary names even though specific reference to this fact is not always made in the text. Therefore, the appearance of a name without designation as proprietary is not to be construed as a representation by the publisher that it is in the public domain.

Dedicated to my mother, Anita Yarost Baxter,
my father, Seymour Baxter, my brothers, Daniel and David,
and to my teachers

Contents

Foreword   xiii
Stuart E. Mervis, MD, FACR

Preface   xv

Acknowledgments   xvi

1 Introduction to Emergency Imaging   **1**
Observing and Interpreting
Reporting
Grading and Measuring
Incidental Findings
Learning Radiology
CT Window and Level
Approximate Radiation Doses for Emergency Studies (mSV)
CT Contrast Administration, Risks, and Adverse Reactions

2 Brain   **9**
Approach
Imaging and Anatomy
Clinical Presentations and Differential Diagnosis
Cerebral Edema Patterns
Anatomic Variants and Incidental Findings
Skull Fracture
Epidural Hematoma
Acute Subdural Hematoma
Subacute and Chronic Subdural Hematoma
Subdural Hygroma
Traumatic Subarachnoid Hemorrhage
Cerebral Contusion
Diffuse Axonal Injury
Pneumocephalus
Cerebral Swelling
Cerebral Herniation
Posttraumatic Atrophy and Encephalomalacia
Hypertensive Hemorrhage
Amyloid Angiopathy
Subarachnoid Hemorrhage
Arteriovenous Malformation
Cavernous Malformation
Anoxic Injury
Cerebral Infarct: Arterial Territories

Venous Sinus Thrombosis and Venous Infarct
White Matter Disease
Cerebritis and Brain Abscess
Herpes Encephalitis
Neurocysticercosis
Bacterial Meningitis
Low- and Intermediate-Grade Gliomas
Glioblastoma
Primary CNS Lymphoma
Cerebral Metastasis
Hydrocephalus

3 Head and Neck   **83**
Approach
Imaging and Anatomy
Clinical Presentations and Differential Diagnosis
Nasal and Naso-Orbito-Ethmoid Fracture
Zygomaticomaxillary Complex Fracture
Le Fort Fractures
Midface Smash Injury
Orbital Wall Fractures
Globe and Orbital Soft Tissue Injury
Temporal Bone Fracture
Mandible Fracture
Laryngeal Fracture
Cervical Vascular Injury
Sinus Obstruction and Inflammation
Nasopharyngeal Masses
Epiglottitis and Croup
Tonsillitis and Mononucleosis
Peritonsillar and Retropharyngeal Abscess
Prevertebral Abscess
Jugular Vein Thrombosis and Septic Jugular Thrombophlebitis
Cervical Adenitis
Lymphoma Involving the Head and Neck
Metastatic Head and Neck Carcinoma
Cervical Developmental Cysts and Masses
Dental Disease and Odontogenic Abscess
Sialolithiasis, Sialodochitis, and Sialadenitis
Orbital Cellulitis and Abscess
Orbital Inflammatory Disease
Dacryoadenitis and Dacryocystitis
Necrotizing External Otitis
Otitis Media and Mastoiditis
Petrous Apicitis

4 Spine   **151**
Approach
Imaging
Clinical Presentations and Differential Diagnosis
Craniocervical Junction Injuries
Atlantoaxial Rotatory Subluxation

C1 Burst (Jefferson) Fracture
Odontoid (Dens) Fracture
Traumatic C2 Spondylolisthesis
Cervical Hyperflexion Injury 1
Cervical Hyperflexion Injury 2
Cervical Hyperextension Injuries
Anterior Compression and Burst Fractures
Flexion-Distraction Injuries
Fracture-Dislocation
Fused-Spine Fracture
Spinal Epidural Hematoma
Discitis and Vertebral Osteomyelitis
Epidural Abscess
Myelitis and Radiculitis
Disc Herniation
Ankylosing Spondylitis
Spondylolysis and Spondylolisthesis
Spinal Cord Infarct
Spinal Dural Arteriovenous Fistula
Spinal Metastatic Disease
Spinal Schwannoma and Meningioma
Ependymoma

5 Chest   **205**
Approach and Analysis
Imaging and Anatomy
Clinical Presentations and Differential Diagnosis
Chest Wall Injuries
Pneumothorax
Hemothorax
Pulmonary Contusion and Laceration
Tracheobronchial Rupture
Traumatic Aortic Injury
Achalasia
Boerhaave Syndrome and Mediastinitis
Aortic Dissection and Nontraumatic Aortic Rupture
Pulmonary Embolism and Deep Venous Thrombosis
Pneumonia
Interstitial Pneumonia
Tuberculosis
Bronchiectasis and Cystic Fibrosis
Septic Pulmonary Embolism and Lung Abscess
Empyema
Pulmonary Arteriovenous Malformation
Pericardial Effusion
Pulmonary Edema
Emphysema
Pneumomediastinum
Lymphoma
Thymoma
Bronchogenic Carcinoma
Pancoast Tumor
Pulmonary Metastases

6 Abdomen and Pelvis   **267**
Approach
Imaging and Anatomy
Clinical Presentations and Differential Diagnosis
Diaphragm Rupture
Splenic Injury
Hepatic Injury
Renal Injury
Pancreatic Trauma
Shock Bowel and Small-Bowel Injury
Bladder and Urethral Injury
Gastric Ulcer/Gastric Outlet Obstruction
Duodenal Perforation
Acute Pancreatitis
Pancreatic Necrosis and Chronic Pancreatitis
Pancreatic Masses and Pancreatic Adenocarcinoma
Acute Cholecystitis
Hepatitis
Cirrhosis and Portal Venous Hypertension
Postsinusoidal Portal Venous Hypertension
Incidental Liver Masses
Hepatocellular Carcinoma
Cholangiocarcinoma
Hepatic Metastases
Hepatic Abscess
Nephrolithiasis
Pyelonephritis and Renal Abscess
Renal Infarct
Renal Masses and Renal Cell Carcinoma
Adrenal Nodules and Masses
Adrenal Hemorrhage
Intussusception
Abdominal Foreign Bodies and Body Packing
Small-Bowel Obstruction I
Small-Bowel Obstruction II
Cecal Volvulus
Sigmoid Volvulus
Acute Bowel Ischemia and Necrosis
Ischemic Colitis
Acute and Perforated Appendicitis
Epiploic Appendagitis and Omental Infarct
Mesenteric Adenitis
Pseudomembranous and Neutropenic Colitis
Crohn Disease
Ulcerative Colitis
Diverticulitis
Benign Pneumatosis Coli
Abdominal Abscess
Abdominal Lymphoma
Peritoneal Carcinomatosis
Sclerosing Mesenteritis
Abdominal Aortic Aneurysm
Retroperitoneal Hematoma
Incarcerated Inguinal Hernia

Benign and Indeterminate Ovarian Cysts
Cystic Ovarian Neoplasms and Ovarian Carcinoma
Ovarian Teratoma
Ruptured Ovarian Cysts
Ovarian Torsion
Tubo-Ovarian Abscess
Ruptured Ectopic Pregnancy
Testicular Torsion and Torsed Appendix Testis
Epididymitis and Epididymo-orchitis
Testicular Carcinoma

7 Musculoskeletal   **399**
Approach
Imaging
Orthopedic Hardware
Clinical Presentation and Differential Diagnosis
Scapular Fracture
Acromioclavicular Separation
Anterior Shoulder Dislocation and Luxatio Erecta
Posterior Shoulder Dislocation
Humeral Head Fracture
Elbow Dislocation
Radial Head Fracture and Essex-Lopresti Fracture-Dislocation
Ulnar Olecranon Fracture
Forearm Fractures
Distal Radius Fractures
Scaphoid Fracture and Scapholunate Dissociation
Perilunate and Lunate Dislocation
Nonscaphoid Carpal Fractures
Metacarpal Neck Fractures
Base of Thumb Fractures
Gamekeeper's Thumb
Finger Deformities
Dorsal and Volar Plate Avulsion Fractures
Pelvis Fractures
Acetabular Fracture
Femoral Neck Fractures
Ligamentous Injuries of the Knee
Patellar Fracture
Quadriceps and Patellar Tendon Rupture
Tibial Plateau Fracture
Baker Cyst
Tibial and Fibular Fractures
Achilles Tendon Rupture
Ankle Fractures
Osteochondral Fracture
Calcaneal Fracture
Talar Fracture and Subtalar Dislocation
Navicular Fracture
Lisfranc Fracture-Dislocation
Metatarsal Fractures
Cellulitis and Necrotizing Fasciitis
Bursitis
Septic Arthritis

Osteomyelitis
Lucent Bone Lesions I
Lucent Bone Lesions II
Skeletal Metastasis
Osteosarcoma and Parietal Osteosarcoma
Paget Disease of Bone
Multiple Myeloma and Plasmacytoma
Avascular Necrosis
Rheumatoid Arthritis and Osteoarthritis
Neuropathic Arthropathy and Gout

8 Pediatrics   **507**
Approach and Analysis
Imaging and Anatomy
Clinical Presentations and Differential Diagnosis
Nonaccidental Trauma
Lung Disease of Prematurity
Bronchiolitis and Acute Pediatric Pneumonia
Aspirated or Swallowed Foreign Body
Necrotizing Enterocolitis
Congenital Diaphragmatic Hernia
Proximal Bowel Obstruction
Hirschsprung Disease
Incomplete and Impacted Pediatric Fractures
Humeral Supracondylar Fracture
Humeral Epicondyle Avulsion Fractures
Slipped Capital Femoral Epiphysis
Hip Effusion
Toddler Fracture
Tillaux and Triplane Fracture

Index   543

Foreword

In the second year of radiology training, most residents across the United States start coverage in the emergency departments (ED) of their institutions. It is extremely common for the resident on this service to be busy giving initial readings, handling clinical and technical questions, filling out study protocols, and discussing and negotiating with other services over work-up decisions. For these novice radiologists beginning their emergency imaging training, it is a rather sudden jump into very cold water at the deep end of the pool, with a shark or two perhaps ramping up the anxiety.

ED imaging is a very demanding undertaking. A huge amount of information must be rapidly acquired before a resident can safely be released into this environment. Yes, there may be an attending radiologist to consult, but most likely he or she is also in "survival mode" and may have little time to answer questions and perhaps only rare opportunities to provide formal teaching. The pace of work in the emergency department is uncontrollable, and there are time limits for many types of studies to be reported and finalized. Surrender is not an option; the resident-in-training has an awesome task to perform to stay afloat.

Thirty-three years ago, when I was a junior resident, coping with ED radiology was quite a bit less challenging. Chest and bone radiographs were by far the most frequent studies. CT was still uncommon; it was time consuming and used mainly for assessing the brain. Occasionally, a barium GI study, sonogram (B-mode), or nuclear-medicine scan would turn up for review. The interpretations were not checked until early the next morning, so I had a few hours to verify my opinions, although with far fewer resources to consult than are available now. I even got three or four hours of sleep most nights. I thought I was working extremely hard, but today's radiology residents work under greater time pressure, handle far more studies, have more and varied responsibilities, and need to know more.

The advent of fast and readily available CT, and the general recognition that patients should receive equivalent medical care anytime they arrive in the ED, prompted the introduction of in-house attending and resident-level coverage 24/7 to quickly provide imaging reports. CT, in particular, provided accurate diagnostic information covering a far wider spectrum of diseases than was available before the extensive deployment of CT. Comprehension of more detailed CT anatomy and recognition of a greater variety of emergency pathology throughout the body was required. CT protocols had to be planned with greater precision to acquire specific information targeted to particular diagnoses. CT developed into the backbone of diagnosis in the ED, and its use has steadily increased given its wide range of applications, greater accuracy for diagnosis, and ready availability.

In recent years, MRI has also been used more frequently to answer diagnostic questions where CT either has little or no role or to clarify and expand upon the information provided by CT. Knowledge of MRI applications, protocols (sequences) required, and the appearance of various pathologies is increasingly necessary as MRI units are placed closer to or within the ED. Of course, radiographs remain the most frequently performed emergency imaging study. Sonograms and nuclear-medicine studies are still commonly evaluated by the on-call resident. Using sonography's various modes can be particularly time consuming to perform and challenging to interpret.

Quite clearly, the relatively young sub-specialty of emergency radiology requires diagnostic competence across many mo-dalities and covers a broad range of trau-matic and nontraumatic pathology. In addition, there are steadily increasing requirements for prompt interpretation of imaging studies to address rapidly pro-gressive and immediately life-threatening illnesses. Greater demands to perform fast and accurate triage, decrease expenses and waiting times, and maintain open beds in the ED require ever-faster study interpre-tation. There is not much time for reflect-ing upon one's report.

In writing *Emergency Imaging: A Practi-cal Guide*, Dr. Alexander Baxter, assistant professor of radiology at New York Univer-sity, had the radiology resident, preparing to cover the ED, in mind. The book he has written encompasses a wide variety of pa-thologies that are likely to be seen in the ED, emphasizing fundamental approaches to interpretation and providing well-estab-lished, useful information about a particu-lar condition. Dr. Baxter has a true passion for teaching and is exceptionally good at it. His knowledge of emergency radiol-ogy is extensive, given his long clinical and academic experience at a busy emergency-trauma center. He is a master at both how to teach effectively and what to teach to give the medical student, radiology resi-dent, and more seasoned radiologist what they need to build or reinforce their basic understanding of the subject and to create a foundation for more advanced learning.

The book attains this goal with a smooth-flowing, consistent literary style. Each chapter starts with a general review of pertinent anatomy, a checklist of struc-tures to focus on in an initial survey, study indications, protocols (mainly CT), special details of anatomy, clinical presentations, imaging correlation, and—for some enti-ties—basic treatment. The book succinctly covers considerable ground, describes the important items one must recognize in or-der to construct a reasonable differential diagnosis, and provides excellent images that clearly illustrate the diagnosis under consideration.

Emergency Imaging: A Practical Guide fills a vital niche in preparing trainees for their entry into the demanding environ-ment of emergency imaging and provides a solid foundation for acquiring more de-tailed knowledge and a deeper understand-ing of the subject. This book also serves as a refresher course for more experienced radiologists to renew their acquaintance with less commonly encountered emer-gency conditions and to pick up current in-formation pertinent to the field. This book would also be very useful to emergency medicine residents and intrepid medical students. The authorship of *Emergency Im-aging: A Practical Guide* is a one-man show and so required tremendous time and fo-cus. Dr. Baxter is to be congratulated for recognizing the need for this book and for his dedication to teaching. His book is the ideal starting point for learning emergency radiology. It will help residents swim con-fidently before jumping into the deep—possibly shark-infested—waters of the ER reading room.

Stuart E. Mirvis, MD, FACR
Professor of Radiology
Department of Radiology and
Nuclear Medicine
University of Maryland
School of Medicine
Past President of the
American Society of Emergency Radiology
Baltimore, Maryland

Preface

Like the oral board examination in Louisville, independent overnight call in radiology residency is a rite of passage that may soon be history. Twenty-four-hour-a-day attending coverage is now the standard at many medical centers, so the beginning resident is less likely to experience the terror of interpreting an unfamiliar or complicated study on his or her own, possibly with a fearsome surgeon breathing down his or her neck. But even with an in-house attending to lean on, the complexity and variety of emergency imaging studies, as well as the pace of work, can still be daunting for the trainee.

Intended as an introduction, a reference tool, and a starting point for further inquiry and study, *Emergency Imaging* provides an overview of the most common conditions encountered in trauma and emergency practice, as well as an approach to imaging study selection and interpretation. It is designed to prepare radiology residents for on-call coverage, build confidence in their interpretation skills, and provide ready access to the practical information they should have on hand in the emergency radiology reading room. This book should also be of value to clinicians who wish to improve their understanding of acute radiology.

I hope that *Emergency Imaging* will contribute to the efforts of residents and more seasoned physicians in their pursuit of first-rate patient care through thoughtful study selection, interpretation, and radiologic consultation.

Acknowledgments

For encouraging me to begin this project and helping me see it to completion, I gratefully acknowledge the support of Michael Selzer, Timothy Hiscock, William Lamsback, J. Owen Zurhellen IV, Kenneth Chumbley, Haskel Fleishaker, Mark Bernstein, Christa Muscato, Carolyn Boltin, Melvyn Feliciano, John McMenamy, Aspan Ohson, Ariel Friedman, and Mariya Kobe.

I offer my sincere appreciation to Trudi Cloyd for her heroic assistance with research and writing during her final year of medical school. And I thank the medical students who generously sacrificed portions of their summer vacations to help with research: Zachary Adler, Fernando Cuadrado, Brianna E. Damadian, Lauren Foster, Rachel Kaplan, Antonio Pires, Yoon Kyoung Choi, and Prabhjot Singh.

In addition, this book benefited from the expert editorial skills of Abby Bussel, the artistic abilities of Monte Antrim, and the technical assistance of Martha Burzynski.

I would also like to acknowledge the physicians who have profoundly influenced my development as a radiologist: Alexander R. Margulis, Steven Ross, Hideyo Minagi, and William D. Robertson.

Finally, this work would not have been possible without the inspiration, influence, and example of my teachers in other disciplines: John Teramoto, Tsutomu Ohshima, Tony Geballe, and Robert Fripp.

1
Introduction to Emergency Imaging

◆ Observing and Interpreting

Some examinations, such as a radiograph of a simple fracture in a long bone, can be appreciated immediately and accurately. Others, especially those involving complex anatomic structures such as the hand, wrist, or foot and most cross-sectional examinations, require a structured approach to ensure that all elements of the study have been reviewed. In reality, most radiologists and other observers use a combination of immediate recognition, or "gestalt," and a mental checklist, and the mix changes with experience. It is much easier to recognize an important finding if one has seen it before, preferably many times before.

Appreciating the significance of an imaging finding is as important as its recognition, and "normality" on a radiograph is a function of many factors, including age, body habitus and composition, radiograph or computed tomography (CT) image quality, and position. Experience and practice leads to both sensitivity in detecting subtle abnormalities and an understanding of whether a finding is truly pathologic.

◆ Reporting

The imaging report is the radiologist's work product. It consists of two major elements: a written description of all observations that support the diagnostic impression and a summary that contains one or several diagnoses and any necessary discussion or recommendations. The format of the report may vary depending on the type of study and the preferences of the radiologist or their institution, but it should always include the following:

- Body part imaged
- Technique
- Indication and relevant history
- Comparison studies (if any)
- Findings
- Impression

It is important to present one's findings and conclusions in a clear, organized, and succinct manner. Unfortunately, many reports are hobbled by wordiness, jargon, and redundancy.

Reports should be complete, but the ratio of "signal to noise" should be as high as possible, especially in the emergency setting. No one has time to wade through excessive, meandering, or unnecessary description of findings not pertinent to the primary goals of the treating emergency physician: acute management, patient disposition, or safe discharge from the emergency department. Although every radiologist will develop a personal style, usually by emulating teachers and colleagues, application of some basic principles will result in reports distinguished by clarity, brevity, and meaning.

Describe findings anatomically, especially when reporting studies of anatomically complex regions, such as the neck and abdomen. Within this context, try to address the findings relevant to the clinical question early in the report, and note incidental findings later.

If many findings—such as multiple facial fractures, intracranial metastases, or enlarged lymph nodes—need to be accounted for on a single report, list each one on a separate line rather than in a densely packed paragraph. Summarize the pattern or condition in the report's impression.

Avoid using "there is" before each finding. "No pneumothorax," for example, delivers the same information as "There is no pneumothorax."

Avoid "is seen," "is noted," "is demonstrated," and the like. These are the equivalent of putting "there is" in front of each finding. Simply state the finding.

Avoid "of the." It is usually possible (and preferred) to put an adjective in front of the noun it modifies. "The neck of the femur" is better described as "the femoral neck."

Avoid abbreviations and jargon. You do not know who will be reading your report. MR can mean mitral regurgitation to one physician and mental retardation to another. It is best to spell out most words and use conventional anatomic terminology: "The first carpometacarpal joint," for example, is understood by anyone who knows basic anatomy. Its synonym, "the basal joint," is known to hand surgeons but not necessarily to psychiatrists or internists, who may be caring for the patient.

While eponyms make for useful shorthand, they should be used in addition to, rather than in place of, a clear anatomic description: "A transverse, extra-articular, fifth metatarsal fracture, one centimeter from the base (Jones fracture)" is preferable to "fifth metatarsal Jones fracture."

Finally, if a word or phrase doesn't add to the meaning of the report, delete it. Radiologists are not meant to create a mood, develop a complex story line, or vividly paint a character. Our aim is to efficiently and effectively interpret the visual evidence presented in order to support an accurate clinical diagnosis and help direct treatment.

◆ Grading and Measuring

When a measurement is necessary to establish a diagnosis, or to provide the approximate size of a mass, it should be recorded in either one dimension (round masses/cysts) or three dimensions (oblong or complex masses). Specific measure-

ments and grading assignments necessary for surgical planning are usually best left to the treating physician, who usually has direct access to images and considerably more detailed clinical information than the radiologist does.

◆ Incidental Findings

"Incidentalomas"—cysts, nodules, osseous lesions, and visceral or other soft tissue masses—are frequently detected on imaging studies. Most are obviously benign, such as simple renal cysts or small ovarian cysts in reproductive-age women, and need not even be described. The radiologist should report any unexpected finding that could potentially endanger the patient in the future or that needs further imaging evaluation. At minimum, any patient with such a finding should be directed to appropriate primary or specialist physician referral. The radiologist should document that this has been communicated to the emergency physician in the report. Common incidental findings will be addressed by anatomic region in each section of this book. The most commonly encountered incidental findings include lung nodules and abdominal visceral cysts or masses.

◆ Learning Radiology

Diagnostic radiology is a broad discipline, and the scope of essential knowledge can be daunting to the student or resident. It is helpful to define learning goals at different stages of training and to remember that learning radiology, like learning anything, is a cyclical process of returning to the beginning again and again. Because one aim of this book is to support the novice radiologist and the learning that takes place in the first year of residency, the following suggestions are presented for consideration.

As a first-year resident, one's focus should be on learning the relevant anatomy for each rotation, learning to communicate results clearly both in reports and verbally, and acquainting oneself with the several hundred conditions likely to be encountered in the emergency setting. These also happen to be the most common diseases one will encounter in any but the most specialized practices. Since the first major step toward independence as a radiologist is beginning overnight call, it makes sense that one's work for the first 6 to 12 months of residency should be directed at preparation for that experience.

Some suggestions for learning in the first year:

- Interpret (and report) as many studies as you can by yourself. Watching other radiologists report studies is a poor substitute for coming to your own conclusions before reviewing them with a more experienced radiologist.
- Read about the diseases you encounter during the workday. Keep a list.
- Follow up uncertain findings (and some of the ones you feel certain about). Speak with clinicians when you can; check pathology and laboratory reports on patients whose studies you have interpreted to be sure of your impression.
- Learn radiographic, CT, ultrasound, and magnetic resonance (MR) anatomy as it applies to image interpretation.
- Practice "taking cases" with a colleague on a regular basis and from the beginning of training. You will learn the most from your fellow residents.
- Read other radiologists' reports, and pay attention to how clearly they express themselves. In your own reports, strive to develop concise written descriptions and terse, clear analysis of your findings.
- Learn the basic physical principles of radiography, CT, ultrasound, MR imaging (MRI), and nuclear medicine.
- Become acquainted with all common and many not-so-common emergent conditions.
- Know the imaging indications and the most appropriate studies for evaluating common conditions.
- Learn the various protocols for CT and MRI examinations and how to modify them to optimize a particular study.

◆ CT Window and Level

CT uses X-rays to create a three-dimensional density map of the patient. As an X-ray source rotates around the patient, the table supporting the patient slides through the scanner, perpendicular to the beam, and density data consisting of overlapping "voxels," or tiny volume units, is acquired based on the X-ray attenuation as it passes through the patient. This data is converted into sectional images in any plane, along a curved path, or as one of several types of three-dimensional reformations. The tissue density value for each voxel is measured in Houndsfield units (HU), after Godfrey Houndsfield, one of the inventors of CT. The densities of air and distilled water are defined as – 1,000 and 0 HU, respectively. While there is no upper limit, medical scanners use a scale of – 1,024 to + 3,171 (**Table 1.1**).

The CT "window" is a representation of the range of tissue densities visible on an image. The window width defines which densities are distributed over the visible grayscale; everything outside of the window is either black or white. The maximum CT window includes all measurable densities and therefore extends over 4,096 HU, more than the ~ 700 shades of gray that humans can distinguish under optimal conditions. The level indicates the center of the window selected and is usually close to the density of the tissue being examined. Consider the following example.

If one wants to evaluate the skull base and calvarium, one assigns a level close to

Table 1.1 Densities of various tissues

Tissue	Density (HU)
Air	– 1,000
Lung	– 500
Fat	– 100 to – 50
Water	0
CSF	15
Soft tissue	10–60
Blood	30–45
Bone	700–3,000

0 and a window of ~ 4,000. In this case, all 4,000 densities are distributed over ~ 700 distinguishable shades of gray. Soft tissues have densities between – 100 and 300, so their densities will be mapped to a relatively small number of gray tones in the middle of the window and will be indistinguishable from each other. The various densities of bone (cortical bone, bone marrow, trabeculae) are distributed over a much larger number of HU, so they will be visible in detail.

To optimally study the subtle differences in densities of the brain, on the other hand, one can a set a level of 30, the density of the brain in HU, and a window of 80, a relatively narrow setting. In this case, only 160 densities are distributed over the visible range, permitting visualization of blood, scalp, white matter, gray matter, and cerebrospinal fluid (CSF). With narrow windows, bone detail is limited, and all bone elements appear white. With these settings fat (– 70) and air (– 1,000) are also both outside of the window margins and will appear black. Widening the window to 150 would increase the visibility of fat as distinct from air (**Fig. 1.1**).

◆ Approximate Radiation Doses for Emergency Studies (mSv)

It is useful to have a sense of the relative radiation doses for common examinations, in comparison to natural background radiation, which is approximately 3–4 millisieverts (mSv) per year. Radiation doses above 10 mSv are associated with increased risk of cancer, with a 5% increased cancer risk at doses above 1,000 mSv (**Table 1.2**).

◆ CT Contrast Administration, Risks, and Adverse Reactions

Contrast material for CT examinations is administered via intravenous (IV) catheter. Rapid administration for arterial and venous visualization (as in pulmonary embolism, mesenteric ischemia, aortic dissection) generally requires a well-functioning, large-gauge peripheral catheter or central introducer sheath. In addition,

Table 1.2 Approximate radiation doses for emergency studies

Whole body doses	mSv
Dental X-ray	0.005
Background radiation, 1 day	0.01
Flight across United States	0.04
Chest X-ray	0.2
Mammogram	0.4
Extremity (per view)	0.5
Pelvis	0.7
Hip	0.8
Abdomen radiograph	1.2
Head CT	2
Ventilation/perfusion scan	2
Lumbar spine radiographs	3.5
Background radiation, 1 year	4
Conventional coronary angiography	5
Chest CT	8
Abdomen CT	10
Pelvis CT	10
Coronary CT angiography	15
Yearly maximum for radiation workers	50
Fetal doses with shielding (unless fetus is in field of view)	
Chest X-ray	< 0.01
Abdomen radiograph	2.4
Pelvis	1.7
Lumbar spine	3.4
Head CT	< 1
Chest CT	< 1
Abdomen CT	10
Pelvis CT	10

some patients are at increased risk for adverse, allergic-like reactions to contrast material. Such reactions range from mild to life-threatening; they can be mitigated by premedication, which reduces the incidence and severity of mild and moderate reactions and theoretically reduces the incidence of severe ones. The following discussion and recommendations are based on the New York University Medical Center and Bellevue Hospital Radiology Department practice policies.

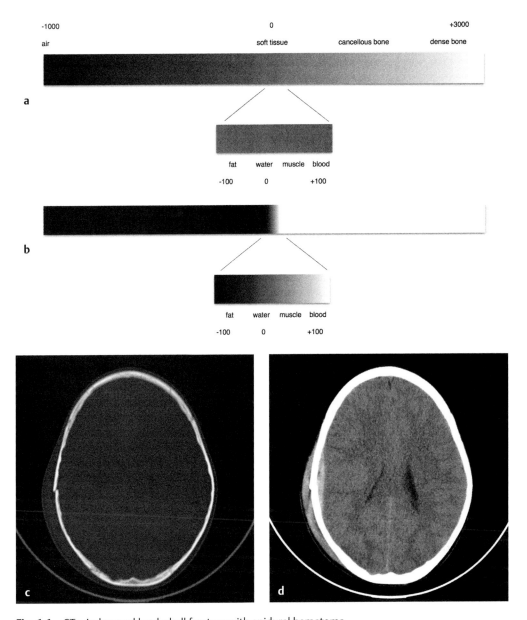

Fig. 1.1 CT window and level: skull fracture with epidural hematoma.
a,c Bone windows. Bone detail is superb, with clear definition of a right temporal bone fracture. The subjacent epidural hematoma is invisible, as it is mapped to the same shade of gray as the adjacent brain.
b,d Soft tissue windows. The epidural hematoma as well as the ventricles, scalp hematoma, gray matter, and white matter are all clearly distinguishable. The skull fracture is visible but less well seen than on wider windows.

IV Contrast Delivery and Maximum Flow Rates

Many CT examinations require rapid injection of contrast material for optimal vessel opacification. Small peripheral IV catheters and some central venous catheters cannot be reliably used for rapid injection. Examples of various catheters and their maximum flow rates are listed here (**Table 1.3**).

Idiosyncratic/Anaphylactoid Reaction to IV Contrast Material

- 0.6% incidence of all reactions (nonionic)
- 0.01–0.02% incidence of severe reactions (nonionic)
- ~ 1/170,000 fatality attributed to contrast injection

Adverse Reaction Classification

(**Table 1.4**)

Risk Factors for Idiosyncratic Reaction and Indications for Premedication

- Prior moderate or severe reaction to intravenous contrast material
- Asthma with active wheezing
- Asthma with history of event requiring intubation in past 90 days
- Any prior life-threatening allergic reaction

Mild or moderate reactions to other allergens (seafood, medications), mild urticarial reactions to contrast material, and mild to moderate asthma do not require premedication with steroids.

Elective Premedication

Recommended premedication consists of prednisone, 50 mg by mouth at 13 hours, 7 hours, and 1 hour before contrast media injection, plus diphenhydramine (Benadryl), 50 mg intravenously, intramuscularly, or by mouth 1 hour before contrast medium.

If the patient is unable to take oral medication, 200 mg of hydrocortisone intravenously may be substituted for oral prednisone.

Table 1.3   IV contrast delivery and maximum flow rates

Peripheral IV catheter	
20-gauge	up to 5 mL/sec
22-gauge	up to 3 mL/sec
24-gauge	up to 1.5 mL/sec
Triple-lumen central catheter	1 mL/sec
PICC line	1 mL/sec
Power PICC	Rate indicated on hub
Introducer sheath	up to 5 mL/sec
Broviac/Hickman	1 mL/sec

Table 1.4   Adverse reaction classification

Mild	Transient, self-limited, and not life-threatening: nausea, cough, headache, dizziness, itching, chills, flushing, chills, sweating, rash, nasal stuffiness
Moderate	Systemic and more severe mild reactions: pulse change, hypotension, hypertension, dyspnea/wheezing, urticaria, bronchospasm, laryngospasm
Severe	Potentially life-threatening: Unresponsiveness, convulsions, anaphylaxis, cardiopulmonary arrest, symptomatic arrhythmia

Emergency Premedication (in Decreasing Order of Effectiveness)

This premedication consists of methylprednisolone sodium succinate (Solu-Medrol) 40 mg or hydrocortisone sodium succinate (Solu-Cortef) 200 mg intravenously every 4 hours until contrast study required plus diphenhydramine 50 mg IV 1 hour prior to contrast injection.

Management of Idiosyncratic Reactions

Epinephrine is contraindicated in severe heart disease.

Mild Reaction

- Most require no specific treatment
- Discontinue injection, maintain IV access
- Monitor, reassure patient
- Diphenhydramine 25–50 mg PO/IV

Moderate Reaction

- Activate medical response team
- Supplemental oxygen
- Epinephrine 1:1,000 IM 0.3–0.5 ml every 5–15 minutes (begin as promptly as possible)
- Diphenhydramine 50 mg IV
- Metaproterenol or Albuterol inhaler for bronchospasm

Severe Reaction

- Activate medical response team
- Epinephrine 1:1000 IM 0.3-0.5 ml every 5-15 minutes (begin as promptly as possible)
- If response to IM epinephrine is inadequate, give epinephrine IV infusion, 2-10 micrograms/min
- Supplemental oxygen
- Nebulized Metaproteranol or Albuteral for bronchospasm
- Consider endotracheal intubation for airway edema/respiratory failure
- Normal saline bolus 1-2 liters

Hypotension and Bradycardia

- Trendelenberg
- Normal saline bolus 1-2 liters
- Atropine IV 0.6-1 mg to total dose of 2 mg (adults)

Seizure

- Protect airway

Contrast-Induced Nephropathy (CIN)

Risk Factors

Patients with certain underlying conditions are more likely to suffer contrast-induced renal injury and should have estimated glomerular filtration rate (eGFR) or serum creatinine levels prior to receiving intravenous contrast in order to better assess their risk. This group includes patients with:

- History of renal disease, prior kidney surgery, transplant, or single kidney
- Immediate family history of renal insufficiency
- Diabetes, collagen vascular disease, sickle cell disease, multiple myeloma, or gout
- Hypertension requiring medication
- Nephrotoxic medications (metformin, nonsteroidal anti-inflammatory drugs [NSAIDs])
- Further risk stratification is based on eGFR or serum creatinine.
- Category I: eGFR > 60 or serum creatinine < 1.5: These patients are normal and do not require any treatment beyond oral hydration
- Category II: eGFR 30–60 or serum creatinine 1.5–2.0: Oral or intravenous hydration 500–1,000 mL before and after CT examination. IV contrast dose should be limited to 75 mL
- Category III: eGFR < 30 or serum creatinine > 2.0: If an alternative study is not possible, the increased risk of CIN versus the benefits of intravenous contrast for the individual patient should be discussed with the referring clinician and documented in the medical record.

Diabetic Patients Taking Metformin (Glucophage)

If renal insufficiency develops after contrast administration, patients are at increased risk of lactic acidosis. Patients taking metformin should not take it for 48 hours after intravenous contrast administration.

Chronic Hemodialysis Patients (Renal Failure)

- No need for urgent dialysis
- Limit amount of contrast to reduce osmotic load

2
Brain

◆ Approach

Noncontrast head CT is one of the most frequently ordered emergency studies. Common indications include headache, suspected cerebral infarct or intracerebral hemorrhage, altered mental status, and trauma.

Images should always be evaluated with windows and reconstruction algorithms optimized for brain, subdural hematoma, and bone. In trauma, multidetector CT from the skull base to the upper thoracic spine can be acquired to image the head, cervical spine, face, and skull base in a single scan. Thin-section reconstructions and reformations in multiple planes or three-dimensional surface renderings can then be extracted from the imaging data obtained.

Noncontrast CT is the initial study for detection of hemorrhage, infarct, intracranial masses, traumatic injuries, and assessment of overall brain volume and quality. A normal noncontrast CT excludes most emergent and surgical conditions. MRI with gadolinium is more sensitive for detection of infectious or neoplastic conditions including metastases, cerebritis, meningitis, and leptomeningeal neoplasm, but it is not typically necessary for acute management. Contrast CT is an alternative if MRI is not available or contraindicated in a particular patient.

Cerebral CT angiography, in which images are obtained during the arterial or early venous phase of contrast enhancement, has largely replaced catheter angiography for primary detection of cerebral aneurysms, arteriovenous malformations (AVM), vascular injuries, and venous or cavernous sinus thrombosis. Conventional angiography is usually reserved for preoperative aneurysm or AVM evaluation, and endovascular therapy. CT perfusion imaging can be useful in identifying the location and extent of vascular compromise in patients with acute stroke symptoms.

On older scanners, brain CT is usually obtained nonhelically to avoid artifacts. Newer multislice CT systems permit adequate imaging of the brain in three planes as well as simultaneous acquisition of high-resolution images of the face and cervical spine in patients with acute head and neck trauma.

Checklist

- Scalp
- Skull
- Epidural space (potential)
- Subdural space (potential)
- Dural sinuses and reflections
- Cortex
- Subcortical white matter
- Basal ganglia
- Ventricles
- Cisterns
- Cerebral vessels
- Pituitary and sella turcica
- Skull base
- Orbits
- Sinuses
- Facial bones

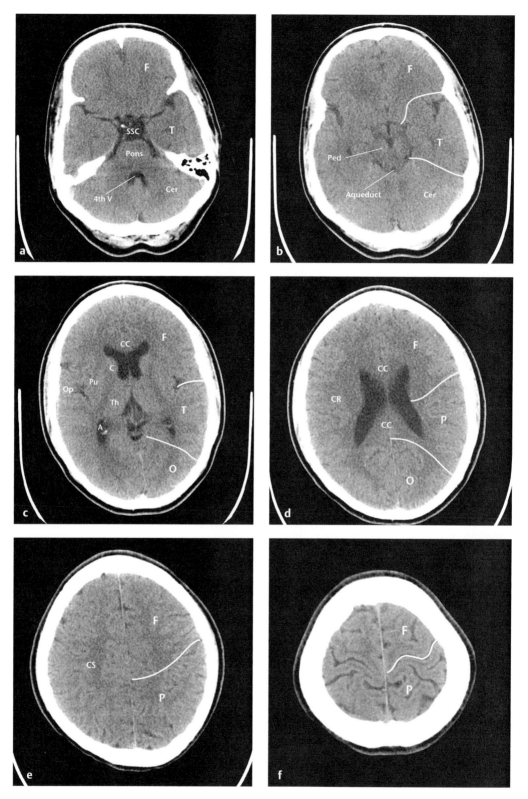

Fig. 2.1a–f   Cerebral anatomy. F: Frontal lobe. P: Parietal lobe. T: Temporal lobe: O: Occipital lobe. Cer: Cerebellum. CS: Centrum semiovale. CR: Corona radiata. CC: Corpus callosum. Th: Thalamus. Pu: Putamen. C: Caudate head. Op: Frontal operculum.

◆ Imaging and Anatomy

Imaging

Head CT (Noncontrast)

Indications: Head injury, altered mental status, seizure, suspected hemorrhage or infarct.

Technique: 5-mm axial images in soft tissue and bone algorithm

Head CT (Noncontrast Helical)

Indications: Head injury with concurrent imaging of the face and cervical spine.

Technique: Helical 0.6-mm dataset with 5-mm axial, 2-mm sagittal, and 2-mm coronal reformations of head, face, and cervical spine. Images obtained from skull vertex to thoracic inlet.

CT Arteriogram

Indications: Subarachnoid hemorrhage. Suspected aneurysm or vascular malformation. Acute cerebral infarct. Penetrating injury.

Technique: Helical 0.6-mm dataset with 2.5-mm axial, 2-mm sagittal, and 2-mm coronal reformations. Images can be obtained from the vertex either to the skull base or to the thoracic inlet depending on the indication.

Contrast: 60–100 mL at 3–4 mL/sec in arterial phase.

CT Venogram

Indications: Suspected venous sinus thrombosis (atypical headache). Trauma to skull base with potential venous sinus disruption.

Technique: Helical 0.6-mm dataset with 2.5-mm axial, 2-mm sagittal, and 2-mm coronal reformations. Images obtained from vertex to skull base.

Contrast: 60–100 mL at 3–4 mL/sec in venous phase (30–45 sec delay).

Anatomy

Effective description and analysis of cerebral pathology requires knowledge of visible cerebral structures (lobes, basal nuclei, ventricles), vascular territories, and arterial and venous anatomy. Cerebral anatomy is shown in **Fig. 2.1**. Cerebral vascular territories and anatomy are seen in **Fig. 2.2**.

◆ Clinical Presentations and Differential Diagnosis

Clinical Presentations and Appropriate Initial Studies

Trauma

Noncontrast head CT is indicated. Head or neck CT angiography should be considered if injury mechanism or initial findings indicate a likely cervical vascular injury.

- Skull fracture
- Epidural hematoma
- Subdural hematoma
- Venous epidural hematoma
- Traumatic subarachnoid hemorrhage
- Contusion
- Diffuse axonal injury
- Skull fracture
- Temporal bone fracture
- Facial bone fracture

Headache

Noncontrast head CT is indicated. Postcontrast head CT or MRI may be considered in immunocompromised patients, in those with underlying malignancy and concern for metastatic disease, and in patients otherwise at risk for brain abscess.

- Subarachnoid hemorrhage
- Venous sinus thrombosis
- Meningitis
- Hydrocephalus
- Cerebral hemorrhage
- Mass (tumor or abscess)
- Sinusitis
- Otitis/mastoiditis

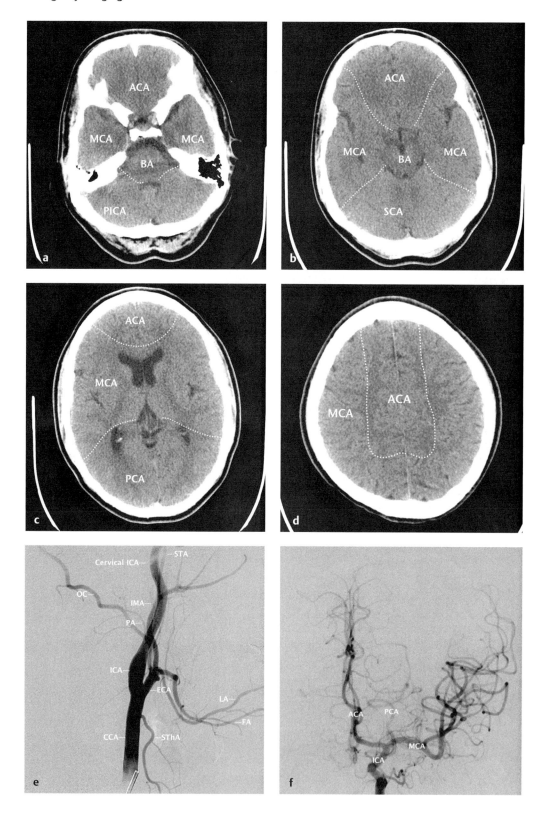

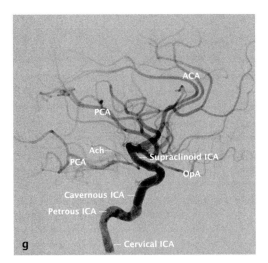

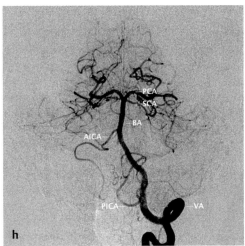

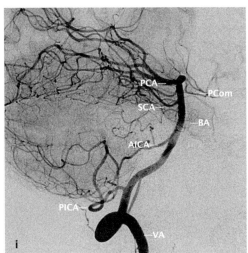

Fig. 2.2a–i Cerebral vascular territories and anatomy. ACA: Anterior cerebral artery. PCA: Posterior cerebral artery. MCA: Middle cerebral artery. Ach: Anterior choroidal artery. CCA: Common carotid artery. ICA: Internal carotid artery. ECA: External carotid artery. SThA: Superior thyroidal artery. LA: Lingual artery. FA: Facial artery. PA: Posterior auricular artery. OC: Occipital artery. IMA: Internal maxillary artery. STA: Superficial temporal artery. BA: Basilar artery. SCA: Superior cerebellar artery. PICA: Posterior inferior cerebellar artery. AICA: Anterior inferior cerebellar artery. PCom: Posterior communicating artery.

Acute Focal Neurologic Deficit

Noncontrast head CT is indicated to exclude hemorrhage in suspected stroke. Noncontrast head CT should be obtained to detect or exclude cerebral hemorrhage. MRI with a diffusion-weighted sequence can confirm the clinical suspicion of infarct in patients whose initial CT appears to be normal. CT or MR angiography and perfusion studies can be obtained to better characterize the extent of ischemia and identify vascular stenoses or occlusion.

- Ischemic infarct
- Lacunar infarct
- Embolic infarct
- Border-zone (watershed) infarct
- Hypertensive hemorrhage
- Amyloid angiopathy with hemorrhage
- Ruptured arteriovenous malformation

Altered Mental Status

Noncontrast head CT is indicated. Postcontrast head CT or MRI may be considered in immunocompromised patients, in those with underlying malignancy and concern for metastatic disease, in patients otherwise at risk for brain abscess, and to evaluate further subtle abnormalities on noncontrast CT.

- Cerebritis (herpes encephalitis)
- Infarct
- Hemorrhage
- Parenchymal volume loss
- Chronic subdural hematoma

Differential Diagnoses

Intraparenchymal Mass

- Glioma
- Metastasis
- Lymphoma
- Abscess
- Arteriovenous malformation

Extraparenchymal Mass

- Meningioma
- Calvarial or dural metastasis
- Epidermoid
- Schwannoma (cranial nerves 5, 8, and 9)
- Arachnoid cyst
- Aneurysm

Sellar and Suprasellar Mass (Mnemonic: SATCHMO)

- Sellar tumor (pituitary adenoma), sarcoidosis
- Aneurysm
- Teratoma (and germ cell tumors)
- Craniopharyngioma
- Hypothalamic glioma
- Meningioma (planum sphenoidale) and metastasis
- Optic glioma

Ring Enhancing Mass (Mnemonic: MAGIC DR)

- Metastasis
- Abscess
- Glioma
- Infarct (evolving)
- Contusion (evolving)
- Demyelinating disease
- Radiation necrosis

Hemorrhagic Metastases (Mnemonic: CT/MR)

- Choriocarcinoma
- Thyroid carcinoma
- Melanoma
- Renal cell carcinoma

Remember that lung and breast carcinoma, even though less frequently hemorrhagic, are much more common and are more likely to be the cause of a hemorrhagic metastasis.

Parenchymal Hemorrhage

- Hypertensive hemorrhage
- Amyloid angiopathy
- Hemorrhagic metastasis
- Herpes encephalitis
- Acute leukemia
- Arteriovenous malformation
- Aneurysm
- Contusion (in trauma)

Subarachnoid Hemorrhage

- Ruptured aneurysm
- Benign perimesencephalic hemorrhage
- Traumatic subarachnoid hemorrhage

Global Cerebral Volume Loss

- Chronic alcohol use
- Anticonvulsants (particularly cerebellar)
- Dehydration
- Steroid use
- Chemotherapy
- Remote head injury
- Normal aging

Communicating Hydrocephalus

- Normal pressure hydrocephalus
- Meningitis
- Prior subarachnoid hemorrhage
- Venous sinus thrombosis

Obstructive Hydrocephalus

- Aqueductal stenosis
- Colloid cyst of third ventricle
- Tectal glioma
- Intraventricular tumor

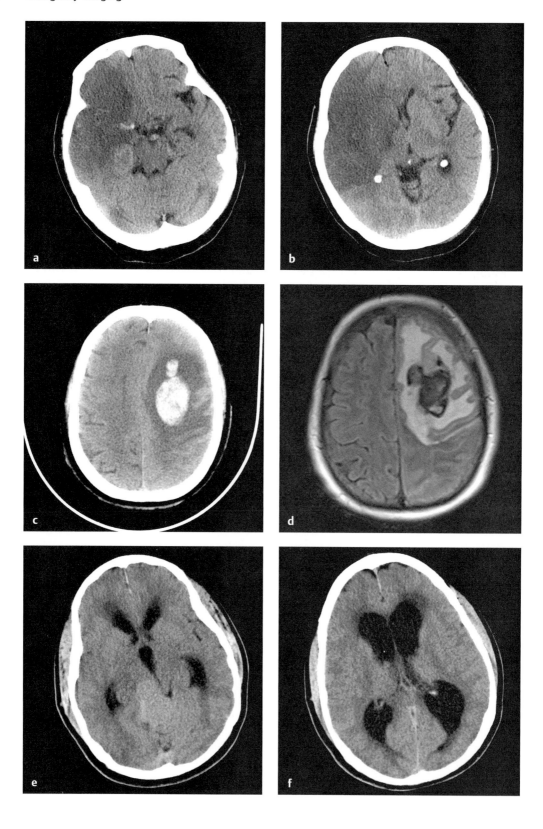

◆ Cerebral Edema Patterns

Localized cerebral edema may be classified as cytotoxic, vasogenic, or interstitial, although overlap is often present. Cytotoxic edema consists of intracellular swelling caused by depletion of adenosine triphosphate (ATP) and consequent sodium/potassium membrane pump failure. Most typical of cerebral infarct and anoxic injury, cytotoxic edema affects both white and gray matter similarly on most imaging studies.

Vasogenic edema, in contrast, preferentially involves white matter and results from conditions that increase intracerebral capillary permeability. Vasogenic edema is often due to brain contusion, severe hypertensive disease, primary and metastatic neoplasms, or inflammatory conditions.

Acute hydrocephalus can cause interstitial edema, as elevated intraventricular pressure leads to transependymal migration of CSF into the periventricular white matter, where it is resorbed via parenchymal capillaries.

On CT, cerebral edema is lower in density than surrounding normal parenchyma. On MRI, signal intensity of edema is lower than that of brain parenchyma on T1-weighted images and higher on T2-weighted images. Diffusion-weighted image (DWI) and apparent diffusion coefficient (ADC) mapping sequences can distinguish between cytotoxic edema (restricted diffusion) and vasogenic or interstitial edema (normal or increased diffusion). Fluid attenuation inversion recovery (FLAIR) sequences suppress intraventricular CSF signal and are sensitive for detecting adjacent areas of interstitial edema (**Fig. 2.3**).

Fig. 2.3a–f
a,b   Cytotoxic edema in cerebral infarction. Extensive right frontal and temporal low-density change with loss of differentiation between gray and white matter, sulcal effacement, and ipsilateral ventricular effacement. The middle cerebral artery is dense, indicating thrombosis.
c,d   Vasogenic edema due to hemorrhagic brain metastasis from lung carcinoma. Left frontal white matter hemorrhage with surrounding low attenuation edema that spares the cortical gray matter. FLAIR MRI shows a hemorrhagic nodule with extensive surrounding high-signal edema limited to the white matter.
e,f   Interstitial edema in hydrocephalus due to fourth-ventricle obstruction by meningioma. Acute hydrocephalus with low-density transependymal CSF resorption, most conspicuous at the frontal, occipital, and temporal horns of the lateral ventricles.

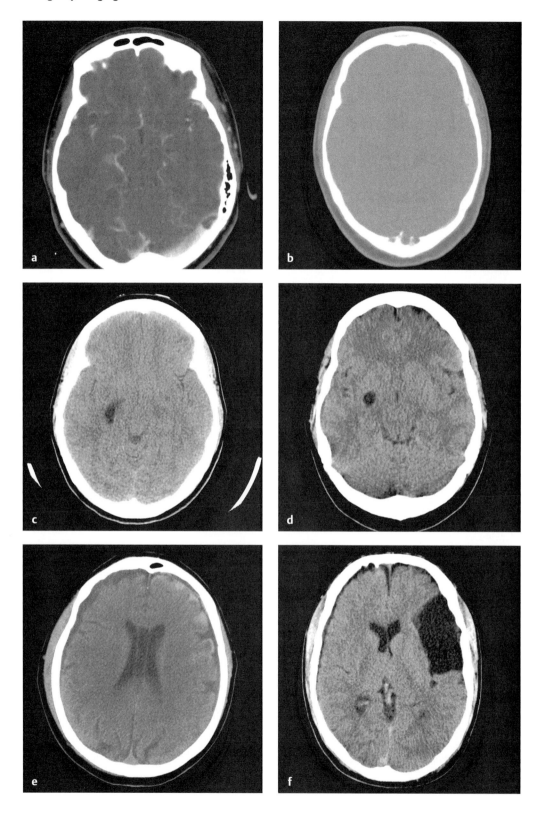

◆ Anatomic Variants and Incidental Findings

Common incidental findings on head CT include arachnoid cysts, prominent arachnoid granulations, choroid plexus and choroidal fissure cysts, remote lacunar infarcts, focal encephalomalacia from prior infarct or trauma, and prominent perivascular spaces. The ventricles may be slightly asymmetric, and the septum pellucidum may contain a central CSF-filled cavity (cavum septum pellucidum). Unless symptomatic, these conditions usually do not require specific follow-up (**Fig. 2.4**).

Fig. 2.4a–f
a,b Arachnoid granulation. When visible, arachnoid granulations, which resorb CSF into the venous system, appear as filling defects in the opacified venous sinuses. They may also cause smooth erosion of the bone adjacent to the sinus. (**a**) Round filling defect in opacified left transverse sinus. Round osseous erosions near the internal occipital protruberance/torcular Hirophili.
c Choroidal fissure cyst. These small CSF attenuation cysts arise in the choroidal fissure and appear lateral to the midbrain or cerebral peduncle on axial images.
d Enlarged perivascular space. 8-mm CSF attenuation space located in the right posterior putamen.
e Cavum septum pellucidum. A developmental variant due to failed embryonic fusion of the leaves of the septum pellucidum, it is present in ~15% of individuals. This CT image also shows cortical contusions, traumatic subarachnoid hemorrhage, and subacute bifrontal frontal subdural hygromas.
f Arachnoid cyst. CSF attenuation, extra-axial collection due to duplication in the arachnoid membrane, which compresses the adjacent brain and may smoothly expand the overlying calvarium. These are usually asymptomatic; however, larger cysts may predispose to hemorrhage in minor trauma or can cause symptoms by compression of the brain. Epidermoids can have a similar appearance on CT, but they have characteristically high signal on FLAIR MRI.

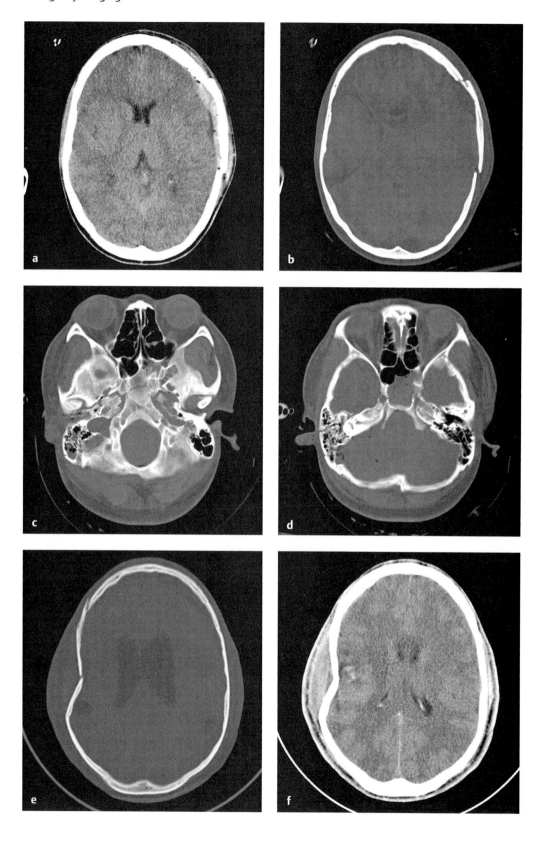

◆ Skull Fracture

A calvarial fracture does not reliably predict underlying brain injury, and a normal skull radiograph does not exclude intracranial injury. Calvarial fractures that are depressed more than 5 mm are usually elevated surgically. Epidural hematoma is associated with fractures that traverse the course of the middle meningeal artery. Skull base fractures are associated with high-energy trauma and with more severe brain injury; the most common locations include the petrous temporal bone, the basiocciput, the sphenoid bone, and the ethmoid bone.

Anterior skull base fractures traverse the paranasal sinuses and orbit, and they can disrupt the cribriform plate and optic canals. Clinical consequences include CSF rhinorrhea, periorbital ecchymosis ("raccoon eyes"), and olfactory or optic nerve damage. Trauma to the central skull base, usually from lateral impact, results in petrous temporal bone fractures and may be associated with CSF otorrhea, hemotympanum, mastoid ecchymosis ("Battle sign"), facial nerve palsy, vertigo, tinnitus, and conductive or sensorineural hearing loss. Fractures through the clivus can injure the sixth cranial nerve. Posterior skull base fractures can injure the dural venous sinuses, resulting in posterior fossa epidural hematoma or dural sinus thrombosis and venous infarct. If the fracture extends to the occipital condyles, it can lead to craniocervical instability.

Most skull base fractures are identified on noncontrast head CT obtained for evaluation of head trauma. High-energy impact and fractures that traverse the carotid canals or cavernous sinus can be associated with carotid or vertebral injury, including dissection and pseudoaneurysm. Vascular injury places the patient at increased risk for secondary embolic cerebral infarct, which can be prevented with anticoagulation. Because of this risk, CT angiography with helical thin-section imaging is generally advised in this group (**Fig. 2.5**).

Fig. 2.5a–d
a,b Calvarial fracture. Left frontal calvarial fracture with small subjacent epidural hematoma and minimal intracranial air. The fracture fragment is elevated one-half calvarial width relative to the remainder of the skull.
c,d Skull base fracture. Nondisplaced longitudinal right temporal bone fracture that traverses the basisphenoid (clivus) and basiocciput. Blood is present in the sphenoid sinus and the right mastoid air cells. A small amount of air is present in the posterior fossa.
e,f Depressed skull fracture. Right parietal calvarial fracture with 1.8-cm depression and subjacent cortical contusion.

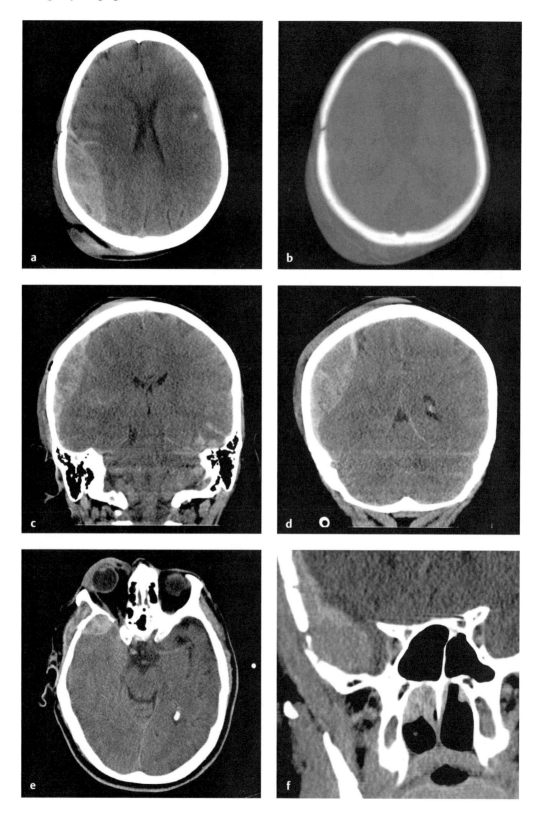

◆ Epidural Hematoma

Most epidural hematomas (EDH) are of arterial origin and result from calvarial fractures that cross branches of the middle meningeal artery. Hemorrhage under arterial pressure separates the outer layer of the dura from the skull, creating an extraparenchymal intracranial mass that compresses the adjacent brain, leading to ischemia and potential compartmental herniation. Epidural hematomas can enlarge rapidly and, if not treated, are often rapidly fatal. With early evacuation, however, the prognosis is good; the skull absorbs most of the energy of impact as it fractures, sparing the underlying brain parenchyma from direct injury.

An acute EDH is a smooth, hyperdense biconvex extraparenchymal blood collection, limited by the coronal sutures, to which the dura is especially adherent. Hyperacute, active bleeding has an inhomogeneous, swirling appearance due to a mixture of clotted and unclotted blood.

Venous epidural hematomas, which account for approximately 10% of EDHs, are the consequence of dural venous sinus disruption or, rarely, diploic vein or arachnoid granulation rupture. They are low-pressure hemorrhages that typically do not enlarge over time and rarely require evacuation. In contrast to arterial hematomas, traumatic venous EDHs often occur in children and are not necessarily associated with skull fractures. They are most commonly seen in the middle cranial fossa adjacent to the greater wing of the sphenoid bone, where venous EDHs are due to disruption of the sphenoparietal venous sinus. They also may follow injury to the sagittal or transverse sinuses and can traverse the tentorium at the occiput or the falx at the vertex (**Fig. 2.6**).

Fig. 2.6a–f
a–d Arterial epidural hematoma. Hyperdense, right parietal, lenticular, extraparenchymal hematoma with maximal thickness 2.7 cm. Ipsilateral cortical sulcal and lateral ventricular compression with minimal subfalcine shift. Contralateral anterior temporal lobe hemorrhagic contusion. Right parietal vertex scalp hematoma and laceration.
e,f Venous epidural hematoma. Lenticular (1-cm) extraparenchymal mixed-density hemorrhage adjacent to the right sphenotemporal buttress with mild compression of the anterior temporal lobe. Right preseptal periorbital and temporal scalp hematoma. The underlying brain parenchyma is normal, and the perimesencephalic cisterns are patent.

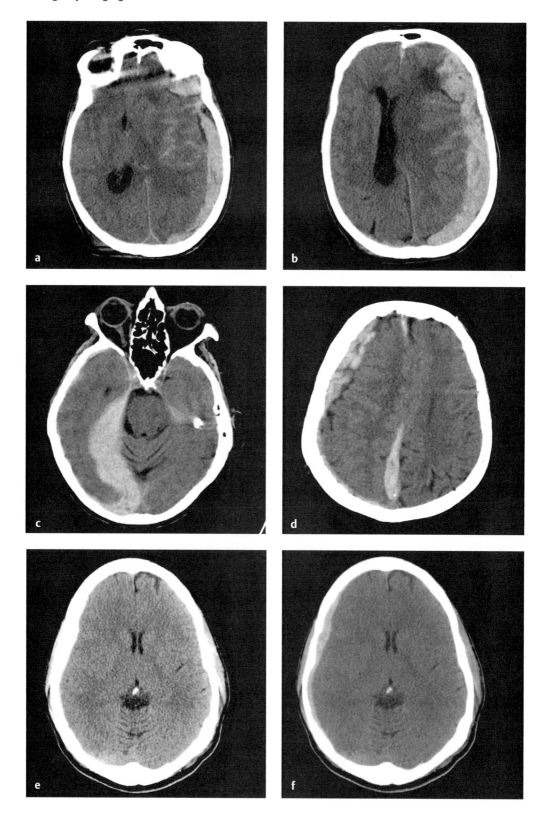

◆ Acute Subdural Hematoma

Acute subdural hematomas (SDHs) occur when cortical veins that traverse the subdural space are torn under cerebral acceleration or rotation. Blood accumulates between the inner (meningeal) layer of the dura, which is firmly attached to the skull, and the smooth arachnoid membrane loosely adherent to the surface of the brain. Uncommonly, a primary parenchymal or subarachnoid hemorrhage can disrupt the arachnoid membrane and rupture into the subdural space. SDH is associated with a skull fracture in less than 50% of cases and is typically a "contrecoup" injury that results from recoil of the brain away from the inner surface of the skull opposite the site of impact.

Especially in younger patients, an acute SDH indicates significant energy transfer and is frequently associated with severe parenchymal brain injury, brain herniation, and cerebral ischemia. SDH due to minor trauma is more common in the elderly and in patients with cerebral atrophy. Parenchymal volume loss and enlarged CSF spaces allow the brain to move more freely in the calvarium and compromise the ability of the brain to tamponade low-pressure hemorrhages. In such patients, enlarged extracerebral space limits the degree of parenchymal compression and ischemia.

Acute SDHs are crescentic, hyperdense, and usually homogeneous. They can extend along the entire hemisphere and are confined by the falcine and tentorial dural reflections. In contrast to most EDHs, SDH is not limited by calvarial sutures. Venous hemorrhage is usually more gradual than arterial bleeding, and SDHs can develop more slowly than EDHs. Nonetheless, large SDHs can cause acute and severe neurologic deterioration and often require urgent evacuation. Hematoma thickness or subfalcine shift of 2 cm or greater is associated with a particularly poor prognosis.

The density of subdural clot can overlap with that of calvarial bone on narrow CT windows optimized for evaluation of brain parenchyma, and small subdural hematomas can be difficult to detect. To avoid this error, head CT obtained for trauma should always be viewed at both narrow and wide (subdural) window settings (**Fig. 2.7**).

Fig. 2.7a–f
a,b Acute subdural hematoma. 1.8-cm hyperdense left holohemispheric subdural hematoma with traumatic subarachnoid hemorrhage, 1.6-cm subfalcine shift, compression of the left lateral ventricle, and trapping of the right lateral ventricle.
c,d Large right subdural hematoma with prominent frontal, parafalcine, and tentorial hyperdense collections.
e,f Window and level in detecting subdural hematoma. (**e**) CT window = 80 (brain) shows subtle effacement of right frontal sulci, but otherwise apparently normal brain. (**f**) CT window = 170 (subdural). A 5-mm right frontotemporal subdural hematoma is now clearly evident.

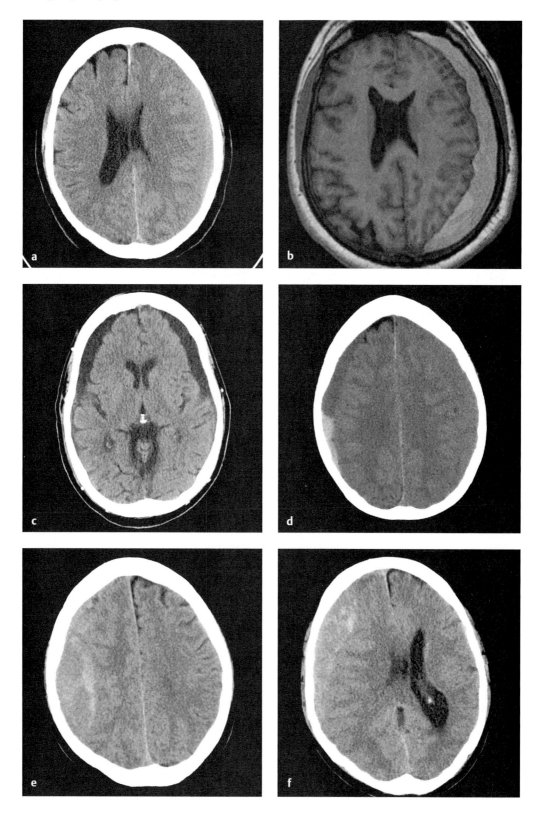

◆ Subacute and Chronic Subdural Hematoma

SDHs evolve over time. Hyperacute hemorrhage, seen in the rare patient imaged immediately after injury, can be hypodense or mixed-density. Most patients are imaged after coagulation has taken place, and acute SDHs are typically hyperdense and crescentic. As an acute SDH ages, protein degradation occurs, extracellular fluid shifts into the hematoma, and density decreases.

SDHs that are 2 to 3 weeks old may be isodense to the adjacent cortex and difficult to detect, especially when they are small or bilateral. MRI or CT+C is more sensitive than NCCT for identification of these subtle hematomas. SDHs of any age can be complicated by rehemorrhage, which can convert a small, well-tolerated subacute SDH into a larger, symptomatic mass.

Three weeks or more after hemorrhage, a SDH is considered chronic. By this time, most simple hematomas are hypodense compared with brain and approach the density of CSF. Unevacuated hematomas incite a local inflammatory response that leads to formation of a fibrinous capsule and fragile, vascularized membranes. These can rupture spontaneously or with minor trauma, and patients who have had a previous SDH are at increased risk of hemorrhage. Delayed bleeding into the subdural space complicates up to one-third of chronic SDHs and appears as hyperdense clot within the lower-density hematoma. Rehemorrhage into a chronic SDH may also appear convex rather than crescentic due to confinement by inflammatory membranes.

Blood fluid levels can be seen in chronic or subacute SDH complicated by rehemorrhage, following lysis of the initial hematoma. Acute or subacute SDH in patients who are taking anticoagulants or are otherwise coagulopathic can also show blood fluid levels (**Fig. 2.8**).

Fig. 2.8a–f
a,b Subacute subdural hematoma. (**a**) CT left holohemispheric subdural hematoma, near isodense to cerebral cortex. Effaced left sulci and lateral ventricle with slight left to right subfalcine shift. (**b**) MRI T1-weighted image more clearly shows extent of subdural hematoma.
c Chronic subdural hematoma. Low-attenuation subdural fluid collections with minimal dependent blood products. Underlying cerebral volume loss and moderate symmetric compression of the frontal brain parenchyma.
d Chronic subdural hematoma with rehemorrhage. Left, isodense SDH. Right, low-density SDH with layering blood products.
e,f Complex subdural hematoma. Rehemorrhage with mixed density and lenticular shape due to confinement of clot by membranes.

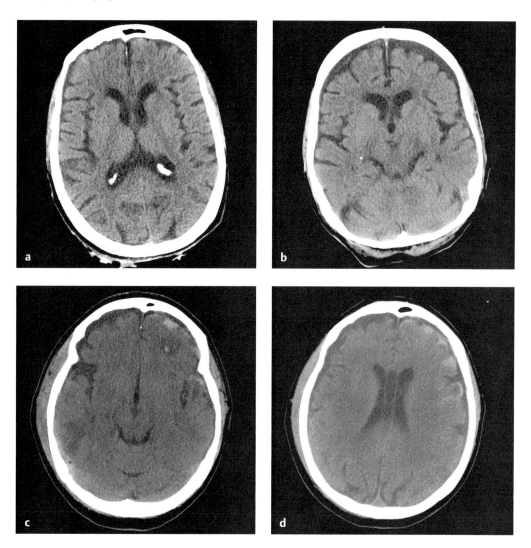

◆ Subdural Hygroma

Subdural hygromas are due to CSF that leaks into the subdural space via either a tear or an irritation of the arachnoid. Subdural hygromas are usually bilateral, located over the anterior frontal or temporal lobes, and develop 2 to 3 days after acute head trauma.

Depending on CSF absorption and post-traumatic brain swelling, subdural hygromas can fluctuate in size over time. Atrophy or encephalomalacia affords a potential space for the development of hygromas, whereas parenchymal expansion and fluid reabsorption will speed resolution of the hygroma.

Subdural hygromas have the same CT density as CSF and can be indistinguishable from chronic subdural hematomas. When isolated and identified in the setting of acute trauma, subdural hygromas are considered a benign consequence of head injury, since most are small and clinically insignificant, and do not require surgical intervention. Subdural hygromas are commonly seen in conjunction with other brain injuries, such as contusion, traumatic subarachnoid hemorrhage, and extra-axial hematomas (**Fig. 2.9**).

Fig. 2.9a–d
a,b Subdural hygroma. (**a**) CT at time of injury. Mild underlying ventricular and sulcal prominence. (**b**) CT 48 hours later. Interval appearance of symmetric, low-attenuation bifrontal subdural fluid collections. **c,d** Subdural hygroma associated with cortical contusion, epidural hematoma, and traumatic subarachnoid hemorrhage. Low-attenuation bifrontal subdural collections. High-attenuation subarachnoid hemorrhage fills the left frontal sulci. Left inferior frontal hemorrhagic contusion. Small right temporo-occipital epidural hematoma containing air.

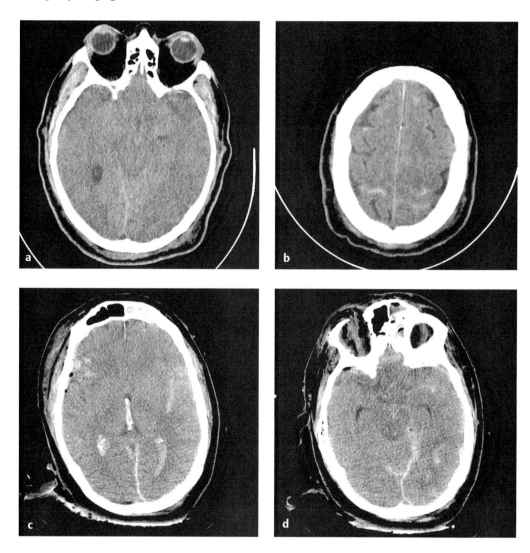

◆ Traumatic Subarachnoid Hemorrhage

Traumatic subarachnoid hemorrhage (SAH) is a consequence of either direct pial vascular injury or extension from a hemorrhagic cortical contusion, parenchymal hematoma, or extra-axial hematoma. Although traumatic SAH is often seen in association with other brain injuries, it can be subtle, particularly if it is the only finding in minor head trauma. Blood that collects between the pia and the arachnoid membrane fills cerebral sulci and forms fine serpentine juxtacortical high-density collections. Hemorrhage is also common in the perimesencephalic cisterns. Over a period of days, blood becomes isodense to brain and ultimately resolves.

Traumatic SAH may be limited to cortical sulci, the interpeduncular cistern, or the posterior perimesencephalic cisterns. Extensive hemorrhage in the suprasellar and middle cerebral artery cisterns, especially in the absence of other traumatic brain injuries (contusion, subdural hematoma, epidural hematoma) or with minor trauma, is more consistent with subarachnoid hemorrhage due to a ruptured aneurysm. It is important to keep in mind that the accident leading to a patient's head injury may have been precipitated by loss of consciousness due to an aneurysmal hemorrhage. CT or conventional angiography can be performed to address this possibility.

SAH is associated with increased morbidity and mortality in trauma, reflecting its potential to induce vasospasm and its association with more severe mechanisms of head injury. Subarachnoid blood is also toxic to the underlying cortex and can interfere with normal CSF absorption, which can lead to later complications of chronic hydrocephalus or superficial siderosis (**Fig. 2.10**).

Fig. 2.10a–d
a,b Isolated traumatic subarachnoid hemorrhage. Generalized cerebral swelling with effacement of perimesencephalic cisterns and cortical sulci. Subarachnoid hemorrhage in the interpeduncular and ambient cisterns. Hemorrhage fills numerous frontal and parietal convexity sulci.
c,d Traumatic subarachnoid hemorrhage associated with other cerebral injuries. Generalized cerebral swelling, right frontal cortical contusions, pneumocephalus, clot within the ventricles, and small tentorial subdural hematoma. Traumatic subarachnoid hemorrhage in the interpeduncular cistern and left Sylvian fissure.

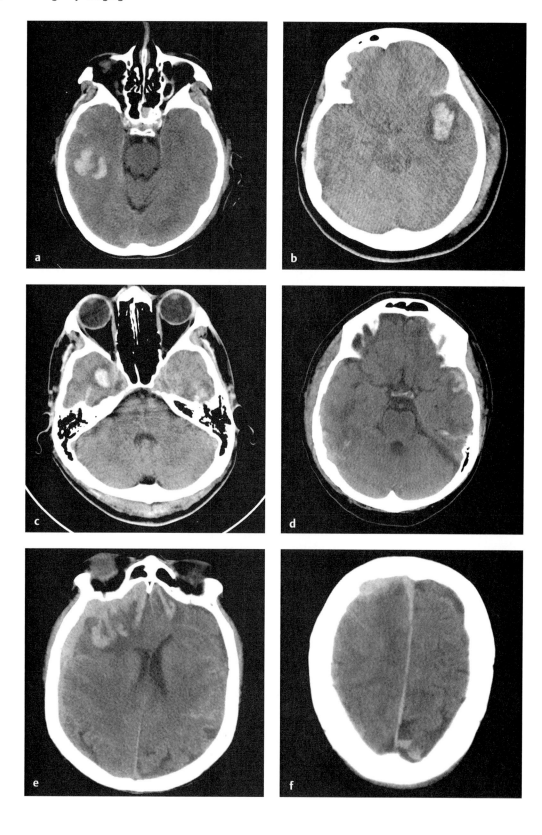

◆ Cerebral Contusion

Cortical contusions result when the brain impacts upon the irregular contours of the orbital roofs, petrous ridges, and sphenoid wings in acute acceleration injury. As a result, most contusions are located in the cortex and immediate subcortical white matter of the inferior frontal lobes, anterior or inferior temporal lobes, posterior cerebellum, dorsal occipital lobes, and frontal and parietal convexities. They may be either coup or contrecoup in location, although the latter are more common. Contusions typically carry a better prognosis than diffuse axonal injury (DAI) unless associated with significant brain swelling.

CT is the first and often only investigation in the emergency setting; MRI is more sensitive for detection of small hemorrhages, which can be important for accurate prognosis. Contusions may be subtle or imperceptible immediately following an acute injury. Delayed hemorrhage, occurring at 12 to 48 hours, is known as posttraumatic apoplexy and reflects hypocoagulability that often develops following head trauma and resolution of acute swelling that serves to tamponade small vascular injuries (**Fig. 2.11**).

Fig. 2.11a–e
a Hemorrhagic right temporal contusion. Right temporal hematoma with adjacent traumatic subarachnoid hemorrhage. Blood within the left sphenoid sinus indicates associated central skull base fracture.
b Nonhemorrhagic right and hemorrhagic left contusions. Low-attenuation edema within the right temporal lobe and hematoma surrounded by vasogenic edema in the left temporal lobe. Generalized brain swelling with cisternal effacement and traumatic subarachnoid hemorrhage in the interpeduncular and quadrigeminal plate cisterns.
c,d Bilateral contusions. Bilateral temporal hemorrhagic and left inferior frontal nonhemorrhagic contusions.
e,f Right frontal and left parietal vertex hemorrhagic contusions. Associated right frontal subdural hematoma, traumatic subarachnoid hemorrhage, and right sided swelling with convexity sulcal effacement.

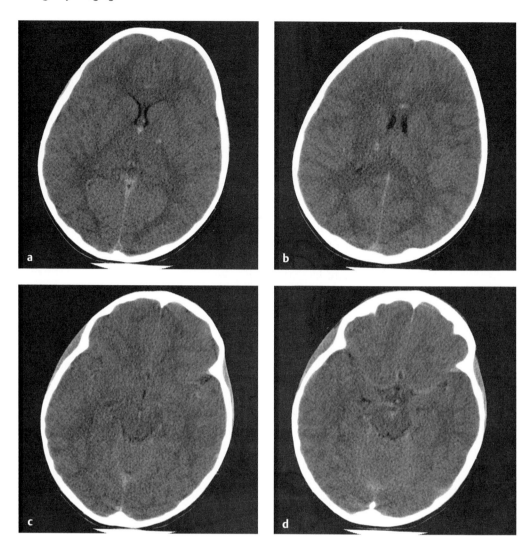

◆ Diffuse Axonal Injury

Diffuse axonal injury (DAI) is the cerebral neuronal damage that occurs when the brain is subjected to severe rotational and translational forces in trauma. Because gray and white matter densities are not identical, differential movement of the cortex relative to white matter during rapid acceleration shears traversing axons and perforating vessels. DAI is a devastating injury, usually the consequence of high-velocity motor vehicle accidents, and the patient typically suffers an immediate loss of consciousness and remains in a persistent vegetative state.

On CT imaging, DAI is revealed by small petechial hemorrhages from laceration of tiny perforating vessels. These are located at the gray-white junction of the cerebral hemispheres, the basal ganglia, the corpus callosum, or the dorsolateral midbrain. The depth of the hemorrhage roughly correlates with trauma severity.

CT can be normal in DAI, and while MRI is more sensitive for detection of micro-hemorrhages, both techniques are likely to underestimate the extent of axonal injury. In patients who survive significant head injury, later Wallerian degeneration of sheared axons, brain atrophy, and ventricular enlargement reveal neuronal damage that is often not apparent on initial CT (**Fig. 2.12**).

Fig. 2.12a–d
a–d Diffuse axonal injury. Punctate hemorrhages at the gray-white matter junction involving the anterior corpus callosum, right thalamus, and left posterior limb of internal capsule. Associated traumatic subarachnoid hemorrhage within the interpeduncular cistern and left quadrigeminal plate cistern.

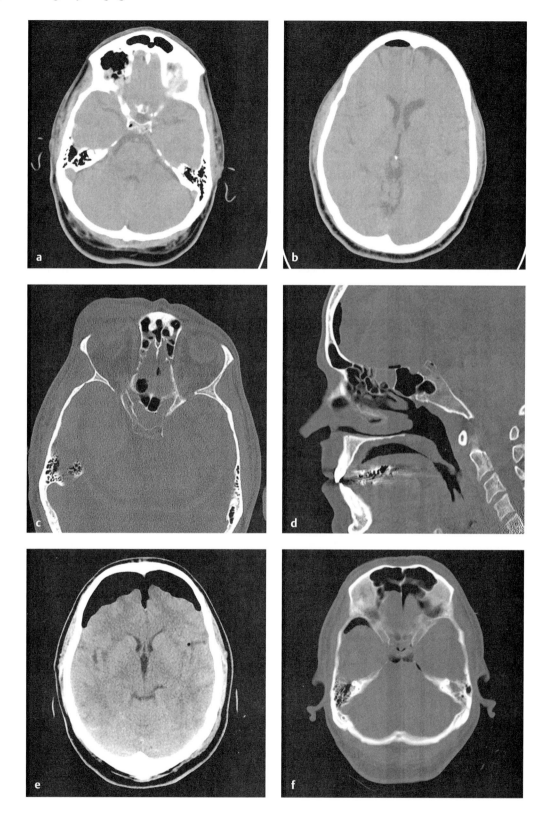

◆ Pneumocephalus

Intracranial air is always seen after craniotomy and also occurs in a small percentage of head trauma patients. If a skull base or calvarial fracture traverses one of the facial sinuses or the mastoid air cells, air is often present in the subdural or subarachnoid space. Rarely, a dural laceration can act like a one-way check valve, permitting inflow of air, but preventing its egress. By this mechanism, intracranial air pressure can exceed tissue pressure and compress the brain. In the supine patient, this is most evident over the nondependent frontal lobes and tends to have a peaked appearance (Mount Fuji sign).

Most cases of pneumocephalus resolve spontaneously and can be observed. Antimicrobial therapy is indicated to prevent meningitis when a disrupted sinus or mastoid air cell communicates with the intracranial cavity. When associated with neurologic deterioration, tension pneumocephalus can be treated with burr hole decompression (**Fig. 2.13**).

Fig. 2.13a–f
a–d Pneumocephalus following facial trauma with orbital roof and ethmoid fracture. Small amount of air anterior to the right frontal lobe, between the ethmoid bone and the olfactory cortex, and within the right superior orbit. This air is not under tension, but it indicates that the skull base periosteum has been breached and that the subdural space communicates with one of the facial sinuses (in this case the ethmoid air cells). The patient is therefore at increased risk of CSF leak or meningitis.
e,f Tension pneumocephalus due to temporal bone fracture. Bifrontal subdural air collections with mild compression of the frontal parenchyma. Opacified left mastoid air cells are consistent with an acute temporal bone fracture. Air in the cisterns and left sylvian fissure indicate arachnoid injury.

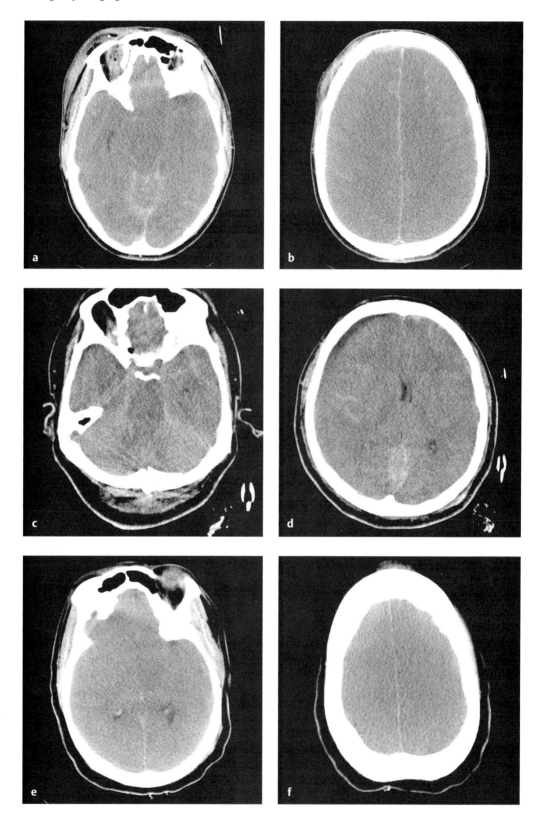

◆ Cerebral Swelling

Cerebral swelling may be due to traumatic injury or one of many nontraumatic etiologies, including intracranial neoplasm, infection, various metabolic derangements, and hypoxic-anoxic injury.

In severe head trauma, cerebral tissue damage, often associated with systemic hypovolemia, hypoxia, and hypercarbia, disrupts normal cerebral autoregulation and leads to a toxic cycle of elevated intracranial pressure, ischemia, and further tissue damage. Swelling localized to one cerebral compartment can cause subfalcine, transtentorial, or central herniation; vascular compromise; and ischemia.

CT findings in both traumatic and nontraumatic swelling include global sulcal effacement, small ventricles, and compressed perimesencephalic and suprasellar cisterns. In head trauma, swelling is usually associated with other findings including extra-axial hematomas, contusions, subarachnoid hemorrhage, and ventricular trapping (**Fig. 2.14**).

Fig. 2.14a–f
a,b Traumatic cerebral swelling. Small right frontal extra-axial hematoma and diffuse traumatic subarachnoid hemorrhage. Global cisternal and sulcal effacement with poor gray-white differentiation. Associated right frontal scalp soft tissue swelling, orbital roof fracture, intraorbital hematoma, and intraorbital air.
c,d Traumatic cerebral swelling in another patient. Poor gray-white differentiation, sulcal and perimesencephalic cisternal effacement, right frontal subacute subdural hematoma/hygroma, and traumatic convexity subarachnoid hemorrhage.
e,f Cerebral swelling due to anoxic injury. Complete loss of gray-white differentiation. No visible sulci or cisterns.

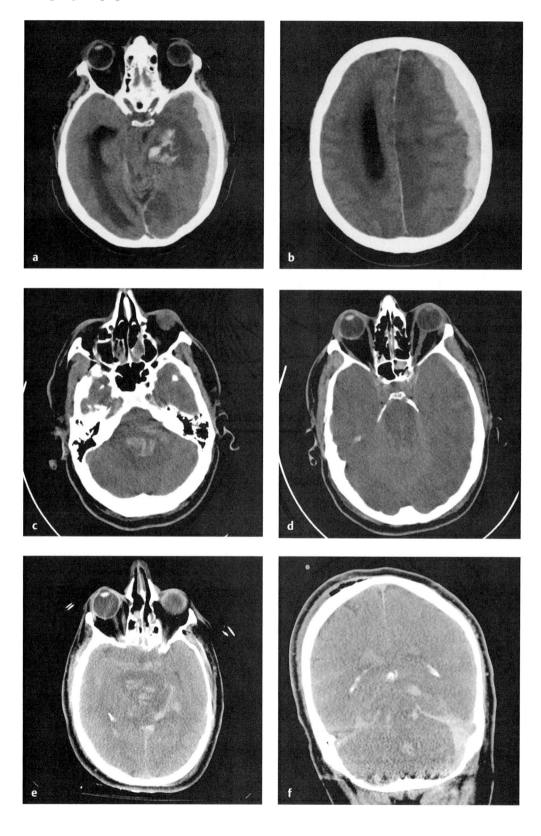

◆ Cerebral Herniation

Cerebral herniation is defined by displacement of swollen or compressed brain across the falcine and tentorial dural reflections, through a calvarial defect, or through the foramen magnum. Causes include subdural or epidural hematomas, parenchymal hemorrhage, tumors, and focal cerebritis or abscess. Depending on location, direction, and severity, herniated brain can compress cranial nerves and descending and ascending brainstem fiber tracts, obstruct intraventricular CSF flow, and occlude cerebral arteries.

The most common pattern is subfalcine herniation, in which the cingulate gyrus herniates under the falx. Contralateral hydrocephalus (ventricular trapping) results from obstruction of the lateral ventricle at the foramen of Monro. Compression of the anterior cerebral artery branches, when displaced across the falx, can cause an ipsilateral superior frontal or cingulate gyrus infarct, which may manifest clinically as contralateral leg weakness.

Brain herniation through the tentorial notch can be either downward (central), upward (due to posterior fossa hemorrhage), or lateral (uncal). Uncal herniation is more common than other transtentorial herniations. As the herniating medial temporal lobe compresses parasympathetic fibers on the periphery of the third cranial nerve, the ipsilateral pupil becomes fixed and dilated. Further compression forces the contralateral cerebral peduncle against the tentorial dural reflection and injures descending motor fibers, causing ipsilateral hemiparesis. The posterior cerebral artery can also be compressed in uncal herniation, causing an ipsilateral temporal/occipital infarct with visual field defects opposite the injured hemisphere.

Downward (central) herniation occurs in severe bilateral hemispheric injuries. Inferior brainstem displacement compromises its vascular supply and can lead to ischemic or reperfusion injury. Cross-sectional imaging findings include cisternal effacement, compression of the cerebral peduncles, and ventral or ventrolateral brainstem hemorrhage (Duret hemorrhage) located near the midline at the pontomesencephalic junction.

Upward transtentorial herniation can occur with cerebellar hemorrhage, low occipital trauma, or infratentorial masses. Like downward transtentorial herniation, it can result in brainstem ischemia and hemorrhage.

Signs and symptoms of herniation often develop rapidly and include somnolence or stupor, agitation, neurologic deficits, cranial nerve palsies, and "Cushing triad" (hypertension, bradycardia, and irregular respiration) (**Fig. 2.15**).

Fig. 2.15
a,b Acute subdural hematoma with subfalcine and uncal herniation. Hyperdense, crescentic left holohemispheric SDH with hemorrhagic temporal contusion. Uncal herniation with complete cisternal effacement, displacement of the left lateral ventricular temporal horn to the midline, and trapping of the left lateral ventricle. Left posterior cerebral artery and anterior cerebral artery occlusion with traumatic cerebral infarcts involving the left occipital lobe (PCA distribution) and left superior frontal gyrus (ACA distribution).
c,d Downward transtentorial herniation with Duret hemorrhage. Diffuse cerebral swelling with cisternal effacement, poor gray-white differentiation, and large central pontine hemorrhage.
e,f Upward transtentorial herniation due to traumatic cerebellar hemorrhage. Diffuse cerebellar swelling with upward transtentorial herniation, complete cisternal effacement, multiple pontine hemorrhages, and low-attenuation brainstem change.

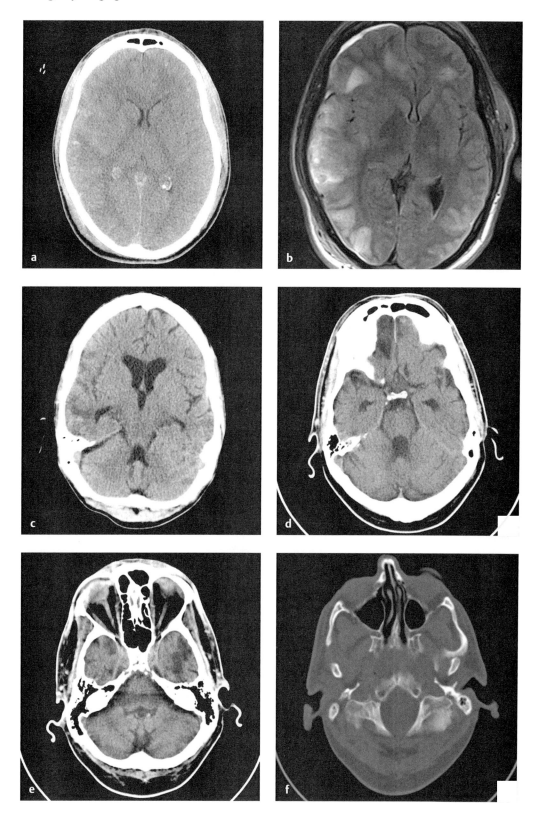

◆ Posttraumatic Atrophy and Encephalomalacia

Survivors of significant head trauma suffer a variety of neurologic symptoms including cognitive impairment, headache, epilepsy, and persistent focal motor or sensory deficits.

Nonenhanced head CT shows generalized volume loss, which can develop in as little as 4–6 weeks. Focal encephalomalacia involving the inferior frontal lobe, the anterior and inferior temporal lobe, the posterior cerebellum, and the parasagittal convexity are common sequelae of cortical contusions. Other findings supporting re-mote head injury include prior craniotomy, facial fractures, and burr holes.

Remote cerebral infarcts may have a similar appearance but can be distinguished by their distribution, which should correspond to arterial territories. Longstanding demyelinating disease and primary brain degenerative disorders are often associated with volume loss and focal low-attenuation change, but lesions in these conditions are usually seen in the white matter and deep nuclei (**Fig. 2.16**).

Fig. 2.16a–f

a–c   Posttraumatic atrophy following head injury in a 24-year-old. (**a**) Initial CT and (**b**) FLAIR MRI show mild swelling, cortical contusions, and shear hemorrhages but near-normal ventricular size and volume for a young adult. (**c**) CT performed one month after injury shows interval global ventricular and sulcal enlargement as well as focal right-sided encephalomalacia.

d–f   Posttraumatic encephalomalacia. Left inferior frontal and bilateral anterior temporal lobe low-attenuation focal parenchymal changes with mild generalized volume loss, indicated by subtle lateral ventricle temporal tip and fourth ventricle enlargement. This distribution is typical of remote traumatic cortical contusions. (**f**) Healed left zygomatic arch fracture further supports a remote injury.

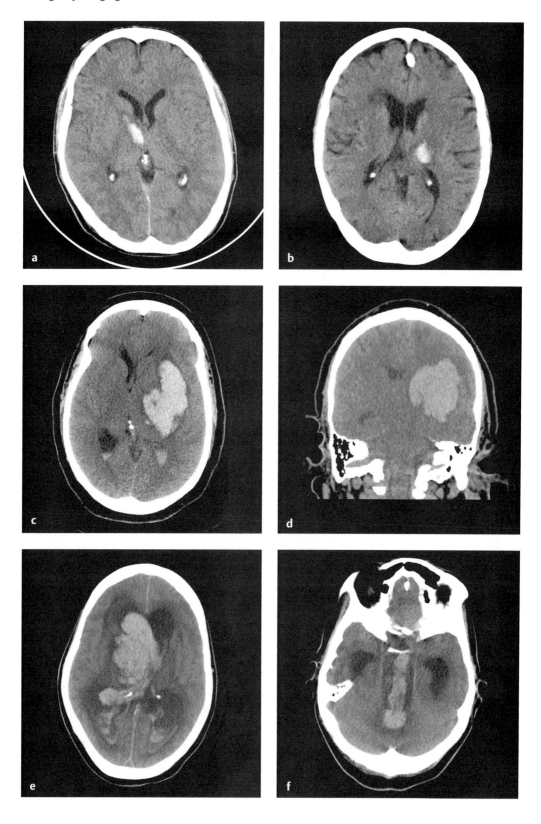

◆ Hypertensive Hemorrhage

Twice as common as subarachnoid hemorrhage, spontaneous intracranial hemorrhage (ICH) comprises 10–20% of strokes, which are clinically indistinguishable from ischemic stroke and subarachnoid hemorrhage. Patients with ICH often present with headache, nausea, and vomiting before a focal neurologic deficit becomes evident. In adults with nontraumatic intracranial hemorrhage, hypertension is the most common etiology.

In long-standing, poorly controlled hypertension, microaneurysms develop in the perforating arterioles, primarily in the lenticulostriate, pontine, and cerebellar distributions. Accelerated atherosclerosis and hyaline arteriosclerosis also play a part in the pathologic changes predisposing to hypertensive ICH. Bleeding usually occurs in the putamen, thalamus, pons, or cerebellum (in order of decreasing frequency), and clinical signs correspond to the location of hemorrhage and function of the involved brain. For example, cerebellar hemorrhage often manifests as dizziness, vomiting, truncal ataxia, and gaze palsies.

Noncontrast CT is the most appropriate initial imaging study in patients with clinical stroke symptoms. If a parenchymal hemorrhage is the cause, the size of the bleed as well as any ventricular extension or secondary hydrocephalus are easily assessed. Acute hemorrhage (within four hours) appears as a well-defined area of high attenuation and may persist for up to a week. As the bleed ages, the margins become less distinct and a surrounding low-attenuation rim develops, reflecting brain edema or extruded serum. Subacute hematomas may show peripheral enhancement on postcontrast CT or MRI. Very remote hematomas appear as slitlike, CSF-density lesions.

The volume of a parenchymal hematoma (mL) is estimated by multiplying the three dimensions (in cm) and dividing the product by 2. Hematoma volumes > 50 mL are associated with a poor prognosis (**Fig. 2.17**).

Fig. 2.17a–f
a,b Small hemorrhages in two patients. (**a**) Small focal hemorrhage in the right internal capsule genu and anterior thalamus. (**b**) Small left thalamic hemorrhage.
c,d Large left external capsule hemorrhage. Large left-sided hematoma with subfalcine shift, modest intraventricular hemorrhage, and trapping of the right lateral ventricle.
e,f Massive hemorrhage with rupture into the ventricular system and severe hydrocephalus. A large parenchymal hematoma obliterates the right basal ganglia and extends into the ventricles. Clot fills the third and fourth ventricles and causes marked hydrocephalus.

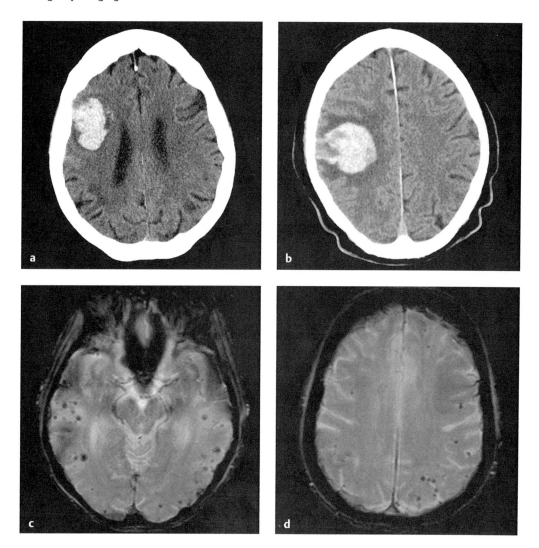

◆ Amyloid Angiopathy

Amyloid angiopathy is due to beta amyloid deposition in cerebral vessels and usually affects adults over age 65. It is a primary cause of cortical and subcortical (lobar) hemorrhage, and this is what brings most patients to clinical attention. Symptoms include sudden focal neurologic deficit, transient ischemic attacks, and variably progressive dementia.

Acute lobar cortical or subcortical hemorrhage against a background of subcortical/periventricular white matter low-attenuation changes and cerebral volume loss are typical CT findings. Microhemorrhages may be present but undetectable on CT. Gradient echo MRI detects these with greater sensitivity.

The differential diagnosis of lobar hemorrhage includes atypical hypertensive bleed, venous thrombosis with infarct, ruptured arteriovenous malformation, ruptured aneurysm, and hemorrhagic neoplasm. In younger and middle-aged patients, CT angiography, MRI with gadolinium and angiography, and conventional angiography can be considered to exclude an underlying hemorrhagic neoplasm or vascular lesion (**Fig. 2.18**).

Fig. 2.18a–d
a,b Lobar hemorrhage. Noncontrast CT shows peripheral, well-defined, acute right frontal lobar hemorrhages in two elderly patients. While a hemorrhagic venous infarct could have this appearance, it would be unusual for either a hypertensive bleed or hemorrhagic conversion of an arterial-distribution infarct. Associated background low-attenuation white matter changes and sulcal prominence indicate chronic underlying small-vessel ischemic change.
c,d Amyloid angiopathy. Gradient echo MRI in a different patient shows multiple punctate low-signal-intensity foci involving the temporal cortices and subcortical white matter. These lesions correspond to local hemosiderin deposition from tiny subclinical hemorrhages.

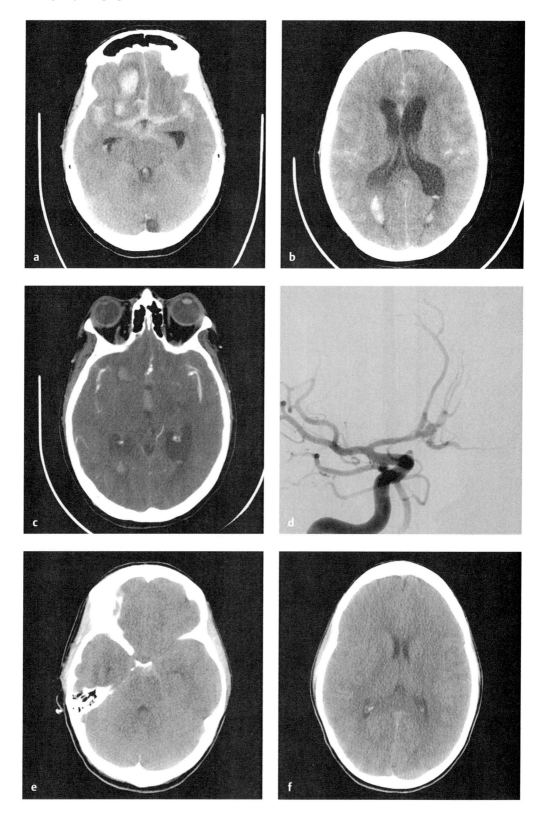

◆ Subarachnoid Hemorrhage

Most acute spontaneous SAH are due to rupture of a saccular aneurysm, usually one arising from the branch points of the cerebral arteries that make up the circle of Willis. Blood fills the adjacent cerebral cisterns and can extend to the sylvian fissures and convexity subarachnoid space. Occasionally the jet of blood can lacerate the adjacent brain, resulting in intraparenchymal, subdural, or intraventricular hemorrhage.

Patients are most often middle-aged and present with the sudden onset of severe headache, accompanied by variable depression of consciousness, meningismus, nausea/vomiting, or photophobia. The most immediate complication is acute hydrocephalus from obstruction of arachnoid granulations and compromise of CSF resorption, which may require urgent ventriculostomy. Vasospasm develops hours to days after acute SAH and can lead to cerebral ischemia and infarct.

CT shows hyperdense blood in the subarachnoid space in > 90% of patients imaged shortly after symptom onset but becomes less sensitive after 24–48 hours. If a lumbar puncture is performed, CSF will show elevated numbers of red blood cells in SAH, but the study may be nondiagnostic in the first 12 hours because of procedure-induced hemorrhage. CSF obtained after 12 hours will be xanthochromic in true SAH, as red cell lysis will have taken place by that time. FLAIR MRI can sensitively identify SAH as increased signal in the subarachnoid space, which normally appears black on this sequence. Conventional or CT angiography is indicated for diagnosis and evaluation of any underlying cerebral aneurysm. These are treated by surgical clipping or endovascular coiling to prevent rehemorrhage. False-negative angiograms may be due to vasospasm, incomplete visualization of the cerebral circulation, or suboptimal technique.

Perimesencephalic nonaneurysmal SAH is due to rupture of small arterioles or venules about the midbrain and pons. Patients present with acute headache but without the depressed sensorium and severe neurologic symptoms of patients with acutely ruptured aneurysm.

Blood is usually small in volume and restricted to the perimesencephalic cisterns. Hydrocephalus or blood extending to the sylvian fissure or convexity sulci is uncommon and would be more typical of a ruptured aneurysm. Given the consequences of failing to diagnose an acutely ruptured aneurysm, high-quality conventional angiography is indicated. Because small aneurysms can be missed due to suboptimal technique or vasospasm, angiography may need to be repeated, particularly if the study is less than perfect or if subtle vascular abnormalities are detected.

Treatment of nonaneurysmal hemorrhage is conservative and consists of symptomatic pain management. Ischemia or rebleeding rarely occurs (less than 1%), and the prognosis is excellent (**Fig. 2.19**).

Fig. 2.19a–f
a–d Subarachnoid hemorrhage due to ruptured anterior communicating artery aneurysm. Nonenhanced CT shows extensive blood within the suprasellar and perimesencephalic cisterns, intraparenchymal hemorrhage, intraventricular hemorrhage, and communicating hydrocephalus due to obstruction at the level of the arachnoid granulations. CTA and conventional angiograms demonstrate an 8-mm aneurysm interposed between the proximal right and left anterior cerebral arteries near their origin.
e,f Benign perimesencephalic subarachnoid hemorrhage. Blood is limited to the prepontine and interpeduncular cisterns; no hydrocephalus.

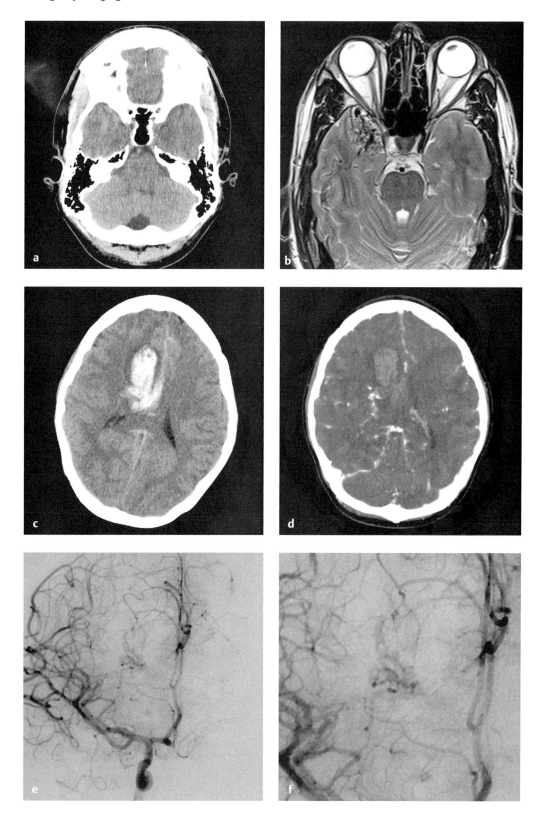

◆ Arteriovenous Malformation

Arteriovenous malformations (AVMs) are developmental anomalies consisting of abnormal arteries and veins without intervening capillaries. They appear as a complex tangle of small vessels, the nidus, with enlarged feeding arteries and draining veins. High-flow, rapid arteriovenous shunting is a physiologic feature, and most AVMs are presumed to enlarge over time. In an individual, an AVM may remain static, grow, or even regress, but the annual risk of hemorrhage for an untreated AVM is approximately 3%, is cumulative, and increases with age. They are typically solitary, and if a patient has more than one, syndromes associated with vascular malformations, such as Wyburn-Mason and Osler-Weber-Rendu (hereditary hemorrhagic telangiectasia), should be considered.

Most AVMs are supratentorial and can be classified as either compact or diffuse with respect to the nidus of anomalous vessels. If the nidus is small and contains little if any interposed neuronal tissue, it is designated as compact. In diffuse AVM a well-formed nidus is absent, and vessels traverse potentially eloquent brain.

It is difficult to detect small unruptured AVMs with noncontrast CT, and the radiologist should be sensitive to the subtle findings of asymmetrically enlarged feeding vessels and draining veins to do so. Up to 25% of AVMs have a calcified nidus, and this is sometimes the only NCCT finding. CT or MR angiography is useful for localizing and determining the vascular supply of most AVMs, but comprehensive evaluation usually requires conventional catheter angiography, which can be performed in concert with therapeutic embolization.

Management depends on the anatomy, size, and location of the AVM. Options include embolization, focused radiotherapy, surgical excision and combinations of these methods. In general, AVMs with superficial venous drainage have a better prognosis than those with deep venous drainage (**Fig. 2.20**).

Fig. 2.20a–f
a,b Incidentally detected arteriovenous malformation. (**a**) NCCT. Focal hyperdensity along the anterior margin of the right anterior temporal lobe with subtle tubular elements. (**b**) T2WI. A small tangle of vascular flow voids in the right anteromedial temporal lobe is supplied by dilated feeding arteries arising from the middle cerebral artery and drained by a large subtemporal cortical vein that courses along the floor of the middle cranial fossa.
c–f Ruptured arteriovenous malformation. (**c**) NCCT. Right frontal parenchymal hemorrhage with intraventricular and subarachnoid extension. (**d–f**) CT and conventional angiograms. Small nidus of enlarged vessels at the posterolateral aspect of the hematoma along the dorsal aspect of the thalamus.

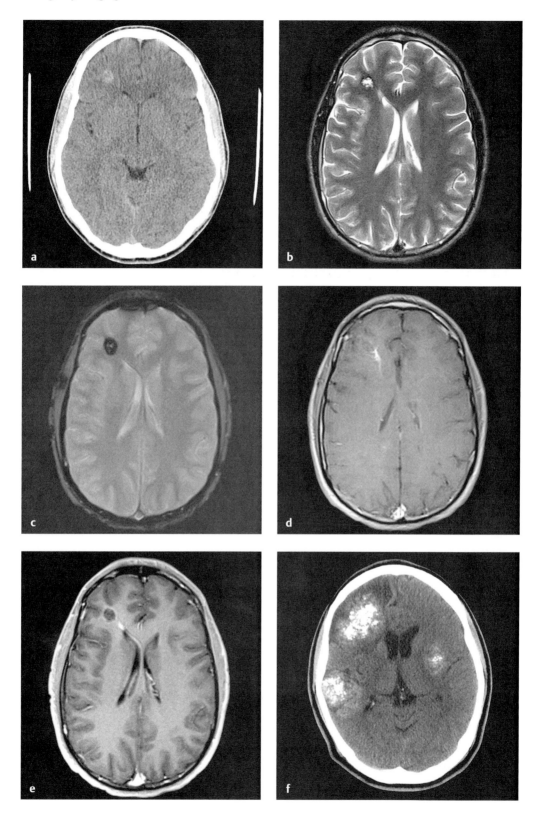

◆ Cavernous Malformation

Cerebral cavernous malformations (also known as cavernous hemangiomas) are compact vascular malformations consisting of thin-walled capillaries without intervening neuronal tissue. On gross examination, they are circumscribed, red, lobulated masses from less than a millimeter to several centimeters in diameter. Most are supratentorial and are found in the frontal and temporal lobes. They are usually solitary, although some patients can have multiple lesions and families have been identified in which several members have multiple lesions.

Occasionally, cavernous malformations are associated with developmental venous anomalies. These are small clusters of venules that drain a small segment of normal brain via a single larger anomalous vein that leads to either a dural sinus or an ependymal vein. Usually seen only on postgadolinium MRI, venous angiomas resemble an umbrella or palm tree.

Most patients are asymptomatic, and most cavernous malformations are found incidentally. Symptomatic patients present with seizures or, if the malformation is located in an eloquent portion of the brain, focal neurologic deficits related to hemorrhage or thrombosis.

CT findings are subtle and nonspecific. When visible, cavernous malformations usually appear as a vague, hyperdense, nonenhancing, subcentimeter parenchymal nodule and are sometimes mistaken for subacute traumatic hemorrhage. MRI is diagnostic and reveals a characteristic mulberry-like collection of blood products in different stages of evolution, often with a rim of surrounding low-signal hemosiderin. Gradient echo imaging is particularly sensitive to blood products and should be obtained when a cavernous malformation is suspected.

Surgical treatment (excision or stereotactic radiosurgery) is reserved for patients with recurrent hemorrhage, intractable epilepsy, or progressive neurologic deterioration (**Fig. 2.21**).

Fig. 2.21a–f
a–e Cavernous malformation with associated developmental venous anomaly. (**a**) NCCT. Vague, 1-cm rounded right frontal hyperdense lesion; no associated edema. (**b**) T2WI. "Mulberry-like," mixed-signal-intensity lesion with surrounding low-signal rim on gradient echo imaging. No associated edema or other parenchymal abnormality. (**c**) GRE. Low signal intensity corresponds to hemosiderin within the malformation. (**d,e**) T1-weighted postgadolinium images show an associated developmental venous anomaly: a small umbrella-like cluster of venules that drain a small segment of frontal lobe parenchyma adjacent to the cavernous malformation. A single draining vein courses along the ventricle and septum pellucidum to join the internal cerebral vein.
f Multiple cavernous malformations. Three large flocculent parenchymal calcifications, up to 4 cm in diameter, located in the right frontal lobe and left insula. Associated right frontal cortical encephalomalacia.

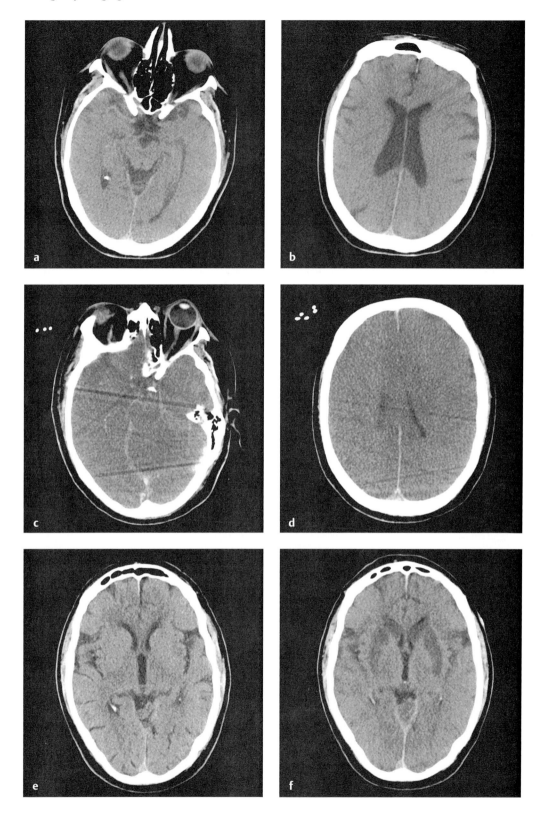

◆ Anoxic Injury

Anoxic (also known as hypoxic-ischemic) cerebral injury results from global lack of oxygen delivery to the brain for an extended period. It is most frequently the consequence of cardiopulmonary arrest, respiratory failure, carbon monoxide poisoning, near-drowning, or asphyxia. Patients typically present to the Emergency Department with a history of prolonged resuscitation efforts.

CT findings in adults with prolonged anoxia, hypoxia, or global hypoperfusion include progressive loss of normal gray-white matter differentiation, generalized cytotoxic edema, and sulcal and ventricular effacement. The brain appears homo-geneous, low in attenuation, and diffusely swollen, with sulcal and cisternal effacement. Because the meninges are supplied by branches of the external carotid artery (ECA), which are usually not compromised, they will often appear dense against adjacent low-attenuation brain and can simulate diffuse subarachnoid hemorrhage.

The basal ganglia, cerebral cortex, thalami, cerebellum, caudate nuclei, and hippocampi are most sensitive to hypoxic ischemic injury, and patients who suffer less severe hypoxia may show low-attenuation CT changes or high-signal T2-weighted MRI changes in these structures (**Fig. 2.22**).

Fig. 2.22a–f
a–d Anoxic injury following prolonged cardiorespiratory arrest. (**a,b**) Initial NCCT. Diminished gray-white differentiation with normal ventricles and sulci. (**c,d**) Follow-up NCCT 24 hours later. Progressive decrease in parenchymal attenuation with complete perimesencephalic cisternal and convexity sulcal effacement. Both lateral ventricles are compressed. Increased apparent density within the subarachnoid space reflects maintained meningeal perfusion rather than true subarachnoid hemorrhage.
e,f Less severe anoxic injury following cardiac arrest and resucutation. Immediate post-arrest CT is normal. Four days later, low attenuation changes are limited to the caudate nuclei and lateral putamina.

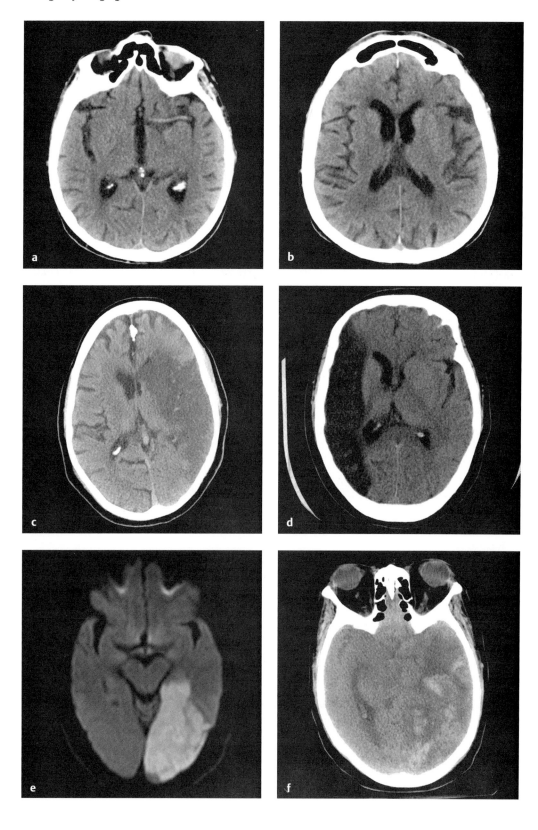

◆ Cerebral Infarct Due to Arterial Occlusion

Ischemic cerebral infarcts result from acute compromise of arterial blood flow to a portion of the brain, with consequent cellular death. The neurologic deficit resulting from the infarct depends on the vessel occluded, the location and extent of the territory it supplies, and the available collateral circulation. For example, a left middle cerebral artery infarct would be expected to result in aphasia as well as contralateral hemiparesis and sensory disturbance.

The sensitivity of nonenhanced CT is limited in the first 12–24 hours after symptom onset; however, subtle signs of early infarct can be seen even within the first 3 hours. A hyperdense cerebral vessel (known as the bright basilar artery or hyperdense middle cerebral artery) indicates thrombosis. Early parenchymal changes are due to ischemic (cytotoxic) cellular swelling and include (1) focal loss of normal gray-white matter differentiation, (2) cortical sulcal effacement, (3) poor basal ganglia definition, and (4) nonvisualization of the "insular ribbon," which is the normally dense insular cortex.

The primary role of CT in acute stroke is to exclude hemorrhage, which contraindicates the use of thrombolytic agents in those patients who present within 3 hours of symptom onset. If readily available, diffusion-weighted MRI is the most sensitive examination for identifying early cerebral infarction, and it can do so within 30 minutes.

Cytotoxic edema increases during the first 3 days after cerebral infarction, and on CT it appears as a well-defined area of low attenuation involving gray and white matter. Corresponding hyperintensity is evident on T2 and FLAIR MRI sequences at this stage. After approximately 2 weeks, an evolving infarct may become less obvious on CT because of a "fogging" effect in which microhemorrhage and cellular repair lead to pseudonormalization of brain density. Diffusion-weighted MRI signal begins to fade around 1 week and is usually nearly normal by 2 weeks. *Hemorrhagic conversion* is a term that refers to spontaneous bleeding within an area of ischemic brain, most commonly in patients with large-territory (middle cerebral or internal carotid artery) infarcts (**Fig. 2.23**).

Fig. 2.23a–f
a,b Early infarct with dense middle cerebral artery and insular ribbon signs. The left middle cerebral artery is abnormally dense. The left insular cortex is isodense to adjacent white matter and hypodense compared with the normal cortex.
c Subacute left middle cerebral artery territory infarct. Cytotoxic edema with homogeneous low-attenuation change involving both gray and white matter in the distribution of the left lenticulostriate vessels and middle cerebral artery. Left hemispheric swelling with effaced lateral ventricle and minimal subfalcine shift.
d Remote right middle cerebral artery territory infarct. This remote infarct is near CSF in density and is associated with volume loss and ex vacuo dilatation of the right lateral ventricle.
e Left posterior cerebral artery distribution infarct. Diffusion-weighted MRI shows marked signal intensity difference between the acute infarct and surrounding brain. DWI is sensitive for acute infarcts within 30 minutes of symptom onset and may remain abnormal for up to 2 weeks.
f Hemorrhagic conversion of a subacute infarct. Multiple areas of hemorrhage within an infarct that involves the left middle and posterior cerebral artery territories. It is due to an internal carotid artery occlusion in a patient whose PCA arose directly from the ICA (fetal origin).

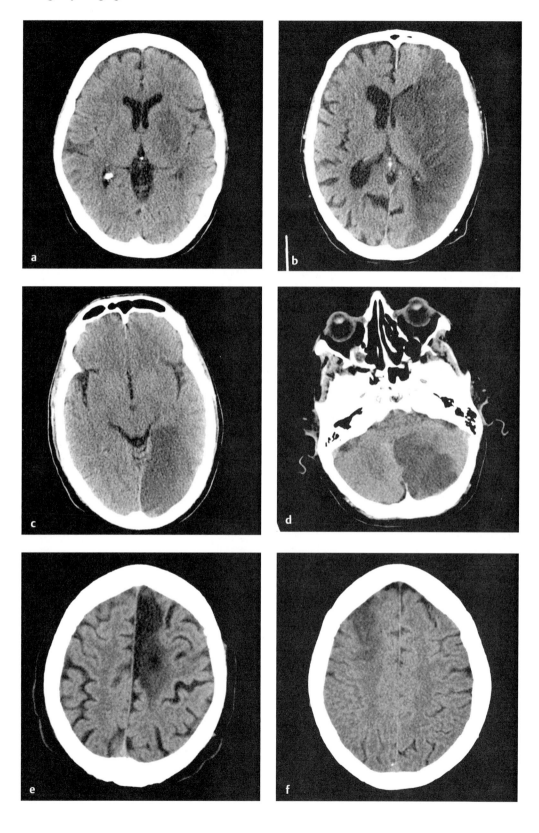

◆ Cerebral Infarct: Arterial Territories

The middle cerebral artery (MCA) is the most frequently involved territory in cerebral infarction. Emboli are the most common cause of occlusion and originate from atherosclerotic plaques in the common or internal carotid arteries, cardiac emboli, or infrequently venous emboli in patients with right to left cardiac shunts (patent foramen ovale). Early imaging signs include hyperdense MCA on noncontrast CT, hypodense basal ganglia, "disappearing" lentiform nucleus, and loss of the normal insular ribbon. Hemorrhage, especially in the basal ganglia and cortex, is common in patients with MCA strokes and may occur 1 to 4 days after onset of infarction.

Lacunar infarctions are common, but many are clinically silent. These are due to occlusion of the small perforating and deep cerebral arterioles and are associated with increasing age and hypertension. Primary small vessel disease, rather than embolization, is the etiology, and lacunar infarcts typically involve the basal ganglia, internal capsule, thalami, and brainstem. Most are discovered incidentally. In acute small vessel infarct, CT findings may be subtle, but diffusion-weighted MRI will usually show an area of high signal, usually less than 1 cm in diameter.

Posterior cerebral artery (PCA) infarcts are less common than ICA or MCA infarction. These may be due to emboli or occlusive disease, or they can follow compression of the PCA in trauma with downward transtentorial herniation. Involvement of the medial occipital lobe produces the characteristic clinical finding of homonymous hemianopsia.

Anterior cerebral artery (ACA) infarcts are uncommon and usually occur with ICA occlusion in patients who have contralateral hypoplasia of the proximal ACA. ACA infarct can also follow subfalcine herniation with "clipping" of the ACA under the falx cerebri. ACA infarcts appear as a region of hypodensity (CT) or hyperintensity (MR T2/FLAIR) involving the cingulate and superior frontal gyri.

Cerebellar and brainstem infarcts are due to emboli, vertebral artery injury, or occlusive vertebrobasilar disease. They can involve the pons, medulla, anterior inferior cerebellum, posterior inferior cerebellum, or superior cerebellum.

Watershed infarcts occur in the borderzones between arterial territories and are seen in patients with limited vascular reserve challenged by hypotension or poor cardiac output. This may be due to atherosclerotic ICA or MCA disease or to vasculopathies such as Moya Moya, in which the proximal MCAs are gradually occluded (**Fig. 2.24**).

Fig. 2.24a–f
a–f Arterial territories delineated by subacute to remote infarcts seen on noncontrast CT. (**a**) Left lenticulostriate. (**b**) Left middle cerebral artery. (**c**) Left posterior cerebral artery. (**d**) Left posterior inferior cerebellar artery. (**e**) Left anterior cerebral artery. (**f**) Right frontal watershed infarct in a patient with Moya Moya disease.

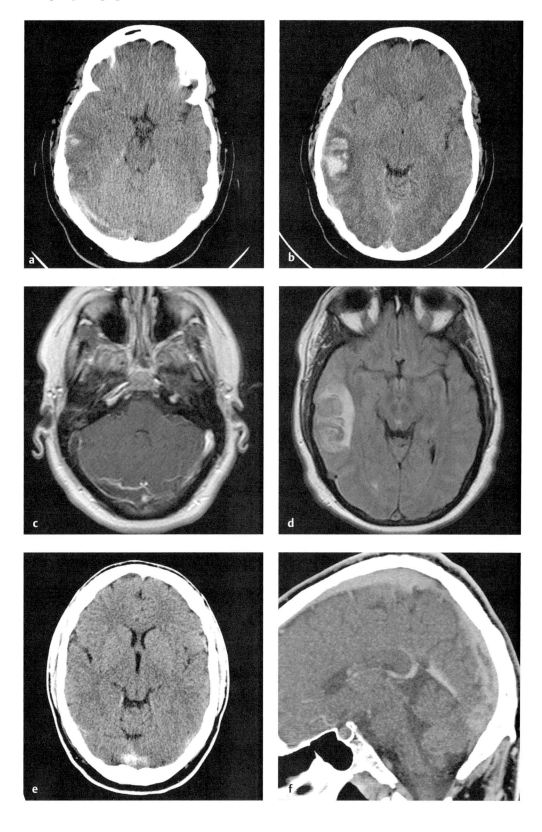

◆ Venous Sinus Thrombosis and Venous Infarct

Venous sinus thrombosis (VST) should be suspected in young and middle-aged adults who present with strokelike symptoms, unusual headache, and visual disturbance. Elevated intracranial pressure from impaired venous outflow typically leads to nausea, vomiting, and headache. Papilledema may or may not be present. The most frequent, but least specific, symptom is headache, often severe and persistent and usually gradually increasing over several days. Headache onset can be abrupt and can clinically mimic acute subarachnoid hemorrhage.

While arterial occlusion or emboli cause infarcts corresponding to well-described vascular territories, venous infarcts tend to involve the cortex or deep nuclei in a nonarterial distribution and are more commonly hemorrhagic. Their location and corresponding clinical findings depend on which dural sinus or cortical vein is occluded.

Predisposing conditions include mastoid or petrous apex infection, polycythemia, malignancy, puerperium, dehydration, oral contraceptive use, head trauma, and inherited prothrombotic disorders such as protein S deficiency. In 20% of patients, no cause is identified.

The diagnosis is made by detecting a hyperdense venous sinus on NCCT or demonstrating nonenhancing thrombus outlined by the enhancing dural sinus walls on CT venography or postgadolinium MRI. The initial study for the patient with suspicious or atypical headache should be NCCT, which can identify a dense dural sinus and exclude competing diagnoses. Findings are often subtle, as the venous sinus can appear dense due to technical factors or hemoconcentration. Confirmation by CT venography, MRI, and or MR venography may be necessary. The most sensitive imaging strategy often involves a combination of these studies (**Fig. 2.25**).

Fig. 2.25a–f
a–d Venous sinus thrombosis with venous infarct. (**a,b**) ~ 3 cm right posterior temporal parenchymal hemorrhage with mild surrounding vasogenic edema and local sulcal effacement. Portions of the right transverse and sagittal venous sinuses are hyperdense. (**c**) The contents of the right transverse and sagittal sinuses are isointense to brain and outlined by enhancing dural sinus walls on this postgadolinium T1-weighted MRI. The left sigmoid sinus opacifies normally. (**d**) FLAIR images show a right posterior temporal cortical/subcortical lesion with associated surrounding edema consistent with a venous infarct. Intermediate signal in the right sagittal sinus.
e,f Partial sagittal sinus thrombosis. Very-high-attenuation material in the torcular herophili and sagittal sinus on nonenhanced CT. Sagittal CT venogram opacifies the internal cerebral veins, vein of Galen, straight sinus, and most of the sagittal sinus. A filling defect in the occipital portion of the sagittal sinus corresponds to intrasinus clot on NCCT.

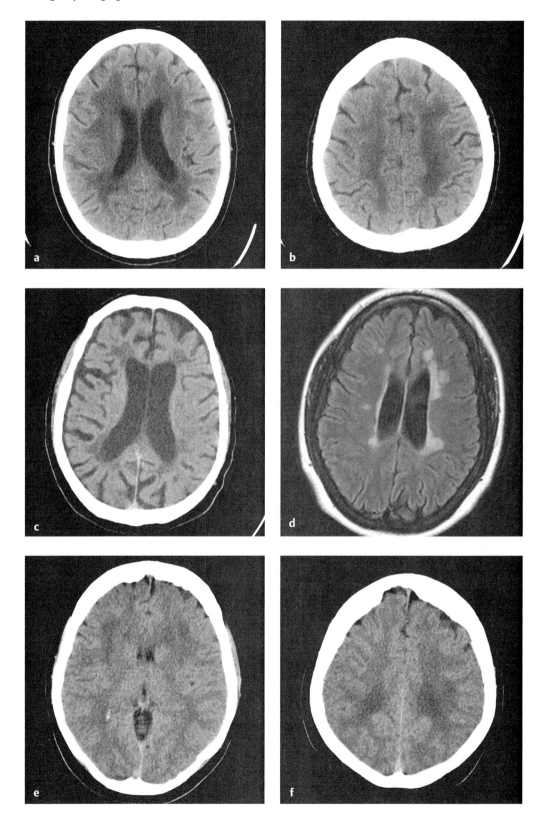

◆ White Matter Disease

Subcortical and periventricular low-attenuation white matter changes are a common finding in patients who undergo head CT scanning for various indications. White matter changes are most common in patients over 60, and in this group small-vessel ischemic or chronic hypertensive disease is usually responsible. In patients under 50, small-vessel ischemic disease is uncommon, and considerations should include a variety of demyelinating diseases.

Small-vessel ischemic disease is a frequent finding on both CT and MRI in older adults and in patients with vascular risk factors, such as hypertension, diabetes, atherosclerosis, and atrial fibrillation. These changes often accumulate over time and can have a variable presentation due to the brain's compensatory mechanisms. Symptoms, if present, are due to either complete or incomplete infarction of subcortical structures, leading to various cognitive, motor, or mood disturbances. The burden of white matter disease does not directly equate with severity of symptoms or even the presence of any clinically detectable abnormality. When symptomatic, patients can present with neurologic deficits ranging from mild subjective cognitive complaints to frank dementia and Parkinsonism.

Demyelinating disease, which may be inflammatory, infective, ischemic, or toxic in etiology, encompasses a number of conditions characterized by destruction of or damage to normally myelinated axons. They include multiple sclerosis (MS), acute disseminated encephalomyelitis (ADEM), osmotic demyelination, human immunodeficiency virus (HIV) encephalitis, progressive multifocal leukoencephalopathy (PML), and posterior reversible encephalopathy syndrome (PRES), among others. The clinical presentation may vary but often includes neurologic deficits, paresthesias, and weakness.

While CT will often show low-attenuation white matter changes similar to those seen in small-vessel ischemic disease, MRI is more sensitive for detecting lesions that can be subtle or even invisible on CT. MS lesions are generally hyperintense on T2 and FLAIR sequences and hypointense on T1-weighted images. They are typically small and irregular but may coalesce into larger lesions that can mimic brain tumors (tumefactive MS). Frequent sites of involvement include periventricular white matter, the corpus callosum, the brainstem, and subcortical white matter. Perilesional vasogenic edema is not characteristic of MS.

HIV encephalitis, or central nervous system (CNS) infection by HIV, typically occurs shortly after primary infection and may present with headache, stiff neck, drowsiness, confusion, or seizures. Both CT and MR findings of HIV encephalitis are insensitive, especially early in infection. Hypodensity or generalized volume loss may be present, but more frequently the CT will be normal. MRI may demonstrate an increased signal T2/FLAIR or smaller demyelinative lesions. With the initiation of highly active antiretroviral therapy (HAART), prognosis is good, with reversal of neurologic symptoms in many patients (**Fig. 2.26**).

Fig. 2.26a–f

a,b Small vessel ischemic disease. Diffuse, severe low attenuation periventricular and subcortical white matter changes. Mild underlying cerebral volume loss.

c,d Multiple sclerosis. (**c**) Generalized volume loss with periventricular low-attenuation white matter changes on nonenhanced CT. In an older patient, this appearance is indistinguishable from small-vessel ischemic or hypertensive disease. In the patient under 50 years, consider demyelination. (**d**) Periventricular, radially oriented areas of high signal intensity on FLAIR imaging.

e,f HIV encephalitis. Subcortical low-attenuation changes that are nonspecific and overlap with other causes of generalized demyelination or small-vessel ischemic disease.

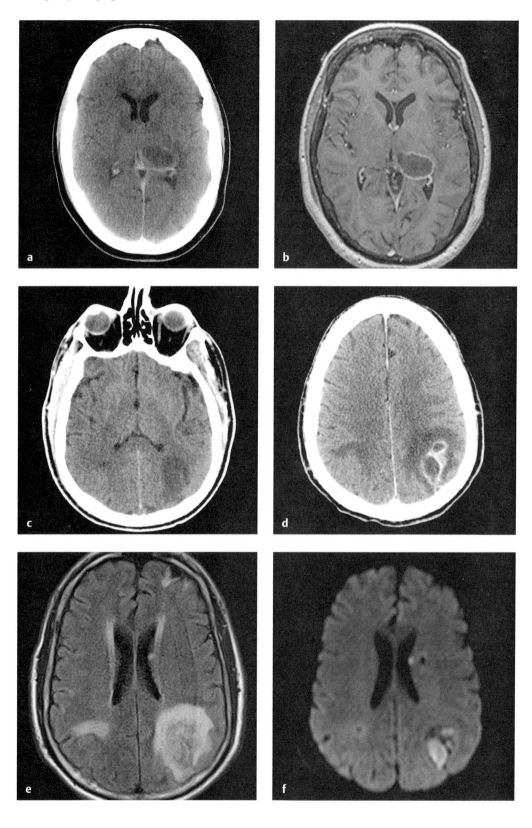

◆ Cerebritis and Brain Abscess

When an area of focal cerebritis organizes into a pus-filled cavity surrounded by granulation tissue and a fibrous capsule, it is termed a brain abscess. Patients do not typically appear acutely toxic and often present with nonspecific symptoms such as headache, fever, vomiting, confusion, or obtundation. Meningeal or focal neurologic findings (hemiparesis, seizures, or papilledema) are present in fewer than half of patients.

Brain abscesses are caused by several mechanisms, including direct extension of a skull base or deep facial infection (otitis media, mastoiditis, or sinusitis), hematogenous seeding (endocarditis, pulmonary arteriovenous shunt), or direct inoculation following open skull fracture or craniotomy. In at least 15% of cases, no source of infection is identified. Discovery of a brain abscess in an immunocompetent patient without evidence of infection elsewhere should suggest the possibility of pulmonary arteriovenous shunting, which can be seen in hereditary hemorrhagic telangiectasia (Osler-Weber-Rendu syndrome).

On noncontrast CT, a brain abscess appears as an area of indistinct low attenuation with variable surrounding vasogenic edema. The differential diagnosis includes atypical infections such as toxoplasmosis, cysticercosis, primary or metastatic neoplasm, subacute infarct or contusion, and demyelinating disease. Postcontrast CT and MRI show characteristic uniform peripheral enhancement. Diffusion-weighted MRI permits distinction from primary brain tumors; pus within a brain abscess shows very high diffusion-weighted signal, whereas brain tumors are typically hypointense. Established abscesses may also show adjacent "daughter" lesions (**Fig. 2.27**).

Fig. 2.27a–f
a,b Brain abscess, gram-positive cocci. (**a**) Postcontrast CT shows a solitary, well-defined, low-attenuation mass with thin enhancing rim centered in the left thalamus. (**b**) Low-signal-intensity mass on T1-weighted postgadolinium images shows thin, well-defined, enhancing rim. Minimal adjacent low-signal white matter change corresponds to vasogenic edema.
c–f Brain abscess. (**c,d**) Pre- and postcontrast CT shows a bilobed, peripherally enhancing mass in the left parietal lobe and a smaller area of vasogenic edema in the right parietal white matter. (**e,f**) Diffusion-weighted MRI shows typical high signal within the center of the abscess. FLAIR images show the larger left parietal abscess and smaller right parietal focal area of vasogenic edema.

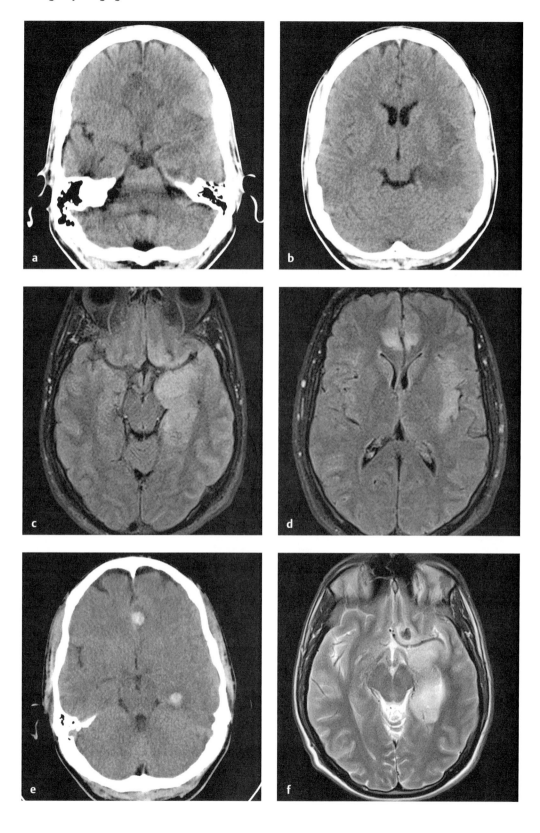

◆ Herpes Encephalitis

Herpes simplex encephalitis (HSE) is the most common cause of sporadic viral encephalitis. Its clinical manifestations range from mild headache, stiff neck, and fever to profound encephalopathy and coma. The virus migrates to the CNS from a facial infection via either the trigeminal or the olfactory nerve, and cerebritis develops in the inferior frontal and medial temporal lobes. Patients often experience malaise, fever, headache, and nausea that progresses to encephalopathy with lethargy, confusion, and delirium. Psychiatric symptoms and seizures are also common. Because HSE can mimic any toxic or infective encephalopathy and early CT findings are often absent or extremely subtle, the diagnosis may be delayed.

CT aids in the evaluation of encephalitis by excluding brain abscess, neoplasm, and other competing diagnostic considerations and can directly support the diagnosis of HSE. In adults, nonenhanced CT frequently shows edema and swelling of the cingulate gyri, the medial temporal lobe, and the inferior frontal lobe, sometimes associated with focal hemorrhage. MRI, particularly T2 and FLAIR sequences, is much more sensitive for detecting the characteristic edema pattern of HSE and should be considered in the encephalopathic patient with a normal CT and no clear metabolic explanation.

Because the consequences of delayed treatment of HSE can be devastating, CSF should be obtained for definitive diagnosis by polymerase chain reaction (PCR), and presumptive antiviral therapy should be instituted as the laboratory and imaging workup proceeds (**Fig. 2.28**).

Fig. 2.28a–f
a–d Herpes encephalitis. (**a,b**) Nonenhanced CT shows subtle low-attenuation parenchymal change in the anterior cingulate gyrus and insula. (**c,d**) FLAIR MRI better defines high-signal edema within the olfactory cortex, cingulate gyrus, medial temporal lobe, and insula. Enlargement of the medial temporal lobe indicates focal swelling.
e,f Herpes encephalitis presenting with intraparenchymal hemorrhage on NCCT. Two ~ 1-cm hemorrhages in the left inferior frontal and posterior temporal lobes with minimal surrounding vasogenic edema. Brain parenchyma is otherwise normal. (**f**) T2-weighted MRI shows a swollen medial left temporal lobe with increased T2 signal that extends to the left inferior frontal lobe (gyrus rectus), where a 1-cm low-intensity nodule corresponds to one of the focal hemorrhages visible on CT.

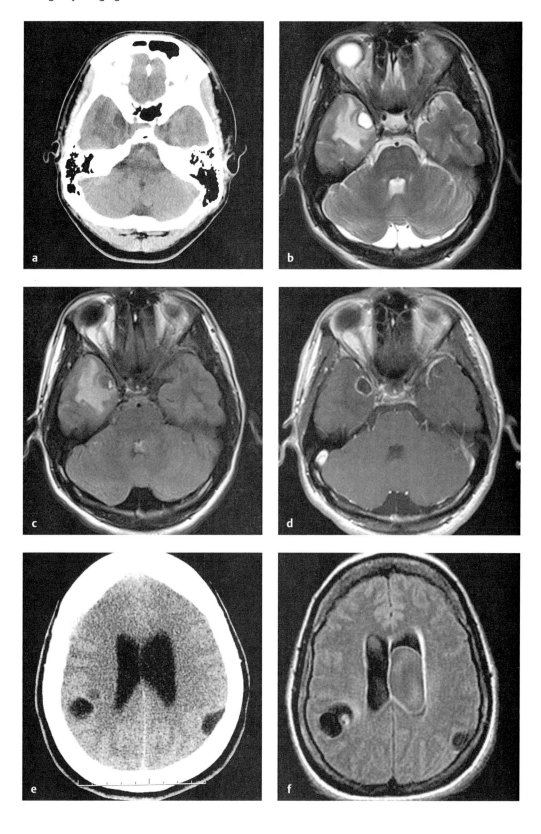

◆ Neurocysticercosis

Cysticercosis—systemic infestation by the larval form of the pork tapeworm *Taenia solium*—is endemic to Central America, South America, Asia, and Africa. The incidence in the United States has been steadily rising as a result of immigration and international travel. Infestation can involve almost any tissue, and neurocysticercosis is the leading cause of adult-onset epilepsy worldwide. Obstructive hydrocephalus, meningoencephalitis, stroke, headache, and altered mental status are other manifestations.

Clinical and imaging findings depend on the stage of the disease. The encysted larva enjoys immunologic invisibility as long as it is alive, and most patients are asymptomatic at this stage. As the larva dies, it elicits an immune reaction that leads to focal cerebritis and seizure. The encysted larva with surrounding cerebritis appears on CT as a low-attenuation lesion with peripheral enhancement and surrounding vasogenic edema. As acute inflammation resolves, the cyst retracts and appears as an enhancing parenchymal nodule with diminishing adjacent edema. Over time, the lesion calcifies.

The racemose form of neurocysticercosis consists of thin-walled "grapelike" cysts in the subarachnoid, intraventricular, and cisternal CSF spaces. Because the CT attenuation of unruptured cysts corresponds to CSF, an intraventricular cyst may be nearly undetectable and a subarachnoid cyst may be indistinguishable from a small arachnoid cyst. MRI imaging with FLAIR sequences readily differentiates the higher-signal cyst contents from normal CSF. Cysts that obstruct normal CSF flow can cause acute hydrocephalus (**Fig. 2.29**).

Fig. 2.29a–f
a–d Neurocysticercosis. (**a**) NCCT. 1-cm right anterior temporal cyst with surrounding vasogenic edema. (**b**) T2-weighted MRI. High-signal cyst with surrounding vasogenic edema. (**c**) FLAIR. The cyst is of intermediate intensity, indicating complicated fluid, and contains a 3-mm hyperintense nodule (larva). Surrounding vasogenic edema. (**d**) T1-weighted MRI + gadolinium. Near-CSF-signal-intensity cyst with thin enhancing rim and surrounding edema.
e,f Neurocysticercosis. (**e**) NCCT. Right parietal intraparenchymal and left parietal subarachnoid cysts. (**f**) FLAIR shows an additional intermediate-signal cyst within the left lateral ventricle, not visible on nonenhanced CT.

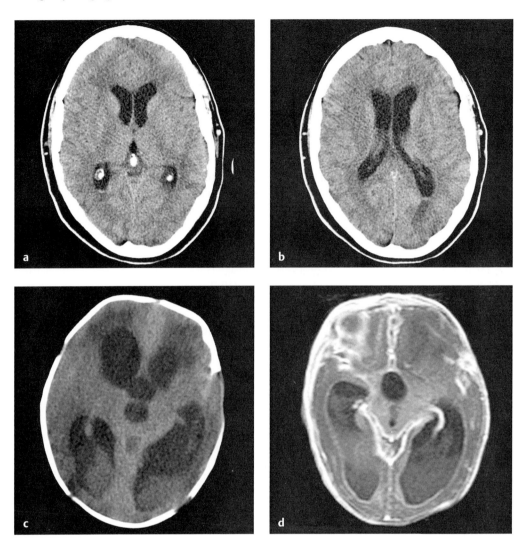

◆ Bacterial Meningitis

Acute bacterial meningitis is most commonly due to *Streptococcus pneumoniae, Neisseria meningitidis,* or group B streptococcus. Patients present with headache, stiff neck, and variable encephalopathy as a result of meningeal inflammation and adjacent cerebral edema. Potential complications include cerebral ischemia, sepsis, and hydrocephalus due to impaired CSF resorption. Viral meningitis, tuberculosis, cryptococcus, and coccidioidomycosis are nonbacterial infections that can mimic bacterial meningitis. Noninfectious considerations include neurosarcoidosis, meningeal carcinomatosis, and CNS lymphoma.

CT findings are often normal and, when present, subtle. They include mild hydrocephalus, sulcal effacement, and (rarely) hyperdense subarachnoid or intraventricular pus. Meningeal enhancement can be seen if contrast is administered.

FLAIR sequences are particularly sensitive to abnormal CSF and can be useful in the early detection of elevated CSF protein seen in meningitis. Oxygen therapy and subarachnoid hemorrhage can have a similar appearance.

The primary role of CT in suspected meningitis is not to establish the diagnosis but to exclude subarachnoid or intraparenchymal hemorrhage and ensure the safety of diagnostic lumbar puncture, which would be contraindicated by significant supratentorial edema or intracerebral mass (**Fig. 2.30**).

Fig. 2.30a–d
a,b Bacterial meningitis in an adult. Noncontrast CT. Mild ventricular enlargement; hyperdense debris fills the occipital horns of the lateral ventricles.
c,d Bacterial meningitis in an infant. (**c**) NCCT. Severe hydrocephalus with transependymal CSF resorption and intraventricular debris. (**d**) T1-weighted MRI with gadolinium. Diffuse leptomeningeal enhancement. Hydrocephalus.

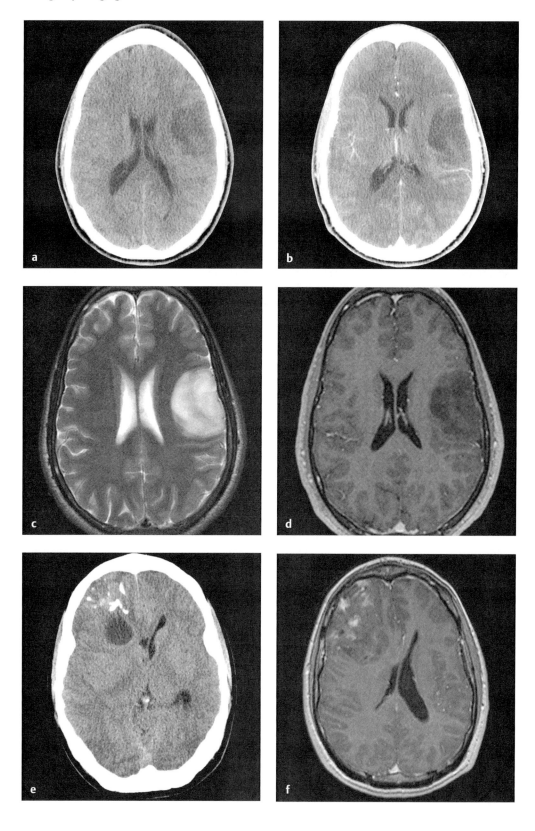

◆ Low- and Intermediate-Grade Glioma

Low-grade gliomas are primary CNS tumors, the majority of which are either astrocytomas, oligodendrogliomas, or mixed oligoastrocytomas. They are a common cause of a first seizure in previously healthy adults. Headache and sensory or motor deficits are other presenting symptoms. In contrast to malignant gliomas, which are usually discovered in older patients, low-grade tumors frequently occur in the third and fourth decades.

On CT, a low-grade astrocytoma appears as a nonenhancing, poorly defined, homogenous low-density tumor. The characteristic MRI appearance is that of a diffuse, non-enhancing mass, hypointense to brain on T1-weighted images and hyperintense on FLAIR and T2-weighted images. Most low-grade astrocytomas do not induce vascular proliferation and therefore do not enhance on CT or MRI. Oligodendrogliomas and mixed tumors comprising both astrocytes and oligodendrocytes may be histologically benign with modest neovascularity.

Anaplastic astrocytomas and anaplastic oligodendrogliomas are intermediate-grade neoplasms that arise from low-grade gliomas as a result of additional mutations in tumor-suppressing genes as the preexisting tumor ages. Like high-grade gliomas, they form blood vessels and will enhance with IV contrast administration. They are not necrotic, which is the pathologic hallmark of glioblastoma. Anaplastic gliomas are typically more heterogeneous than low-grade tumors on both CT and MRI (**Fig. 2.31**).

Fig. 2.31a–f
a–d Low-grade mixed oligoastrocytoma. CT shows a homogeneous low-attenuation mass involving the right frontal cortex and white matter. The mass is high in signal on T2-weighted MRI and low in signal on T1-weighted MRI, and it does not enhance after administration of MR or CT contrast material.
e,f Anaplastic oligodendroglioma. Partially calcified, partially cystic right frontal mass (CT) with scattered foci of enhancement on postgadolinium T1-weighted MRI.

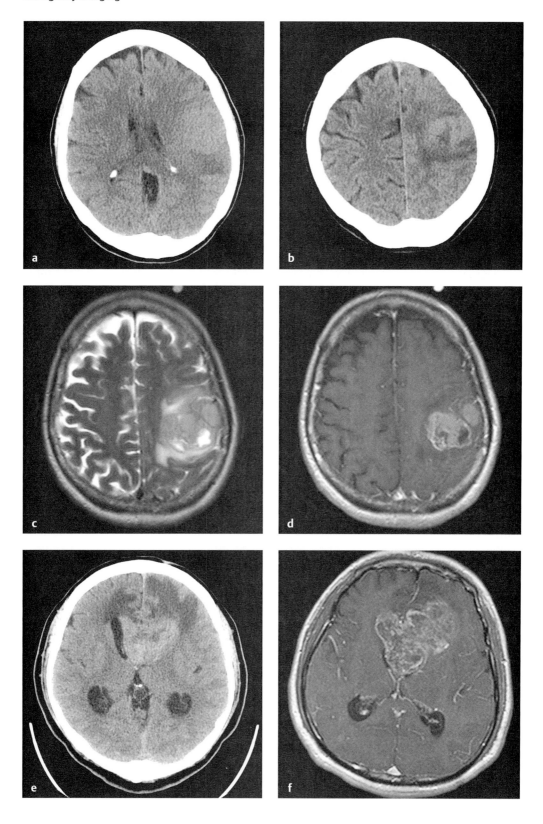

◆ Glioblastoma

Glioblastoma multiforme (GBM) is the most common adult primary brain tumor. It is a high-grade malignancy with poor prognosis; the average survival with treatment is 15 months or less. Most are discovered in the sixth and seventh decades, and patients usually present with a slowly progressive localizable neurologic deficit, symptoms of increased intracranial pressure (headache, nausea, vomiting, cognitive impairment), or new-onset seizure. Tumor cells migrate along white matter tracts and can traverse the corpus callosum to involve both hemispheres ("butterfly glioma"). Neovascularity and necrosis are defining pathologic features.

Most malignant astrocytomas are sporadic, but certain genetic syndromes are associated with an increased incidence, including neurofibromatosis type 1 and Li-Fraumeni and Turcot syndromes.

The emergent diagnosis of GBM and other brain tumors is often made by non-enhanced CT, which shows an irregular hypodense parenchymal mass with surrounding vasogenic cerebral edema. If contrast is administered, the margins invariably show enhancement. MRI may be the initial study, especially in patients who do not present to an emergency department.

Once diagnosed, MRI with gadolinium and multiplanar images is the most appropriate examination for comprehensive preoperative evaluation. The typical appearance is that of a heterogenous mass within the hemispheric white matter, with irregular, enhancing margins and central low T1 or high T2 signal corresponding to necrosis. Infiltrating glioma cells have been identified well beyond the apparent margins of the primary tumor, and discontinuous foci can develop, indicating migration along white matter tracts or spread via the CSF spaces (**Fig. 2.32**).

Fig. 2.32a–f
a–d Glioblastoma. (**a,b**) NCCT shows a 4-cm left posterior frontal cortical mass with ill-defined borders, adjacent vasogenic edema, sulcal effacement, and minimal subfalcine shift. (**c**) On T2-weighted MRI the mass is heterogenous with areas of cystic change. Vasogenic edema is more apparent. (**d**) On postgadolinium T1-weighted MRI there is heterogeneous tumor enhancement with surrounding edema and central low signal intensity change (necrosis).
e,f Glioblastoma "butterfly glioma." (**e**) NCCT shows a hyperdense mass that involves the genu of the corpus callosum and extends into the white matter of both frontal lobes. Large amount of associated vasogenic edema. The frontal horn of the left lateral ventricle is compressed with mild enlargement of the right frontal horn and ventricular atria. (**f**) Postgadolinium T1-weighted MRI shows heterogenous enhancement with central low signal changes (necrosis).

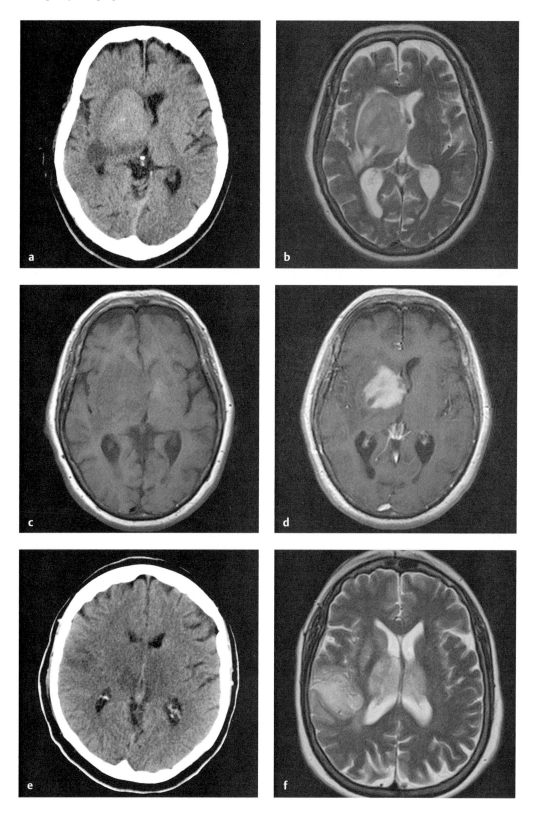

◆ Primary CNS Lymphoma

Primary CNS lymphoma is an uncommon tumor strongly associated with HIV/AIDS and other immunocompromised conditions, and most are non-Hodgkin and B-cell type, with peak incidence in the fifth decade. Signs and symptoms are usually nonspecific and include focal neurologic dysfunction, seizure, and headache.

In most patients CNS lymphoma develops rapidly and involves the deep cerebral nuclei or periventricular white matter. The mass is usually bulky and well demarcated with mild to moderate surrounding cerebral edema. In immunocompromised patients, primary CNS lymphoma may be multifocal, ring-enhancing, and difficult to distinguish from toxoplasmosis. In general, toxoplasmosis will always show ring enhancement when > 1 cm, whereas larger lymphomatous masses often, but do not necessarily, enhance homogeneously. When meningeal spread is identified, it is usually due to metastatic disease from an extracerebral primary site.

CNS lymphoma is characteristically hyperdense on CT because of the high lymphoblastic nuclear to cytoplasmic ratio. Enhancement in nonimmunocompromised patients is usually homogeneous, sometimes described as having a "lamb's wool" appearance. MRI shows one or more well-demarcated, homogeneously enhancing, round or oval masses that are usually slightly hypointense to white matter on T1-weighted images and of variable intensity on T2-weighted scans.

Treatment consists of steroids and chemotherapy after surgical biopsy. One feature of CNS lymphoma is that it may regress so rapidly and dramatically to steroid treatment that the diagnostic biopsy may be negative after as little as 24 hours. Prognosis is dependent on the grade and is usually worse in immunocompromised patients (**Fig. 2.33**).

Fig. 2.33a–f
a–d Primary CNS lymphoma. ~ 4-cm diameter hyperdense mass centered in the right putamen with compression of the right lateral ventricle and adjacent vasogenic edema. MRI shows relatively low signal intensity on T1-weighted images, mildly increased signal intensity on T2-weighted images, and avid contrast enhancement.
e,f Multifocal CNS lymphoma. Subtle right frontal and thalamic low-attenuation changes on nonenhanced CT. T2-weighted MRI is much more sensitive and shows high signal changes in both thalami and the right inferior parietal lobe.

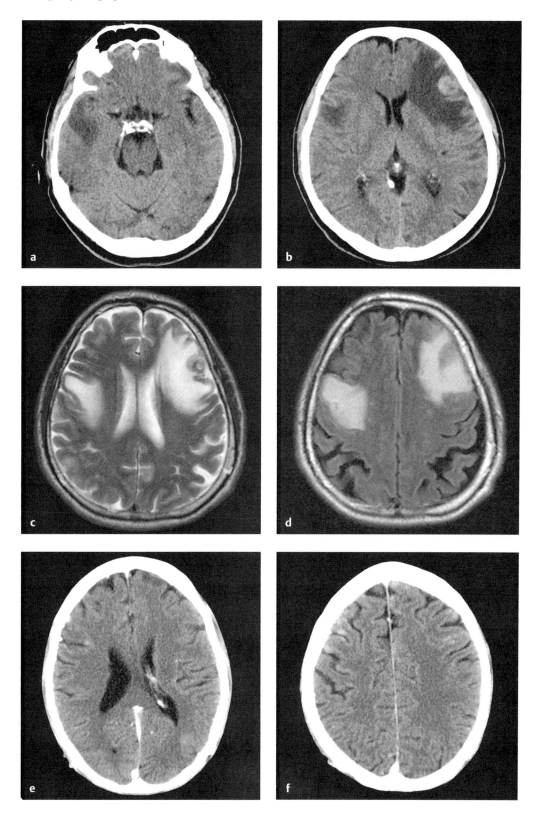

◆ Cerebral Metastasis

Brain metastases are common in advanced malignancy and are most frequently seen in patients with lung cancer, breast cancer, melanoma, renal cell carcinoma, or gastrointestinal adenocarcinoma. Patients often present with subacute headache, seizure, or focal neurologic impairment.

Most cerebral metastases are bloodborne, and their pattern of distribution is a consequence of regional intracerebral blood flow. Approximately 80% are found in the cerebrum, most often in the middle cerebral artery territory; 15% occur in the cerebellum, and 5% in the brainstem. Leptomeningeal metastases involve the surface of the brain and spinal cord and are the result of cortical or meningeal seeding.

Brain metastases are usually well demarcated with pronounced surrounding vasogenic edema. Enhancing nodules are usually less than 2 cm in diameter and located in the subcortical and cortical parenchyma near the gray-white matter junction. Because of their juxtacortical location, even small metastases can cause acute neurologic abnormalities, particularly seizures. Primary glial tumors, which arise deep to the cortex, are usually much larger than metastases when they become symptomatic.

On nonenhanced CT, metastases may be iso- or hypodense to adjacent brain and are usually revealed by their surrounding vasogenic edema rather than the mass itself. Metastases are typically hyperintense on T2 and FLAIR MRI and will usually enhance following CT or MR contrast administration. Some are characteristically hemorrhagic: choriocarcinoma, thyroid carcinoma, melanoma, and renal cell carcinoma. These should be considered in patients with unexplained parenchymal hemorrhage, particularly at the gray-white junction. The mnemonic CT-MR (choriocarcinoma, thyroid carcinoma, melanoma, renal cell carcinoma) can aid in their recollection. Lung and breast carcinoma metastases should be considered as well, because even though they are less likely to bleed, they are far more common (**Fig. 2.34**).

Fig. 2.34a–f
a–d Parenchymal metastases from lung carcinoma. (**a,b**) 2-cm left frontal cortical mass with marked associated vasogenic edema. A second focus of edema involves the right frontal operculum. Minimal left-to-right subfalcine shift. The brain is otherwise normal. (**c,d**) T2 and FLAIR images show corresponding extensive vasogenic edema.
e,f Leptomeningeal metastases from lung carcinoma. Multiple small nodules and focal linear cortical enhancement on postcontrast CT.

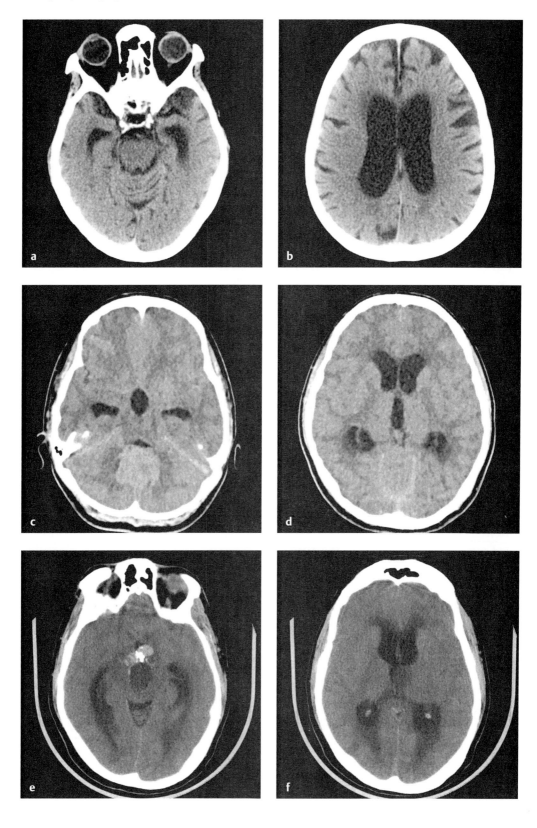

◆ Hydrocephalus

Communicating hydrocephalus consists of enlargement of all cerebral ventricles due to impairment of CSF resorption by dural arachnoid granulations. It may be acute or chronic. Causes include trauma, subarachnoid hemorrhage, meningitis, and prior surgery. In patients with chronic communicating hydrocephalus, a cause may not be identified, and patients come to clinical attention when hydrocephalus is incidentally discovered on studies obtained for minor trauma or in the evaluation of cognitive impairment.

Distinguishing between communicating hydrocephalus and global cerebral atrophy may be difficult and depends on estimation of ventricular size in relation to sulcal enlargement. Generalized cerebral atrophy may be due to chronic alcohol or anticonvulsant use, prior trauma, and neurodegenerative disorders such as Parkinson disease, Alzheimer dementia, and long-standing multiple sclerosis.

Normal-pressure hydrocephalus is a clinical syndrome, usually seen in patients over 50 years old, in which communicating hydrocephalus is associated with gradual development of urinary incontinence, gait disturbance, and memory loss. Even though these patients have a normal CSF opening pressure, some patients' symptoms may improve with therapeutic lumbar puncture, and patients in this group sometimes benefit from ventriculoperitoneal shunt placement.

Obstructive hydrocephalus, or noncommunicating hydrocephalus, refers to dilation of ventricles proximal to a mechanical block by tumor, blood clot, developmental web, periventricular parenchymal hemorrhage, or other mass. The most frequent sites of obstruction are the foramina of Monro, the third ventricle, the sylvian aqueduct, and the fourth ventricle.

Obstructive hydrocephalus may be acute or chronic. In acute obstructive hydrocephalus, CSF passes through small tears in the stretched ventricular ependymal lining and is absorbed by capillaries in the adjacent brain parenchyma (transependymal CSF resorption). This appears as low-attenuation parenchymal changes adjacent to the dilated lateral ventricles and does not occur in chronic or slowly developing hydrocephalus.

Temporal horn enlargement may be the earliest manifestation of acute ventricular obstruction. The width of the third ventricle is a sensitive and reliable indicator of changes in ventricular volume on serial examinations (**Fig. 2.35**).

Fig. 2.35a–f
a,b Chronic communicating hydrocephalus. Ventricular enlargement out of proportion to sulcal size. This appearance would be characteristic of a patient with clinical findings of normal-pressure hydrocephalus or could be due to remote meningeal inflammation, most often from subarachnoid hemorrhage or meningitis.
c,d Chronic obstructive hydrocephalus due to a cerebellar medulloblastoma. A hyperdense mass fills the fourth ventricle. The third and lateral ventricles are enlarged but do not show transependymal CSF resorption.
e,f Acute obstructive hydrocephalus due to craniopharyngioma. Partially calcified, solid, and cystic suprasellar mass. Lateral ventricular enlargement; normal third ventricle and cortical sulcal effacement are due to obstruction at the foramina of Monro. Subtle low-attenuation parenchymal changes adjacent to the ventricles indicate transependymal CSF resorption.

3
Head and Neck

◆ Approach

Head and neck conditions evaluated in the emergency department include facial trauma, blunt neck injury, orbital and periorbital inflammatory disease, neck masses, pharyngitis, and dental or neck abscesses. Most imaging involves face or neck CT, usually without contrast in the setting of trauma or with contrast for suspected inflammatory or neoplastic disease.

Facial trauma is common, and in this setting the radiologist's goals are to describe fractures and their displacements, identify specific fracture patterns, anticipate injuries to adjacent soft tissue structures, and communicate findings effectively to the surgeon. In the face, the most important fracture patterns include nasal and naso-orbito-ethmoid (NOE), zygomatico-maxillary (ZMC) complex fractures, Le Fort fractures, orbital wall fractures, and mandibular fractures.

Noncontrast CT is the primary imaging study for facial trauma, and multiplanar reformations are essential for accurate interpretation. Three-dimensional reconstructions aid in surgical visualization and should be included if available. All facial fractures should be individually listed in the report and assigned to whichever fracture pattern they most closely correspond. It is unusual for an acute fracture to involve a sinus wall without intrasinus hemorrhage. Intraorbital air indicates an orbital wall fracture and potential for complicating orbital infection. If the pterygoid plates are intact, all of the Le Fort fractures are excluded.

Facial Trauma Checklist

First Look

- Blood in sinuses?
- Blood in mastoid air cells?
- Pterygoid fracture?
- Orbital emphysema?
- Orbital hematoma or fat stranding?

Bone Survey

- Frontal sinus
- Nasal bones
- Ethmoid air cells
- Medial orbital walls (with attention to the nasolacrimal duct and attachment of the medial canthal ligament)
- Orbital rim
- Zygomatic arch
- Zygomaticofrontal suture
- Lateral orbital wall
- Orbital floor
- Orbital roof
- Pterygoid plates (involvement of the pterygoid plates defines the Le Fort fractures)
- Maxillary alveolus
- Maxillary sinus walls
- Mandible and temporomandibular joints
- Teeth
- Sphenoid sinus
- Carotid canals
- Mastoid air cells
- Petrous temporal bone (cochleae, vestibule and semicircular canals, ossicles)

Soft Tissue Survey

- Superficial soft tissues
- Nasal septum
- Sinus contents
- Orbital fat (with attention to any orbital stranding, emphysema, or subperiosteal hematoma)
- Globes
- Optic nerves
- Extra-ocular muscles
- Brain (pneumocephalus, hemorrhage)

Indications for Neck CT Angiogram in Trauma

Blunt neck trauma is associated with clinically occult vascular injury in up to 3% of hospitalized patients. Early detection of vascular injury and therapeutic anticoagulation or endovascular occlusion can significantly reduce the incidence of stroke in this group. The Denver Modified Blunt Cerebrovascular Screening Criteria define a high-risk group of trauma patients for whom urgent CT angiographic imaging is indicated:

- Direct signs of vascular injury (hemorrhage, bruit, hematoma)
- Focal neurologic deficit or CT demonstrating acute cerebral infarct.
- Le Fort II or III fracture
- Cervical spine fracture
- Basilar skull fracture involving carotid canal
- Severe brain injury (diffuse axonal injury, GCS < 6)
- Hanging injury
- Neck contusion

Patients with penetrating injuries who do not undergo immediate surgical exploration should be imaged by CTA or conventional angiography. Typical vascular injuries in both blunt and penetrating trauma include dissection, occlusion, pseudoaneurysm, and arteriovenous fistula. Urgent CTA should also be considered in patients who present with focal neurologic findings, as vascular dissection with minimal or no trauma is an important cause of stroke, particularly in younger adults.

Approach to Inflammatory or Neoplastic Conditions

Suspected inflammatory or neoplastic conditions of the face and neck should be evaluated using postcontrast CT. Because of its anatomic complexity, neck CT interpretation is aided by grouping related structures.

Nontraumatic Face/Neck Checklist

Airway and Related Structures

- Nasal cavity
- Nasopharynx
- Oropharynx
- Hypopharynx
- Larynx
- Trachea
- Lung apices
- Esophagus
- Thyroid gland

Soft Tissues and Bones

- Muscles
- Blood vessels
- Lymph nodes
- Cervical spine and skull base

Oral Cavity and Salivary Glands

- Tongue
- Tongue base
- Mandible, maxilla, and dentition
- Floor of mouth
- Submandibular glands
- Parotid glands

Orbits

- Globes
- Muscles
- Optic nerve
- Orbital fat
- Orbital walls

Everything else

- Skull base
- Brain
- Temporal bones

Temporal Bone Approach

Like the face and neck, the temporal bone is a complex structure, and a repeatable anatomic method is useful in order to avoid errors. One practical approach is to:

1. Address structures from outside to inside, beginning with the auricle and ending with the ossicles.
2. Evaluate the mastoid bone.
3. Address structures from inside to outside, beginning at the cerebellopontine angle, evaluating the internal auditory canal, cochlea, vestibule, and semicircular canals and ending with the facial nerve. The facial nerve, carotid canal, and jugular bulb canals can be dehiscent, and they should be described if so, as these anatomic variants can complicate surgery if not detected preoperatively.

Outside to Inside

- Auricle
- External auditory canal
- Tympanic membrane
- Tympanic cavity (hypo-tympanum and epitympanum)
- Sinus tympani and pyramidal eminence
- Ossicles and scutum

Mastoid Bone

- Mastoid air cells
- Mastoid antrum
- Tegmen tympani
- Tegmen mastoideum

Inside to Outside

- Cerebellopontine angle and brainstem
- Internal auditory canal
- Cochlea, vestibule
- Semicircular canals
- Vestibular aqueduct
- Petrous bone mineralization
- Facial nerve
- Carotid canal
- Jugular bulb

◆ Imaging and Anatomy

Imaging

Face CT (Noncontrast Helical)

Indications: Facial, orbital, or mandibular trauma.

Technique: 0.6-mm dataset with 1–2-mm axial, 2-mm sagittal, and 2-mm coronal reformations of head, face, and cervical spine. Oblique sagittal images, 1 mm, along the course of the optic nerve may be obtained for evaluation of orbital pathology. Images obtained from orbital roof to hyoid (unless obtained in conjunction with head and cervical spine CT).

Face CT (Helical + Contrast)

Indications: Orbital cellulitis, suspected facial abscess, mass.

Technique: 0.6-mm dataset with 1–2-mm axial, 2-mm sagittal, and 2-mm coronal reformations of head, face, and cervical spine. Oblique sagittal images, 1 mm, along the course of the optic nerve may be obtained for evaluation of orbital pathology. Images obtained from orbital roof to hyoid (unless obtained in conjunction with head and cervical spine CT).

Contrast: 60–100 mL at 1–2 mL/sec with 100-second delay.

Neck CT (Helical + Contrast)

Indications: Neck mass, abscess, adenopathy.

Technique: 0.6-mm dataset with 2–3-mm axial, 2-mm sagittal, and 2-mm coronal reformations of head, face, and cervical spine. Images obtained from orbital roof to thoracic inlet.

Contrast: 60–100 mL at 1–2 mL/sec with 100-second delay.

Neck CT Arteriogram

Indications: High-energy blunt trauma, suspected arterial dissection, penetrating injury.

Technique: 0.6-mm dataset with 2-mm axial, 2-mm sagittal, and 2-mm coronal reformations of head, face, and cervical spine. Images obtained from orbital roof to thoracic inlet.

Contrast: 60–100 mL at 3–4 mL/sec in arterial phase.

Temporal Bone CT

Indications: Skull base fracture, auditory or vestibular dysfunction, hemotympanum in trauma, mastoiditis, otitis media or externa.

Technique: 0.6-mm dataset with 0.6-mm axial, 1-mm sagittal, and 1-mm coronal reformations of the temporal bone in bone algorithm. Images obtained from petrous apex to C1.

Contrast (optional depending on indication): 60–100 mL at 3–4 mL/sec in venous phase (30–45-second delay).

Anatomy

Interpreting neck CT is aided by an understanding of the various deep compartments that are separated by investing fascia. Because the differential diagnosis of a neck mass depends primarily on its location, this approach is useful for establishing the likely nature of an inflammatory or neoplastic processes. These compartments include

- Pharyngeal mucosal space
- Parapharyngeal space
- Retropharyngeal space
- Pre- (or peri-) vertebral space
- Carotid space
- Parotid space
- Masticator space
- Submandibular space
- Sublingual space

Because the fascia investing each of these spaces acts as a barrier to the spread of infection and because each contains specific tissues, locating a process to one space or another goes a long way toward making a diagnosis of head and neck disease.

The pharyngeal mucosal space (PMS) consists of the mucosa lining the upper aerodigestive tract and associate lymphatic tissues. Pharyngitis, tonsillitis, and most squamous cell carcinomas of the head and neck will be located in the PMS.

The parapharyngeal space (PPS) is important not for what it contains, which is mainly fat and small blood vessels, but because it is easily identified by its low density and displaced by masses in the adjacent pharyngeal mucosal space, carotid space, masticator space, and retropharyngeal space.

The retropharyngeal space (RPS) is a potential space containing lymph nodes located behind the dorsal PMS. It is an important route of spread for infections of the PMS, including tonsillitis and peritonsillar abscess. Infections involving the RPS can arise by contiguous spread from adjacent spaces and by suppuration of draining lymph nodes in the RPS. RPS infections can also extend inferiorly to the chest, leading to mediastinitis, a severe and potentially fatal condition.

The prevertebral space (PVS) is defined by the fascia that invests the vertebrae and prevertebral muscles. Infections and tumors located in the PVS usually arise from the disk or vertebral body. Because the PVS is contiguous with the epidural space, infection of the PVS can potentially lead to an epidural abscess.

The carotid space (CS) contains the carotid artery, jugular vein, lymph nodes, the carotid body, and the ninth and tenth cranial nerves. Pathologies specific to this space include carotid body tumors, CN9 and CN10 schwannomas, vascular disease (arteritis and thrombophlebitis), and arterial injuries and anomalies including pseudoaneurysms and arteriovenous fistula.

The parotid space (PS) surrounds the parotid gland, a number of lymph nodes, the proximal parotid duct, and the seventh cranial nerves. Parotitis, parotid sialadenitis, benign and malignant salivary gland tumors, lymphoepithelial cysts (seen in HIV-positive patients), and lymphadenitis occur here.

The masticator space (MS) contains portions of the mandible and the masseter, temporalis, and pterygoid muscles, as well as blood vessels and nerves. Most infections in this space are of dental origin. Neoplasms arising from muscle and bone can also occur in the MS.

The submandibular space (SMS) is located inferior and lateral to the mylohyoid muscle. It contains the submandibular glands, second branchial cleft cysts, and lymph nodes. The sublingual space (SLS) is superior and medial to the mylohyoid and contains mi-nor salivary glands as well as portions of the submandibular gland and duct. Infections in these spaces are usually odontogenic or submandibular in origin. Neoplasms tend to arise from minor salivary glands or the mandible (**Fig. 3.1** and **Fig. 3.2**).

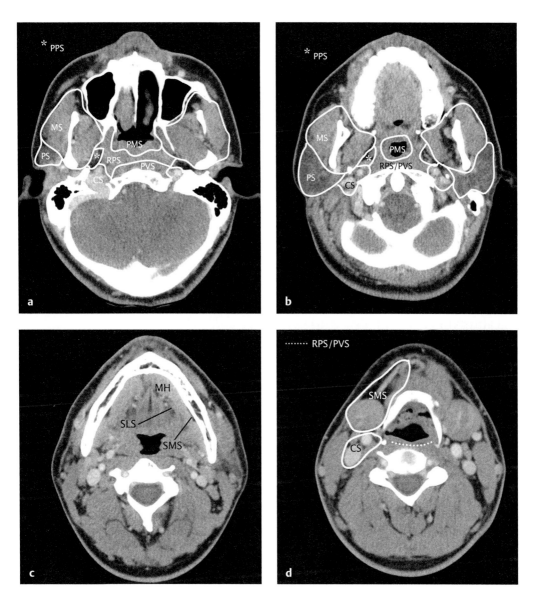

Fig. 3.1a–d Neck compartment anatomy. PMS: pharyngeal mucosal space. PPS: parapharyngeal space. RPS: retropharyngeal space. PVS: pre- (or peri-) vertebral space. CS: carotid space. PS: parotid space. MS: masticator space. SMS: submandibular space. SLS: sublingual space.

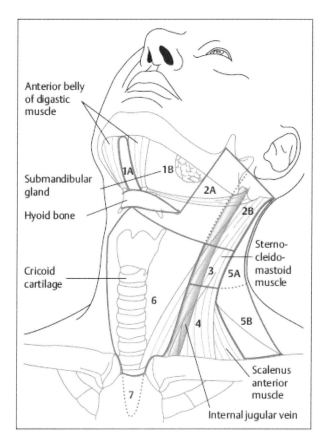

Fig. 3.2 Cervical lymph node levels. Level 1A nodes are submental and located between the digastric muscles. Level 1B nodes are submandibular and located lateral to the digastric and anterior to the posterior aspect of the hyoid bone. Level 2A, 2B, 3, and 4 are nodes of the jugular chain. Level 2 nodes are above the hyoid, Level 3 nodes are between the hyoid and cricoid cartilages, and level 4 nodes are below the cricoid. Level 2B nodes are posterior to the jugular vein but anterior to the margin of the sternocleidomastoid. Level 5 nodes are all posterior to the sternocleidomastoid margin and make up the spinal accessory chain, with level 5A nodes above the cricoid and level 5B nodes below it. Level 6 and 7 nodes are paratracheal and paraesophageal.

◆ Clinical Presentations and Differential Diagnosis

Clinical Presentations and Appropriate Initial Studies

Trauma

- CT Face or Neck without Intravenous Contrast
  - Frontal sinus/orbital roof fracture
  - Nasal or nasal septal fracture
  - Naso-orbito-ethmoid fracture
  - Zygomaticomaxillary complex fracture
  - Le Fort fracture
  - Orbital wall (blowout) fracture
  - Globe rupture
  - Orbital hematoma
  - Temporal bone fracture
  - Skull base fracture
  - Carotid or vertebral vascular injury
  - Larynx fracture

Infection/Inflammation

- CT Face or Neck with Intravenous Contrast
  - Tonsillitis/pharyngitis
  - Parapharyngeal or retropharyngeal abscess
  - Dental or periodontal disease with abscess
  - Sialadenitis
  - Orbital cellulitis
  - Infectious or reactive adenopathy (suppurative adenitis, mycobacterial disease, mononucleosis)

Mass

- CT Face or Neck with Intravenous Contrast
- MRI with Gadolinium
  - Lymphoma
  - Metastatic head and neck carcinoma
  - Parotid or submandibular neoplasm
  - Developmental cysts (thyroglossal duct cyst, branchial cleft cyst)

Differential Diagnosis

Clival/Skull Base Mass

- Metastasis
- Chordoma
- Chondrosarcoma

Nasopharyngeal Mass

- Prominent lymphatic tissue (normal in patients < 30, consider HIV in patients > 40)
- Prevertebral space infection (osteomyelitis/diskitis)
- Nasopharyngeal carcinoma
- Juvenile nasopharyngeal angiofibroma (adolescent males)
- Lymphoma
- Tornwaldt cyst

Pharyngeal Mucosal Space Mass

- Tonsillitis/abscess
- Squamous cell carcinoma
- Lymphoma

Retropharyngeal Mass

- Abscess/phlegmon
- Adenopathy/nodal metastasis
- Lymphoma

Prevertebral Space Mass

- Osteomyelitis/diskitis
- Abscess
- Chordoma/skull base chondrosarcoma/ vertebral metastasis

Parotid Space Mass

- Parotitis (diffuse enlargement)
- Benign salivary gland neoplasm, 80% (pleomorphic adenoma, Warthin tumor)
- Malignant neoplasm, 20% (mucoepidermoid, adenoid cystic carcinoma)
- Intraparotid lymph node
- Lymphoepithelial cyst (HIV)

Carotid Space Mass

- Paraganglioma
- Schwannoma
- Carotid pseudoaneurysm/dissection

Jugular Foramen Mass

- Schwannoma
- Meningioma
- Paraganglioma

Masticator Space Mass

- Odontogenic abscess
- Primary bone or muscle neoplasm (sarcoma)
- Osteomyelitis

Submandibular Space Mass

- Odontogenic abscess
- Submandibular sialadenitis/abscess
- Salivary gland neoplasm
- Obstructed minor salivary gland (ranula)
- Lymphadenopathy

Mandibular Cystic Lesion

- Periradicular cyst (in carious teeth)
- Dentigerous cyst (around crown of unerupted tooth)
- Aneurysmal bone cyst
- Ameloblastoma
- Giant cell tumor

Sinus Disease with Bone Destruction

- Invasive fungal sinusitis (mucormycosis, actinomycosis)
- Carcinoma
- Lymphoma
- Wegener granulomatosis

Thyroid Mass

- Benign nodule
- Carcinoma
- Parathyroid adenoma
- Distal thyroglossal duct cyst

Multiple Enlarged Cervical Lymph Nodes

- Lymphoma
- Mycobacterial disease
- Metastatic head and neck carcinoma
- Lymph node hyperplasia

Low Attenuation Lymph Nodes

- Mycobacterial disease
- Metastatic head and neck carcinoma

Ocular Mass

- Retinoblastoma
- Melanoma
- Retinal detachment

Intraconal Orbital Mass

- Cavernous malformation
- Optic nerve meningioma
- Optic glioma
- Inflammatory pseudotumor
- Metastasis
- Lymphoma
- Hematoma

Extraconal Orbital Mass

- Orbital abscess
- Lacrimal gland tumor or inflammation
- Dermoid
- Lymphoma
- Metastasis
- Hematoma

Orbital Muscle Enlargement

- Thyroid orbitopathy
- Idiopathic orbital inflammation (pseudotumor)

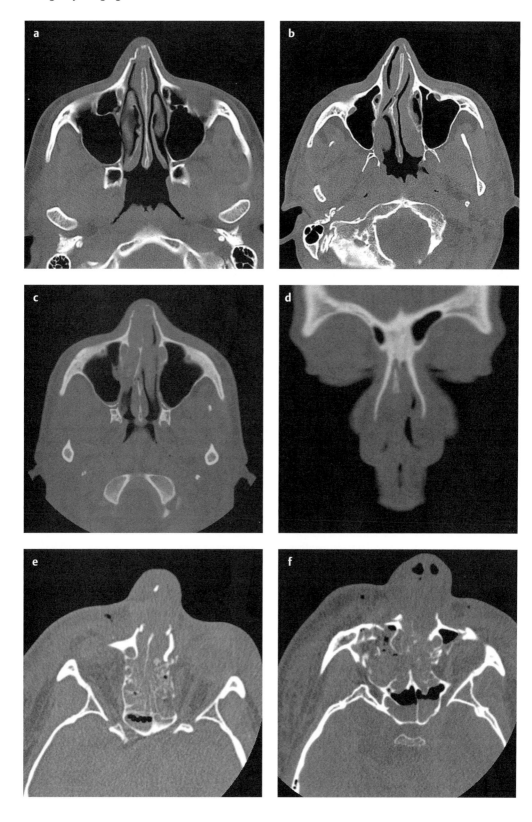

◆ Nasal and Naso-Orbito-Ethmoid Fracture

Nasal fractures result from direct impact, and deformity, laceration, or ecchymosis are often evident on examination. Epistaxis and CSF rhinorrhea indicate potentially severe injuries to the ethmoid bones or nasal septum.

Plain radiographs are rarely helpful. At best, they serve to document the presence of a fracture. If there is clinical concern for septal fracture or adjacent facial bone injury, or if operative reduction is planned, CT scanning is preferred and provides more comprehensive evaluation. Nasal fractures are often detected when CT is obtained for more severe injuries, and they often make up a part of a larger facial fracture complex. Most are oriented perpendicular to the nasal bridge, cross the nasomaxillary suture, and traverse the groove for the nasociliary nerve.

Because most simple nasal bone fractures are managed conservatively, clinical examination should include a search for septal deformity or hematoma. Although not specific for fracture, nasal septal hematomas are associated with significant morbidity and may lead to septal perforation or necrosis if untreated. Other consequences of failing to recognize a septal fracture are delayed nasal obstruction and cosmetic deformity. CT findings include fracture through the vomer or perpendicular ethmoid plate, and swollen paraseptal soft tissues. Treatment for significantly displaced septal fractures is surgical.

Naso-orbito-ethmoid (NOE) fractures are complex fractures of the nasal bones and the upper central mid-face due to direct impact to the nasal bridge. Fragments of the nasal bones, ethmoid air cells, and medial orbital walls are compressed and displaced posteriorly toward the sphenoid sinus. Cribriform plate and ethmoid roof fractures, when present, can be associated with anosmia, pneumocephalus, or CSF leak. Comminution and lateral displacement of the lacrimal bone can result in ocular, nasolacrimal duct, or nasofrontal duct injury. The medial canthal ligament, which anchors the globe, can be disrupted, with consequent enophthalmos, telecanthus, or ptosis. Traumatic nasolacrimal duct obstruction may require surgical repair.

CT scans should include reformations in three planes, with particular attention to the nasolacrimal ducts, attachment of the medial canthal ligament, and integrity of the anterior skull base. Three-dimensional reformations are valuable for surgical planning (**Fig. 3.3**).

Fig. 3.3a–f
a Nasal bone fracture. Minimally depressed right nasal bone fracture. The nasal septum and turbinates are normal.
b Nasal septal fracture. Osseous septal fracture without associated hematoma. Bilateral minimally displaced nasal bone fractures.
c,d Nasal septal fracture with hematoma. Anterior septal soft tissue thickening. Osseous septal fracture.
e,f Naso-orbital-ethmoid fracture. Severely comminuted nasal, ethmoid, and bilateral medial orbital wall fractures, with posterior telescoping of the ethmoid fragments. Left ethmoid and orbital roof fractures. Extensive facial soft tissue swelling with associated bilateral intraorbital hematomas.

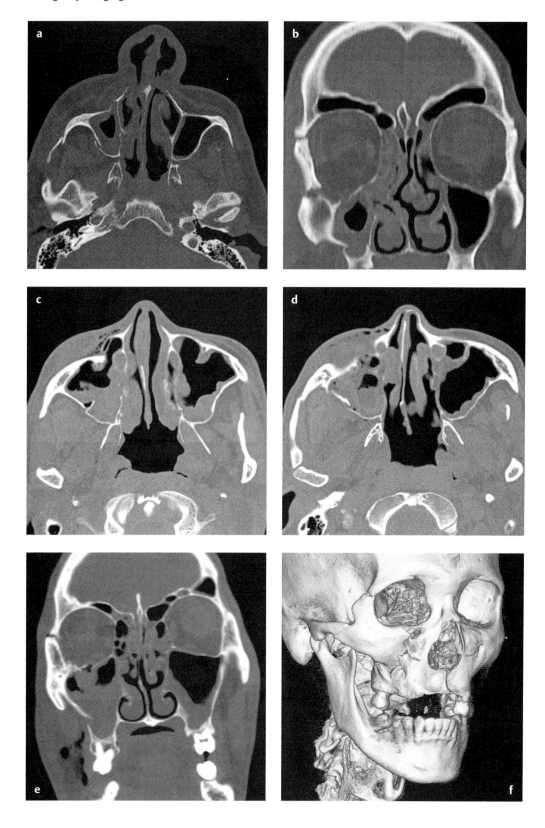

◆ Zygomaticomaxillary Complex Fracture

The zygomaticomaxillary complex (ZMC) fracture results from a direct blow to the cheek and comprises the following fractures: (1) zygomatic arch, (2) lateral orbital wall (or diastasis of the zygomaticofacial suture), (3) inferior orbital rim and floor, and (4) anterolateral maxillary sinus wall. As they involve all four zygomatic articulations, the ZMC fractures effectively separate a malar fragment from the lateral facial skeleton. ZMC fractures can be variably rotated or depressed. Clinical findings include a palpable step-off at the inferior orbital rim or zygoma, subcutaneous emphysema, and hyperesthesia or anesthesia over the cheek (CN V2 distribution). Diplopia on upward gaze may be due to orbital edema or impingement of the inferior rectus muscle by an orbital floor bone fragment. Other clinical findings include pain with mastication from associated mandibular coracoid process and temporalis muscle impingement.

CT with multiplanar reformations locates the fracture components, the degree of malar fragment displacement and rotation, and any associated soft tissue or ocular injuries. The infraorbital canal (containing the maxillary nerve), orbital contents, nasolacrimal duct, and medial canthal ligament attachment should be specifically examined (**Fig. 3.4**).

Fig. 3.4a–f
a,b Zygomaticomaxillary complex fracture. Minimally displaced right zygomatic arch, anterior and posterolateral maxillary sinus wall, orbital rim, and orbital floor fractures. Right zygomaticofrontal suture diastasis.
c–f Zygomaticomaxillary complex fracture. Posterior displacement of the malar fragment with soft tissue emphysema. Right zygomatic arch, anterior and posterolateral maxillary sinus wall, orbital rim, and orbital floor fractures. Right zygomaticofrontal suture diastasis. 3D reconstruction shows the malar fragment.

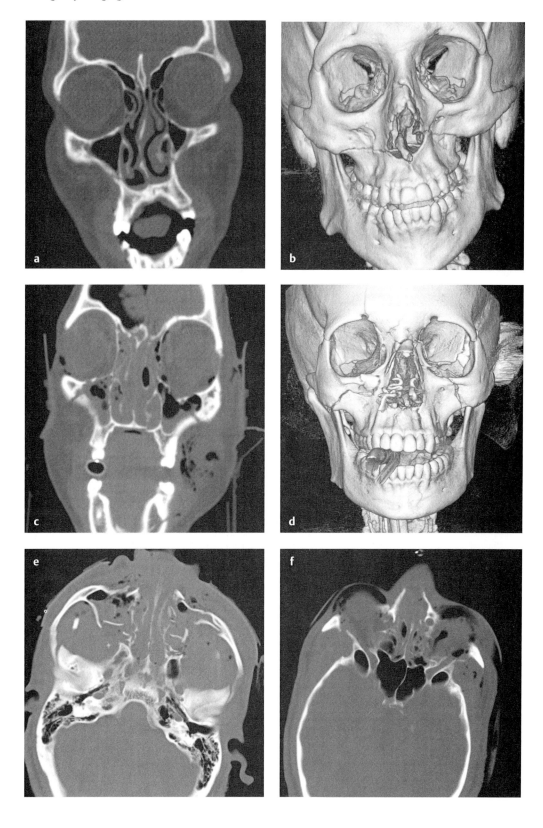

◆ Le Fort Fractures

The sine qua non of a Le Fort fracture is involvement of the pterygoid plates, and all Le Fort fractures effectively separate a portion of the midface from the cranium. Le Fort I, II, and III patterns often occur in combination and can overlap with other complex fracture patterns such as midface smash, naso-orbito-ethmoid, and ZMC (**Fig. 3.5**).

The Le Fort I fracture is a horizontal maxillary fracture that traverses the pterygoid plates, inferior maxillary sinus, and nasal septum, separating the teeth and maxillary alveolus from the upper face. This injury can often be diagnosed on physical exam based on isolated mobility of the hard palate. Le Fort I fractures always involve the inferior maxillary sinus walls and do not extend to the orbits or upper nasal bones.

Le Fort II is a pyramidal midface fracture that involves the maxillary antra and inferior orbital rims, intersecting at the glabella. The fracture follows an oblique course from the bridge of the nose to the pterygoid plates and separates the maxilla, anterior nasal bones, and anterior orbital floor and rim from the remainder of the skull. Le Fort II fractures do not involve the lateral orbital walls or zygomatic arches. The absence of an infraorbital rim fracture excludes a Le Fort II injury.

Le Fort III fractures separate the entire midface from the cranium and involve the pterygoid plates, the orbital walls, and the zygomatic arches. The fracture passes horizontally and posteriorly through the nasofrontal suture, frontomaxillary suture, lateral orbital wall, zygomatic arches, and pterygoid plates. Zygomatic arch fracture, best visualized on axial CT images, is unique to a Le Fort III fracture, and its absence excludes the diagnosis (**Fig. 3.6**).

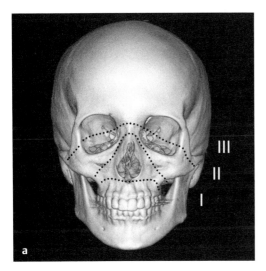 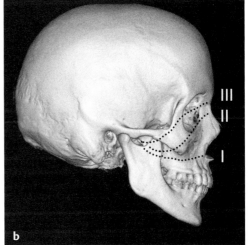

Fig. 3.5 Le Fort I, II, and III patterns.

Fig. 3.6a–f
a,b Le Fort I. Transverse fracture of the maxilla with involvement of the inferior maxillary sinuses and nasal septum. The orbits and upper maxillae are intact.
c,d Le Fort II. Pyramidal fracture of the inferior orbital rims, anterior maxillary sinus walls, and nasal bridge.
e,f Le Fort III. Severely comminuted bilateral pterygoid, orbital wall, and zygomatic arch fractures. Extensive orbital emphysema. Severe comminution reflects overlap with midface smash pattern.

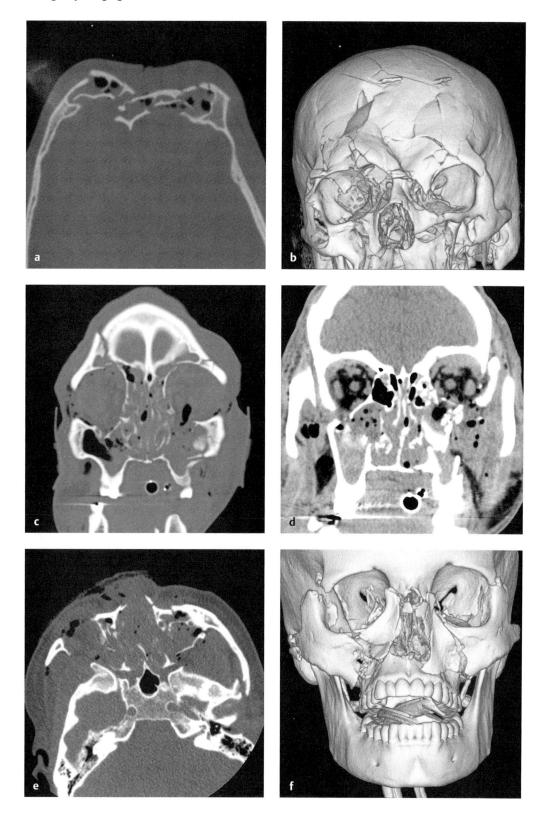

◆ Midface Smash Injury

Midface smash injury is a general term applied to severely comminuted, high-energy impact, facial fractures that are not easily categorized as Le Fort, SMC, or NOE fractures. They can be loosely classified based on the their location as frontal, nasofrontal, or central, but these categories typically overlap. Frontal midface smash injuries are characterized by disruption of the frontal sinus; nasofrontal injuries involve the orbits, orbital apices, and ethmoidal roof; and central smash injuries involve the orbits, maxilla, and mandible. CT shows extensive facial bone comminution, often with posterior fragment displacement. Nonosseous structures that can be injured include upper cranial nerves, globes, extraocular muscles, nasolacrimal ducts, and sinuses (**Fig. 3.7**).

Fig. 3.7a–f
a,b   Frontal type midface smash. Severely comminuted fracture, predominantly involving the frontal sinus, but with associated comminutions of the orbital walls and maxillae.
c,d   Nasofrontal type. Comminuted fractures of the nasal bones, orbital roofs, orbital floors, and frontal bone. Bilateral superior orbital extraconal hematomas. Extensive soft tissue emphysema.
e,f   Central smash injury. Nasal, maxillary, and lateral orbital wall fractures.

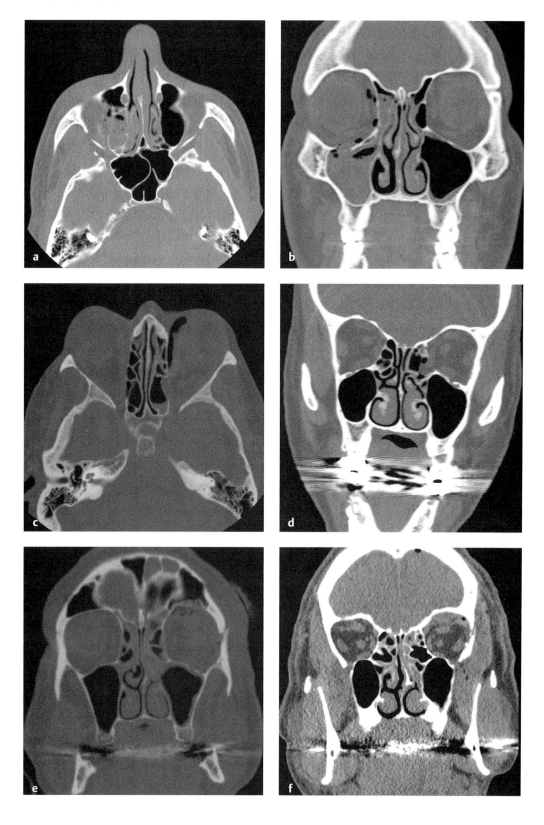

◆ Orbital Wall Fractures

Orbital wall fractures may be due to extension from a calvarial or skull base fracture, or they can follow direct impact from a fist or a ball to the eye socket. In this case an abrupt increase in intraorbital pressure leads most commonly to orbital floor failure with variable orbital fat herniation, inferior rectus or oblique muscle entrapment, orbital emphysema, and intrasinus hemorrhage. These are often referred to as orbital blowout fractures. Clinical findings, when present, include restricted upward and lateral gaze, subcutaneous emphysema, and diminished sensation in the distribution of the infraorbital nerve (V2). Enophthalmos is usually not evident acutely, but it can be seen in unrepaired fractures after initial swelling resolves. Rarely symptomatic bradycardia can result from stretching of the infraorbital nerve (oculocardiac reflex).

Medial orbital wall, or lamina papyracea, fractures often occur in conjunction with floor fractures, but isolated medial wall fractures are much less common than floor fractures or combinations. Most medial orbital wall fractures are small, of little consequence, and discovered on CT obtained for other indications long after an injury. When symptomatic, medial wall fractures are associated with orbital emphysema and potential medial rectus muscle entrapment, which can lead to diplopia on lateral gaze.

Orbital roof fractures are uncommon, and most are due to extension from frontal and calvarial fractures in major head injury.

CT defines the area and location of the fracture as well as any fragment displacement. Orbital fat herniation, extraocular muscle entrapment, and infraorbital canal involvement are easily identified. Muscle entrapment is evident clinically by diplopia on horizontal or vertical gaze, and corresponding CT findings include an acute change in the angle of the muscle as it passes through the orbit or impalement of one of the muscles on a bone spicule. Intraorbital emphysema and retroseptal intraorbital or subperiosteal hematoma should be sought, as the former indicates risk of orbital infection and the latter may lead to increased intraorbital pressures, with secondary globe ischemia or optic nerve damage.

Surgical intervention is usually indicated for severe fractures to prevent late enophthalmos and diplopia. Emergent surgical indications include symptomatic bradycardia and large orbital hematoma (**Fig. 3.8**).

Fig. 3.8a–f
a,b   Orbital floor fracture. Right orbital floor fracture with depression of the lateral orbital floor. The infraorbital canal (V2 branch) is intact. Intraorbital air and intrasinus hemorrhage.
c,d   Medial orbital wall fracture. Left posterior medial orbital wall fracture with intraorbital emphysema and fat and medial rectus herniation into the posterior ethmoid air cells. The medial rectus is tethered at the anterior margin of the fracture.
e,f   Orbital roof fracture. Left orbital roof fracture with extension into aerated frontal sinus. Superior orbital extraconal hematoma and orbital emphysema.

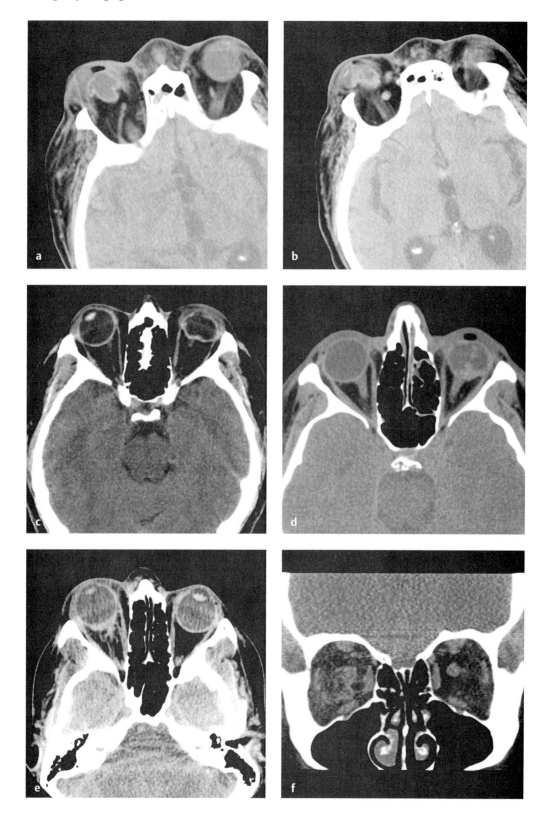

◆ Globe and Orbital Soft Tissue Injury

Open globe injury is a consequence of direct ocular trauma in which the sclera is disrupted and vitreous humor leaks into the adjacent orbital tissue. Although ophthalmoscopy is more sensitive for detection of small ruptures, it is not always possible to examine the globe in acute facial trauma due to periorbital soft tissue swelling, and globe rupture is often identified on CT for face or head injury. The ruptured globe is often small and irregular and can have a flattened contour reminiscent of a "mushroom" or "flat tire." Globe rupture may follow either blunt or penetrating trauma. In blunt trauma, it frequently occurs at intraocular muscle insertions, where the sclera is thinnest.

Some globe ruptures are inapparent on CT. In patients with an apparently intact globe, unilateral posterior lens subluxation (deep anterior chamber) or thickening of the posterior sclera are subtle signs of globe injury. More obvious CT findings include scleral discontinuity, intraocular air

or hemorrhage, lens subluxation, intraocular foreign bodies, and traumatic cataract.

Orbital hematomas are caused by penetrating or blunt orbital trauma. Blood collections within the orbit cause increased intraorbital pressure, which, if not recognized and treated, can lead to compressive optic nerve injury. Retrobulbar hematomas, in particular, have the potential to compress the optic nerve. The clinical presentation is variable, and symptoms related to hematoma formation may not manifest until several days after the acute injury.

CT identifies proptosis, stretching of the optic nerve, and "globe tenting," in which the angle made by two tangents to the globe that intersect at the optic nerve head is less than 130°. While orbital hemorrhage and hematoma are uncommon, traumatic orbital compartment syndrome can lead to vision loss; in such cases prompt lateral canthotomy and cantholysis may prevent blindness (**Fig. 3.9**).

Fig. 3.9a–f
a,b Globe rupture with intraocular lens prosthesis extrusion. Extensive right-sided preseptal periorbital hematoma. The right globe is distorted with a mushroom-like appearance. A tiny linear density superolateral to the anterior globe is an extruded intraocular lens implant.
c Globe rupture. Globe deformity with posterior flattening and reduced volume. The lens is displaced from its normal position.
d Globe rupture with vitreous hemorrhage from drill-bit perforation. Flattened anterior globe, intravitreous hemorrhage, and posterior vitreous versus choroidal hemorrhage.
e,f Intraorbital hematoma. Right intraconal and retrobulbar soft tissue stranding with associated mild proptosis.

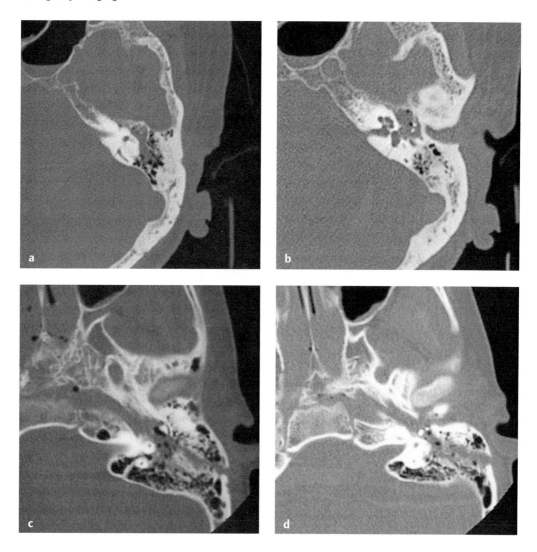

◆ Temporal Bone Fracture

High-energy impact to the lateral skull can result in fractures through the mastoid and temporal bone. They are best described by the fracture orientation relative to the axis of the petrous temporal bone and by involvement of the otic capsule or labyrinth. Patients may have conductive or sensorineural hearing loss, facial paralysis (peripheral seventh-nerve palsy), bruising about the mastoid eminence (Battle sign), or periorbital ecchymosis (raccoon eyes).

Indirect findings are usually evident on noncontrast head CT and include mastoid air cell opacification, fluid within the external auditory canal and middle ear, air in the temporomandibular fossa, and intracranial air adjacent to the petrous bone. High-resolution axial and coronal reconstructions of multiplanar data or dedicated temporal bone CT can provide more detailed anatomic assessment.

Longitudinal fractures do not typically involve the otic capsule. Hemorrhage within the mastoid air cells and tympanic cavity causes an immediate conductive hearing loss that resolves over time. Some patients will have more complicated injuries with ossicular dislocation and/or tympanic membrane disruption. In the case of ossicular dislocation, conductive hearing loss may not resolve without surgical repair. In contrast, fractures that involve the otic capsule are usually transversely oriented and are more likely to result in immediate and irreversible sensorineural hearing loss, CSF otorrhea, and facial nerve injury (**Fig. 3.10**).

Fig. 3.10a–d
a,b Otic capsule–violating (transverse) fracture. The fracture is oriented perpendicular to the axis of the petrous temporal bone and crosses the vestibule, the posterior semicircular canal, and the lateral semicircular canal. The tympanic cavity and epitympanum are completely opacified.
c,d Otic capsule–sparing (longitudinal) fracture. This fracture is parallel to the axis of the temporal bone and results in incudomalleolar dislocation and intratympanic hematoma. The otic capsule is intact.

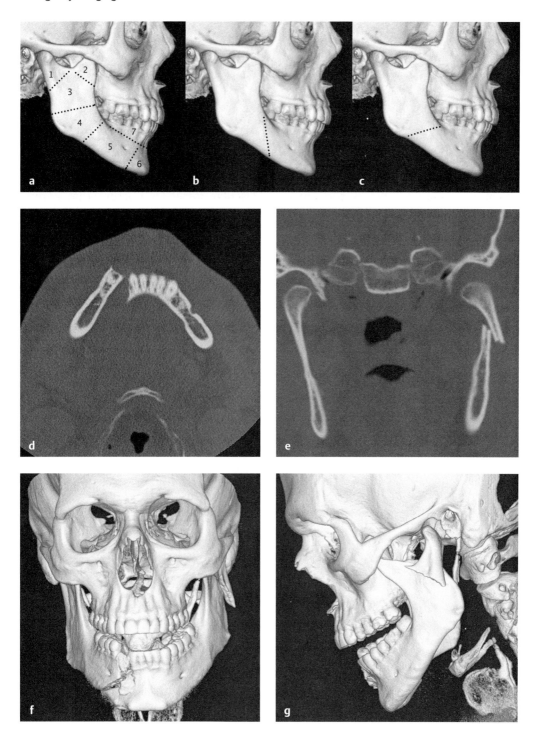

FigFig

◆ Mandible Fracture

Mandible fractures are classified by anatomical location: condyle, coronoid process, subcondyle or ramus, angle, body, symphysis/parasymphysis and alveolus. Because the mandible is functionally a ring, fractures often occur at two sites or at a single bony site with associated temporomandibular joint (TMJ) separation. Frontal impact results in symphyseal fractures, while lateral impact, typical of assault injuries, leads to condylar, angle, or body fractures. Facial swelling, dental malocclusion, trismus, and intraoral bleeding are common clinical findings.

Oblique radiographs or panoramic tomography can identify most mandible fractures. CT, which is usually available in the emergency setting, has the benefit of detecting any associated facial fractures and concomitant intracranial injury. The cortical margin of the entire mandible should be examined for discontinuity.

"Favorable" fractures are located more posteriorly at the superior mandibular margin and more anteriorly at the inferior margin; these fractures tend to be held in alignment by the pterygoid muscles. "Unfavorable" fractures, which have the opposite orientation, are distracted by normal muscular forces. A fracture that enters the root of a tooth is considered an open fracture, and these patients will require antibiotics.

Treatment depends on the location and conformation of the fracture and can consist of either immobilization by maxillomandibular fixation, with arch bars and wiring, or by open surgery with miniplate fixation (**Fig. 3.11**).

Fig. 3.11a–g
a–c Mandible anatomy and fracture orientation: (**a**) (1) condyle, (2) coronoid process, (3) subcondyle or ramus, (4) angle, (5) body, (6) symphysis/parasymphysis, (7) alveolus. (**b**) Favorable orientation. (**c**) Unfavorable orientation.
d–g Left condylar and right parasymphyseal fractures. The left mandibular condyle is laterally angulated and displaced with respect to the left body. The left body and symphysis are displaced to the left as a result of unopposed muscle pull from an "unfavorable" right parasymphyseal fracture.

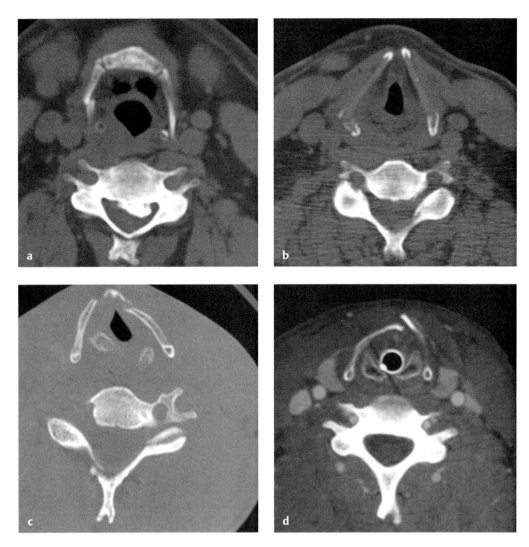

◆ Laryngeal Fracture

Seen in penetrating and blunt neck injuries, laryngeal fractures can lead to life-threatening airway obstruction, compromised airway protection with aspiration, and late vocal dysfunction. The primary goal of emergency management is preservation of the airway, which may require tracheostomy rather than conventional intubation.

Signs of laryngeal injury in the setting of major trauma include subcutaneous emphysema and loss of the normal tracheal prominence. Polytrauma patients with multiple injuries are often intubated prior to CT imaging. In this group, laryngeal fractures can be overlooked and diagnosis delayed for days or weeks, until the patient is extubated and late complications such as dysphonia or aspiration become apparent. Careful CT evaluation of the laryngeal skeleton can detect laryngeal injuries, which can be managed by early tracheostomy and surgical repair.

In patients with less severe injuries, and who are able to cooperate with clinical examination, dyspnea, dysphonia, hoarseness, dysphagia, odynophagia, neck pain, and hemoptysis should prompt laryngoscopy and CT imaging.

On CT, laryngeal fractures may be isolated or can affect several cartilaginous rings. The thyroid cartilage is most often involved and often associated with hyoid or cricoid fractures. Cricoid fractures are frequently bilateral and put the patient at risk for airway collapse due to perforation by an anterior fragment. Other findings include soft tissue asymmetry, subcutaneous and deep space emphysema, submucosal edema, and laryngeal hematoma (**Fig. 3.12**).

Fig. 3.12a–d
a,b Thyroid and hyoid cartilage fractures. (**a**) Right hyoid fracture. (**b**) Right thyroid cornua fracture. Moderate laryngeal edema.
c Thyroid and cricoid cartilage fractures. Bilateral anterior thyroid cartilage fractures, with grossly displaced cricoid fracture and associated soft tissue edema.
d Thyroid and cricoid cartilage fractures in an intubated patient. Anterior thyroid cartilage and posterior cricoid fractures. An endotracheal tube traverses the glottis.

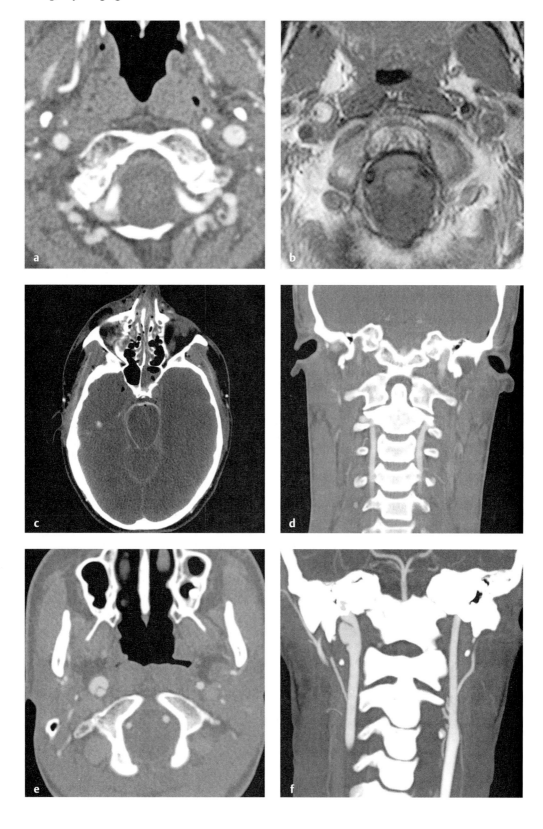

◆ Cervical Vascular Injury

Stretching, twisting, or compression of the neck can result in carotid or vertebral artery dissection, which is characterized by intimal injury, intramural hemorrhage, vascular narrowing, and potential intravascular thrombosis with embolization. When the subendothelium is exposed to intraluminal blood, it induces a coagulation/repair process that can form small clots. These can embolize to the cerebral circulation and lead to an acute arterial distribution infarct. Dissection is an important cause of stroke in patients under 45 years and should be considered in the young or middle-aged adult with new-onset neurologic deficits.

Dissection may follow major blunt neck trauma or trivial injury, including head turning or chiropractic manipulation. Many patients have no history of prior neck trauma. Connective tissue disorders such as Marfan and Ehlers-Danlos syndromes may predispose to spontaneous or minimal-injury dissection. In high-velocity trauma, carotid injury often occurs at the junction of the cervical and petrous segments of the internal carotid artery, where the vessel enters the skull. Patients without a history of acute trauma may have unilateral headache, retro-orbital pain, facial pain, or upper neck pain. Ipsilateral Horner syndrome without anhidrosis or retinal ischemia are more specific findings that should prompt urgent imaging investigation. If a cerebral infarct has already occurred, hemiparesis, hemisensory loss, or aphasia may be the dominant finding.

Carotid pseudoaneurysm is an uncommon complication of neck trauma, especially penetrating injury. Blood that extravasates from a vascular tear accumulates in and is contained by the adjacent tissues, forming a contained outpouching that has the potential for expansion and later catastrophic rupture.

CT without contrast is the initial study obtained in head trauma and suspected acute cerebral infarct, but it is not sensitive for detection of vascular injury. CT angiography (CTA) is the study of choice for detecting either dissection or pseudoaneurysm in the trauma setting. Indications include: Glasgow coma scale score < 6, diffuse axonal injury, severe facial fractures, skull base fractures, upper cervical spine fractures, fractures involving the transverse vertebral foramina, neck hematoma, and hanging mechanisms.

CTA accurately evaluates most acute cervical vascular injuries. Conventional angiography is reserved for cases in which endovascular therapy such as embolization, angioplasty, and placement of stents and stent grafts is contemplated. In carotid artery dissection, CTA shows an eccentric, narrowed, arterial lumen associated with a thick vascular wall, often greater in diameter than that of the contralateral artery. MRI is sensitive for arterial dissection and is often obtained in the patient without a history of significant trauma. On cross-sectional T1-weighted images (optimally with fat suppression), the intramural hematoma appears as an isointense or hyperintense crescent in the vessel wall. After several days, the hematoma becomes hyperintense on T1 MRI (**Fig. 3.13**).

Fig. 3.13a–f
a,b   Carotid dissection. (**a**) CTA shows marked narrowing of the right internal carotid artery (medial to the styloid process and anterior to the jugular vein). The left carotid artery is normal. (**b**) T1-weighted image shows a large, high-signal intramural hematoma with severely narrowed luminal flow void.
c,d   Bilateral traumatic carotid injury. (**c**) Generalized cerebral swelling with absent gray-white differentiation. Normal opacification of the posterior cerebral arteries with complete absence of cavernous carotid artery opacification. (**d**) Marked narrowing of the right and left internal carotid arteries at the skull base.
e,f   Carotid pseudoaneurysm. Choking injury. A 1-cm pseudoaneurysm arises from the cervical portion of the right internal carotid artery.

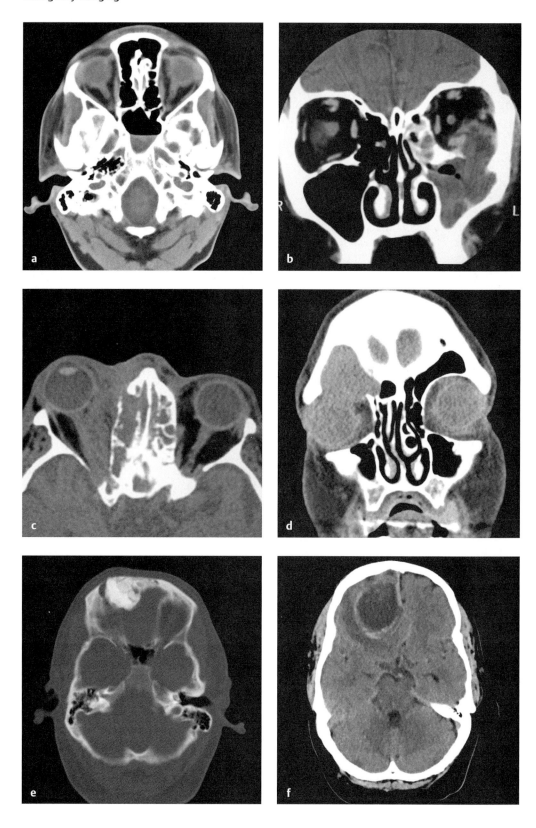

◆ Sinus Obstruction and Inflammation

Acute sinusitis is characterized by inflammation of the lining of the paranasal sinuses and may be allergic in etiology or due to viral, bacterial, or fungal infection. The diagnosis is based upon the entirely clinical findings of facial pain and tenderness, postnasal discharge, congestion, and anosmia. Imaging is not indicated for acute sinusitis but may be obtained to evaluate an atypical headache or to diagnose the uncommon complications of untreated or inadequately treated sinusitis (facial or orbital cellulitis, cavernous sinus thrombosis, or cerebritis). If a CT is obtained, acute uncomplicated sinusitis usually appears as fluid within a sinus.

Invasive sinusitis is associated with bone erosion and inflammatory disease that extends into the adjacent facial soft tissues. Invasive fungal sinusitis, the most common variety, is a disease of immunocompromised patients, most commonly diabetics, neutropenic patients on chemotherapy, or in patients with advanced AIDS. Clinical findings vary but include fever, facial pain, epistaxis, and nasal congestion. Infection that extends from the sinus into the orbit can lead to visual deterioration, proptosis, diplopia, and pain. Cranial nerve III–VI dysfunction indicates cavernous sinus involvement.

On noncontrast CT, the involved sinuses are usually opacified, with hyperostotic or thinned walls, permeative bone changes, and intraorbital or deep facial fat stranding. Intracranial complications include epidural empyema, meningitis, cerebritis, vasculitis, mycotic aneurysm, and vascular thrombosis.

Systemic antifungal therapy and surgical débridement are often necessary for successful management.

Sinus mucocele results from ostial obstruction due to chronic inflammation, allergies, trauma, or underlying neoplasm. Mucous under pressure accumulates in the sinus, expands and thins the walls, and can rupture into an adjacent sinus, the orbit, or the cranium. The frontal and ethmoid sinuses are most frequently involved, but any combination of paranasal sinuses may be affected. Clinical findings include facial deformity, exophthalmos, or diplopia from encroachment upon the adjacent orbit. Cellulitis and facial or intracranial abscess can result from rupture.

CT imaging shows an expanded, completely opacified sinus with remodeling and thinning of at least one wall (**Fig. 3.14**).

Fig. 3.14a–f
a Acute sinusitis. Low-attenuation fluid within the sphenoid sinus. No associated hyperostosis.
b,c Invasive sinusitis due to aspergillosis. (**b**) Aspergillosis. The left maxillary sinus is opacified and inflammatory tissue with enhancing margin extends through in the orbital floor to involve the inferomedial orbit. (**c**) Mucormycosis. Right ethmoid opacification with erosion of the ethmoid walls and extension of inflammatory tissue into the medial intra- and extraconal right orbit and preseptal soft tissues.
d Frontal sinus mucocele. Right frontal sinus opacification with smooth expansion and erosion of the anterior orbital roof. Associated inferior displacement of the globe. Intraorbital soft tissue infiltration indicates cellulitis.
e,f Brain abscess due to frontal sinus obstruction by osteoma. Large frontal sinus osteoma with small ruptured mucocele and complicating right frontal lobe brain abscess.

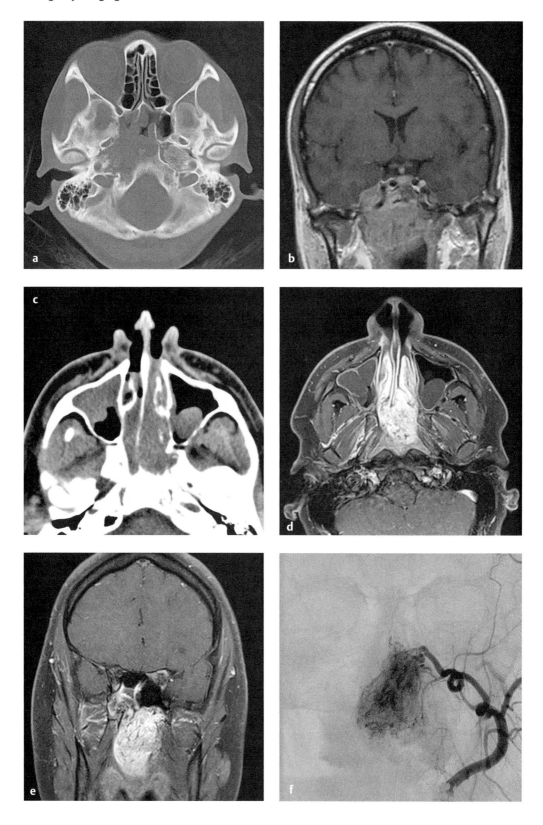

◆ Nasopharyngeal Masses

Nasopharyngeal carcinoma is the most common malignancy of the nasopharynx. It is a squamous cell carcinoma of which some types have been associated with Epstein-Barr virus (EBV) infection. It is more prevalent in Asian, especially Chinese, populations. Clinical findings include cervical lymphadenopathy, serious otitis media with conductive hearing loss, middle ear effusion, nasal obstruction, epistaxis, and cranial nerve dysfunction. The primary tumor is usually located in the fossa of Rosenmüller, near the orifice of the eustachian tube, and for this reason, it should be considered in any adult who presents with a first episode of otitis media.

CT and MR imaging characterize the primary mass and local nodal metastases, which are present in more than half of patients at diagnosis. The primary tumor can extend in any direction, eroding the base of the skull or invading the cranium via the eustachian tube, clivus, or skull base foramina.

Primary treatment is external-beam radiation therapy, which is supplemented with chemotherapy in some cases.

Juvenile nasopharyngeal angiofibroma (JNA) is a locally aggressive, highly vascular, benign tumor of prepubertal and adolescent males. Although JNAs account for only a small fraction of all head and neck tumors, they are the most common benign nasopharyngeal neoplasm. Patients present with chronic obstructive symptoms, epistaxis, facial deformity, anosmia, and headache.

JNAs arise from the walls of the pterygopalatine or sphenopalatine fossa, which are often remodeled and expanded at the time of diagnosis. Extension into the maxillary and ethmoid sinuses is common, and nasopharyngeal angiofibromas often reach a considerable size at presentation. Intracranial involvement is less common but can occur.

CT shows a lobulated, enhancing, non-encapsulated soft tissue mass centered in the sphenopalatine foramen, often bowing the posterior wall of the maxillary sinus. MRI can supplement tumor evaluation and shows the characteristic salt-and-pepper appearance of intratumoral vascular flow voids on most sequences. Arterial supply is almost exclusively from the ipsilateral internal maxillary or ascending pharyngeal arteries, permitting embolization prior to definitive resection (**Fig. 3.15**).

Fig. 3.15a–f
a,b Nasopharyngeal carcinoma. (**a**) Right lateral nasopharyngeal soft tissue mass that has eroded the petrous apex, right lateral clivus, and right lateral sphenoid sinus. (**b**) Coronal postgadolinium T1-weighted image shows the large, enhancing right nasopharyngeal mass invading the clivus and right cavernous sinus and encasing the right cavernous internal carotid artery.
c–f Juvenile nasopharyngeal angiofibroma. (**c**) The posterior left nasal cavity is filled by a modestly expansile soft tissue density mass that is centered at the left sphenopalatine foramen. (**d,e**) T1-weighted postgadolinium MRI better defines a soft tissue mass that fills the nasopharynx and extends into both sides of the posterior nasal cavity. (**f**) External carotid artery angiogram confirms the highly vascular nature of the mass and its vascular supply via an enlarged internal maxillary branch of the left external carotid artery.

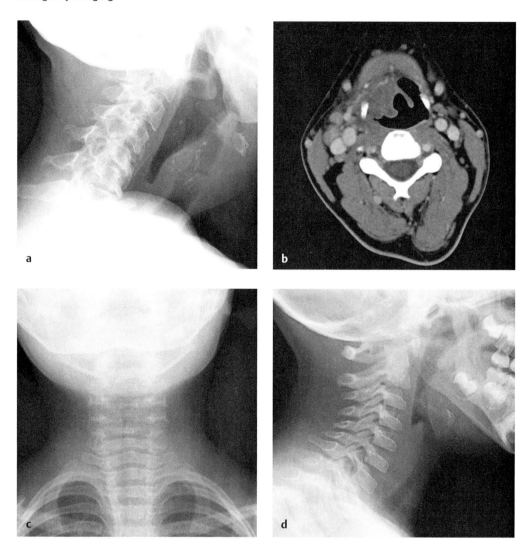

◆ Epiglottitis and Croup

Epiglottitis, acute inflammation of the epiglottitis and arytenoepiglottic folds, can lead to life-threatening airway obstruction. It is usually the result of bacterial infection, and in the past it was commonly caused by *Haemophilus influenzae* (HIB). Since the advent of widespread pediatric HIB vaccination, its incidence has decreased fivefold in children. Today, it is usually due to *Staphylococcus* or *Streptococcus* bacteria. It can occur at any age but is still more common in children than adults. Most patients are between 3 and 6 years old and typically present with dysphagia, stridor, drooling, and high fever.

Portable radiographs should be obtained in the emergency department with as little manipulation of the neck as possible. Lateral radiographs may show the "thumb" sign, a thickening of the epiglottis and arytenoepiglottic folds. The hypopharynx may appear distended. The vocal cords and subglottic airway are usually normal but may appear narrowed on anteroposterior (AP) view in cases of severe inflammation.

Given the potential for acute airway compromise, treatment should be expeditious. If there is clinical decompensation, tracheal intubation should be secured by a specialist and may be difficult due to epiglottic inflammation and enlargement. Emergent cricotracheotomy may be required to maintain airway patency.

Croup, or laryngotracheobronchitis, is an acute upper airway infection seen in younger children (6 months to 6 years) who typically present with barking cough, stridor, and hoarseness. It is more common in males and occurs more frequently in the autumn. Since the advent of immunization against diphtheria, most cases are viral (parainfluenza, influenza, respiratory syncytial virus [RSV], adenovirus, and measles), although bacterial superinfection is possible. Epiglottitis, aspirated foreign body, and retropharyngeal abscess can have similar clinical presentations, and these conditions should be considered and excluded.

The diagnosis is clinical, but neck radiographs are often obtained to exclude epiglottitis or prevertebral edema and can show the "steeple sign" of subglottic edema and narrowing.

Croup is managed medically, with corticosteroids and nebulized epinephrine providing rapid symptomatic relief (**Fig. 3.16**).

Fig. 3.16a–d
a Epiglottitis. Lateral radiograph showing pharyngeal distention, markedly thickened epiglottis and thickened arytenoepiglottic folds. No prevertebral soft tissue swelling.
b Epiglottitis. CT in another patient shows edema of the epiglottis and right arytenoepiglottic fold.
c,d Croup. Narrowed subglottic tracheal air column on frontal view. No retropharyngeal or epiglottic swelling.

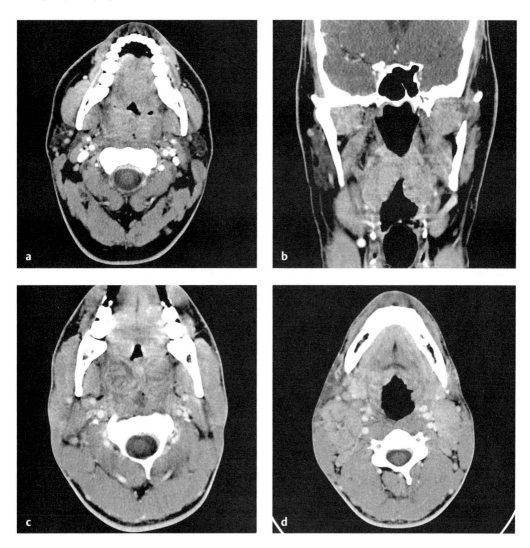

◆ Tonsillitis and Mononucleosis

Tonsillitis is an infection and inflammation of the pharyngeal, adenoid, and/or lingual tonsils, often with concomitant pharyngitis. It is usually viral, with most cases due to adenovirus, herpes simplex virus, Epstein-Barr virus, cytomegalovirus, or adenovirus. Bacterial infections by *Mycoplasma pneumoniae, Corynebacterium diphtheriae, Chlamydophila pneumoniae,* or *N. gonorrhoeae* are less common causes of tonsillitis and pharyngitis. Symptoms include fever, sore throat, dysphagia, odynophagia, and tender cervical lymphadenopathy.

While most patients are treated without imaging, contrast-enhanced CT may be obtained in those with persistent or refractory tonsillitis to identify a complicating peritonsillar or retropharyngeal abscess. CT shows mild posterior pharyngeal soft tissue swelling with linear, striated enhancement of the palatine and lingual tonsils. Mild reactive adenopathy may be present; if pronounced, it should raise the possibility of mononucleosis.

Infectious mononucleosis is a clinical syndrome consisting of fever, pharyngitis, and cervical adenopathy caused most frequently by Epstein-Barr virus. It is most common in adolescents or young adults and can be associated with prolonged and profound fatigue that resolves gradually over months. Physical findings include tonsillar enlargement, palatal petechiae, and a generalized maculopapular rash early in the course of infection, with late transient splenomegaly. Because of these findings, mononucleosis can mimic lymphoma on both clinical examination and imaging studies. Most cases are subclinical and resolve without complication.

Imaging is not necessary to diagnose mononucleosis, but it is often obtained when a neck abscess is clinically suspected. Tonsillar enlargement and striated enhancement are identical to that of simple tonsillitis. Generalized cervical lymphadenopathy is usually present (**Fig. 3.17**).

Fig. 3.17a–d
a,b Tonsillitis. The pharyngeal tonsils are enlarged with subtle striated enhancement. No adenopathy or peritonsillar fluid.
c,d Mononucleosis. The pharyngeal tonsils are enlarged with pronounced striated enhancement. Bulky associated bilateral level IIa and IIb lymph nodes.

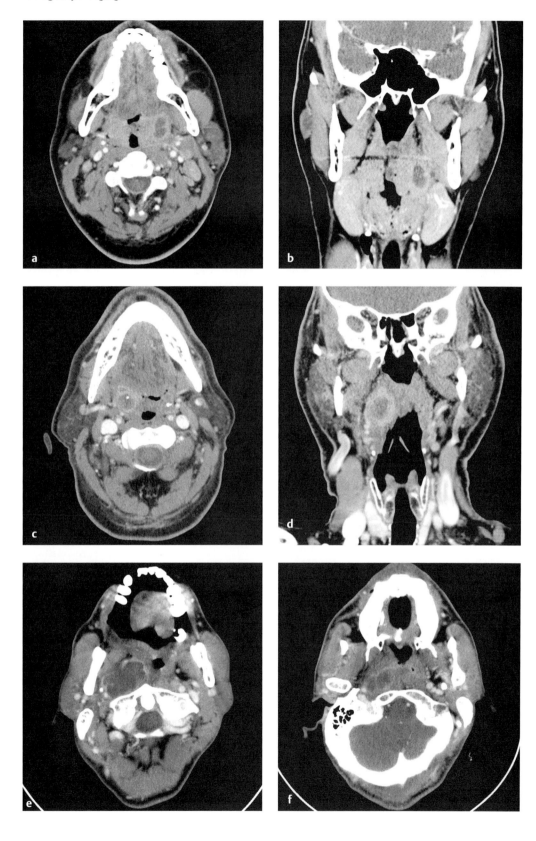

◆ Peritonsillar and Retropharyngeal Abscess

Peritonsillar abscess is a potential complication of tonsillitis. If a bacterial tonsillitis is neglected or inadequately treated, an abscess can develop between the tonsil and the pharyngeal constrictor muscle. Sore throat is an early symptom, with fever, dysphonia, cervical lymphadenopathy, dysphagia, dyspnea, stridor, trismus, and upper airway obstruction. Treatment of an established abscess usually requires a combination of surgical drainage and antibiotic therapy, and most patients recover within a few days without complication. A small number of patients will experience recurrent infection and may ultimately require tonsillectomy.

CT or intraoral ultrasound can differentiate peritonsillar abscess from simple tonsillitis/cellulitis. Contrast-enhanced CT defines a hypodense fluid collection with peripheral rim enhancement at the superior tonsillar pole. Associated findings include asymmetric or striated tonsils, adjacent cellulitis, and reactive lymphadenopathy.

Retropharyngeal abscess is an infection of the retropharyngeal space that results from suppuration of a lymph node draining a primary infection elsewhere in the neck or, less frequently, from direct extension of cellulitis/abscess. Primary infective sites include the nasopharynx, paranasal sinuses, and middle ear.

Retropharyngeal abscesses are frequently seen in the pediatric population with the most cases occurring before the age of 5. Common causative organisms are *Staphylococcus aureus, Haemophilus parainfluenzae,* and β-hemolytic *Streptococcus* group A species. In adults, direct spread from adjacent diskitis, peritonsillar abscess, or inoculation from penetrating trauma are potential etiologies. Clinical presentation is nonspecific, and symptoms include fever, sore throat, neck pain, and limited neck mobility.

Contrast-enhanced CT shows a low-attenuation fluid collection in the retropharyngeal space with peripheral marginal enhancement and adjacent inflammatory stranding. Potential complications include extension into the mediastinum or vertebral column, epidural abscess, and carotid space inflammation.

With early diagnosis and aggressive antibiotic treatment, prognosis is good. Transoral surgical drainage may still be necessary for large or complex abscesses (**Fig. 3.18**).

Fig. 3.18a–f
a,b Peritonsillar abscess. Well-demarcated, ~1 × 1 × 2 cm peripherally enhancing low-attenuation collection located between the left pharyngeal tonsil and pharyngeal constrictor muscle. Poor definition of the adjacent parapharyngeal fat. Mild bilateral tonsillar enhancement and left sided reactive adenopathy.
c,d Peritonsillar abscess. 1-cm peripherally enhancing collection in the superior right tonsillar fossa.
e,f Retropharyngeal abscess. Peripherally enhancing, low-attenuation fluid collection centered anterior and to the right of C1. The parapharyngeal space is displaced anteriorly. The mass contacts and displaces the carotid artery and jugular vein posterolaterally. The epidural space, C1 vertebra, and spinal canal are normal.

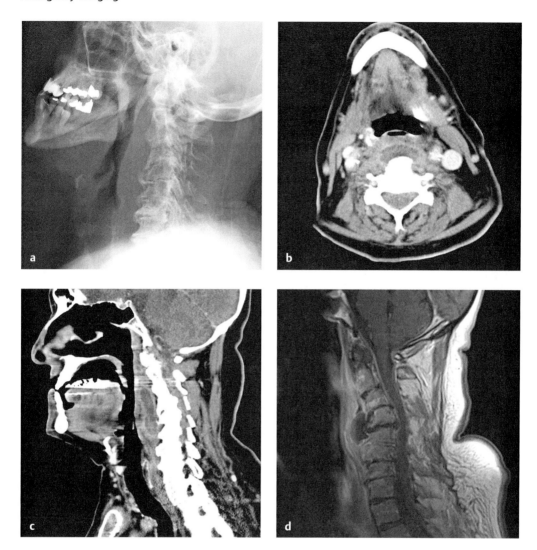

◆ Prevertebral Abscess

Prevertebral space infection is usually due to contiguous spread from primary cervical diskitis or osteomyelitis, penetrating injury, surgical complication, hematogenous spread from an infection elsewhere in the body, or transient bacteremia. *Staphylococcus aureus* is the usual associated organism, but other gram-positive organisms may be identified. Historically, prevertebral abscesses were a frequent complication of spinal tuberculosis, but this is less common today. Clinical signs and symptoms include neck or back pain, fever, dysphagia, radiculopathy or myelopathy, and cranial nerve deficits.

Contrast-enhanced CT or MRI should be obtained for evaluation of any suspected deep neck infection. While increased prevertebral soft tissue thickness may be identified by lateral radiograph, cross-sectional imaging is necessary to evaluate the extent of disease optimally and exclude spinal canal involvement. On CT, a prevertebral abscess appears as a hypodense fluid collection with peripheral enhancement both anterior and adjacent to the longus colli and longus capitus muscles. On MRI, the central portion of the abscess is low in signal on T1-weighted images and high in signal on T2-weighted images with pronounced postgadolinium enhancement. Prevertebral edema and air within the adjacent soft tissues are sometimes present (**Fig. 3.19**).

Fig. 3.19a–d
a–d   Prevertebral abscess. (**a**) Marked prevertebral soft tissue swelling apparent on lateral radiograph. Severe cervical spine degenerative changes. (**b,c**) 1 × 4 × 4-cm fluid collection anterior to C4 and C5 with subtle enhancing margins. (**d**) Postgadolinium T1-weighted MRI demonstrates a low-signal-intensity collection anterior to the C4/5 intervertebral disk with enhancement of adjacent prevertebral soft tissues, posterior longitudinal ligament, and ventral spinal dura, reflecting both prevertebral abscess and a contiguous epidural inflammatory component.

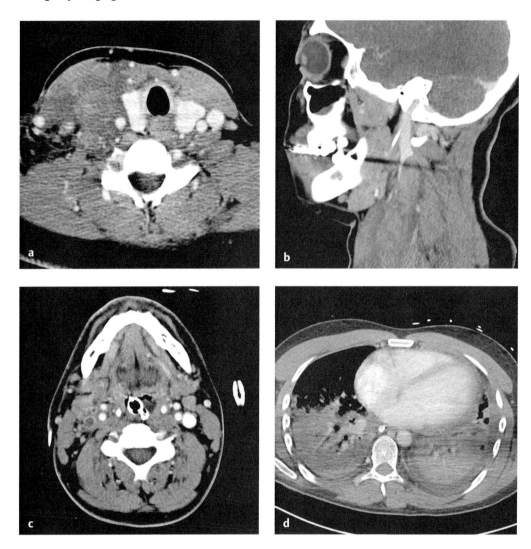

◆ Jugular Vein Thrombosis and Septic Jugular Thrombophlebitis

Jugular vein thrombosis can occur after neck surgery or central venous catheter placement and in patients with an underlying malignancy, hypercoagulable state, or neck cellulitis/abscess. Patients can be entirely asymptomatic or may have local pain and swelling. Complications include sepsis, septic pulmonary embolism and pneumonia, emboli to other organs and tissues, and intracranial propagation of the thrombus with venous sinus occlusion. Ultrasonography shows a dilated and noncompressible jugular vein that does not distend with Valsalva maneuver, while on CT the jugular vein is expanded by nonenhancing thrombus and demonstrates variable mural enhancement.

Treatment is with intravenous antibiotics and systemic anticoagulation. Ligation or resection of the vein is reserved for those patients who fail conservative medical therapy.

Lemierre syndrome is a rare but serious complication of oropharyngeal infection in which an initial anaerobic gram-negative infection (most commonly pharyngitis due to *Fusobacterium necrophorum*) causes jugular vein thrombophlebitis and distant septic embolization. Microemboli disseminate throughout the body, forming abscesses in the lungs and larger joints. Patients typically present days to weeks following an episode of acute pharyngitis with sepsis, high fever, rigors, and malaise. Clinical findings include pain, tenderness, and swelling along the course of the jugular vein with variably associated trismus, hoarseness, or dysphagia.

If the diagnosis of Lemierre syndrome is suspected, CT of the chest should also be performed to identify pulmonary cavities and consolidation. Other potential complications include meningitis, septic arthritis, and renal, hepatic, or splenic abscesses (**Fig. 3.20**).

Fig. 3.20a–d
a,b Jugular vein thrombosis. The right jugular vein is enlarged and does not opacify after intravenous contrast administration. Inflammatory changes reduce the definition of adjacent cervical fat and the medial aspect of the sternocleidomastoid muscle.
c,d Lemierre syndrome (septic thrombophlebitis). (**c**) Right internal jugular vein thrombosis with mild enhancement of the vascular wall. Endotracheal and enteric tubes. (**d**) Bilateral lower lobe consolidation. Mild cardiac enlargement.

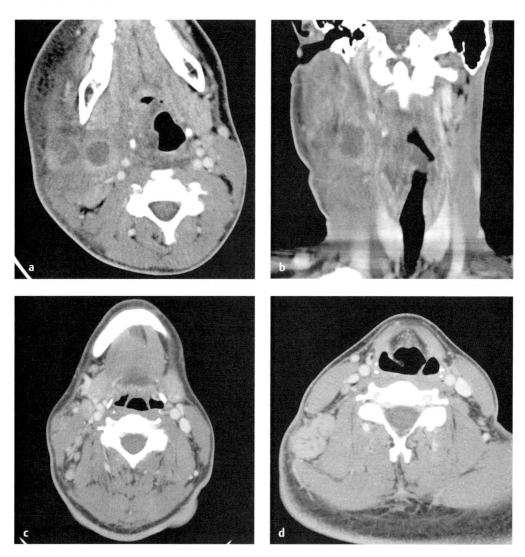

◆ Cervical Adenitis

Suppurative adenitis is a common soft tissue infection usually caused by *Staphylococcus aureus* or *Streptococcus pyogenes* and characterized by inflammation of one or more lymph nodes with distention, edema, and ultimately liquefactive necrosis. Swollen, painful superficial cervical nodes can be appreciated clinically. Deeper nodal involvement in children indicates retropharyngeal suppurative adenitis, which can progress to retropharyngeal abscess.

Contrast-enhanced CT shows hypodense lymph nodes with rimlike enhancement and perinodal inflammatory fat stranding. Adjacent homogeneous lymph nodes are usually reactive rather than infected. While metastatic nodes can have a similar appearance, inflammatory fat changes are less common in malignancy. Coalescent, very low-attenuation lymph nodes, particularly in patients with mild, subacute symptoms, suggest mycobacterial infection.

Mycobacterial adenitis may be the only manifestation of systemic tuberculosis, and this should be considered in the differential diagnosis of any cervical mass, especially in endemic areas or in the immunocompromised patient. Cervical adenitis may also be due to nontuberculous mycobacteria such as *M. avium* complex, *M. bovis*, and *M. africanum*. Mycobacterial disease characteristically causes a subacute cervical lymphadenopathy of more than 3 weeks' duration, and patients present with firm, nontender lymph nodes in the anterior cervical, submandibular, and supraclavicular chains. Lymph nodes are initially nonfluctuant but may suppurate, and sinus tracts may appear.

Early in the course of mycobacterial infection, affected nodes will enhance homogeneously on CT. As the disease progresses, necrosis and conglomeration are common. Healed nodes may calcify. Chest radiographs should be obtained and may show evidence of present or remote tuberculosis. Radiographs are usually normal in nontuberculous mycobacterial infections (**Fig. 3.21**).

Fig. 3.21a–d
a,b Suppurative right level II jugular chain nodes. Two adjacent enlarged, peripherally enhancing nodes with surrounding edema and prominent subcutaneous lymphatics.
c,d Mycobacterial adenitis. Enlarged enhancing right level II and V nodes, the largest of which show areas of early necrosis.

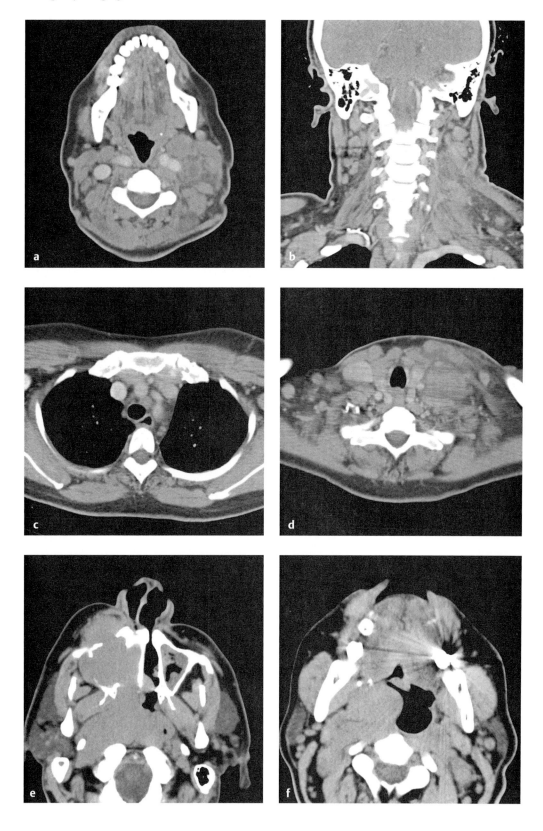

◆ Lymphoma Involving the Head and Neck

Lymphoma, while a systemic disease, often presents with subacute painless cervical lymphadenopathy. Extranodal lymphoma in the head and neck can involve the sinuses, pharyngeal tissues, and orbits. Lymphoma typically has a "liquid" appearance on CT, with homogeneous density and poor marginal definition.

Lymphoma is broadly classified as (1) Hodgkin lymphoma, (2) non-Hodgkin lymphoma (NHL), and (3) immunodeficiency-associated lymphoproliferative disorder. Contiguous nodal involvement is typical of Hodgkin lymphoma, which usually involves the neck and thorax. Non-Hodgkin lymphoma may arise from B-cells, T-cells, or natural killer cells and comprises a more varied group of lymphocytic malignancies. In NHL, low-grade disease may manifest as slowly progressive lymphadenopathy, while high-grade lymphomas may show rapidly enlarging nodes, frequent extranodal disease, and an aggressive course.

Persistent painless cervical nodal enlargement, especially if it involves the posterior triangle (spinal accessory chain) or supraclavicular region, should be investigated. Superficial enlarged nodes can be assessed by ultrasound, and features that indicate malignancy include increased size (greater than 3 cm), rounded shape, decrease in internal echogenicity, and loss of the normally echogenic hilum. Contrast-enhanced CT of the neck, chest, abdomen, and pelvis permits a more comprehensive assessment and should be obtained to evaluate the extent of deep cervical, thoracic, and abdominal adenopathy. In both Hodgkin lymphoma and NHL, the lower jugular chain nodes (levels III and IV) are almost always involved. Multiple nodes of varying sizes are frequently visualized. Nodal necrosis may be, but is not necessarily, present. Lymph nodes that measure less than 10 mm in short axis are generally considered normal or reactive (**Fig. 3.22**).

Fig. 3.22a–f
a–d Lymphoma involving the cervical and axillary lymph nodes. Enlarged, predominantly homogeneous nodes in all groups with asymmetric prominence of the left jugular chain nodes.
e,f Sinonasal B-cell lymphoma. A homogeneous soft tissue mass expands and erodes the right maxillary sinus, with adjacent tonsillar and nasopharyngeal involvement.

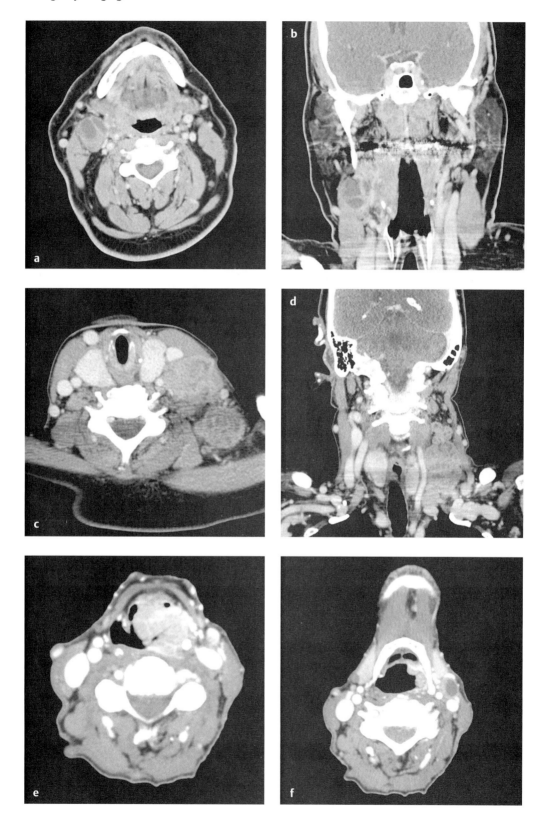

◆ Metastatic Head and Neck Carcinoma

Primary head and neck cancers arise from the mucosa of the oral cavity, the pharynx, and larynx, usually in patients with significant past tobacco or alcohol use. Most are squamous cell carcinomas. The remainder originate in the skin, salivary glands, and thyroid gland, and they include adenocarcinomas, melanomas, and other rare neoplasms. The typical clinical presentation is that of a middle-aged man with a painless neck mass for several months. Nonhealing mucosal ulcers, otalgia, hoarseness, dysphagia, chronic cough, and respiratory difficulties are other common complaints.

The location of the involved lymph node can point to the site of origin of the primary tumor. Lymph nodes in the posterior triangle (2B, 5) drain the nasopharynx, whereas nodes in the upper jugular chain (2A, 2B, 3) are seen with tonsil and base-of-tongue carcinomas. Isolated nodal disease in the lower neck and supraclavicular region (4) points toward the lungs or gastrointestinal tract as the site of origin. Metastatic lymph nodes are typically enlarged, with low-attenuation centers and enhancing capsules. Primary mucosal neoplasm may not be easily identified on CT but is usually found on endoscopic examination. Description of nodal location on CT should include both the chain and the CT level. Indistinct or shaggy nodal margins indicate extracapsular spread. In the setting of known malignancy, lymph nodes larger than 1 cm in short axis are considered abnormal (**Fig. 3.23**).

Fig. 3.23a–f
a,b   Metastatic squamous cell carcinoma. Enlarged, centrally necrotic, right level 2A (jugular chain) and 2B/3 (spinal accessory chain) lymph nodes.
c,d   Metastatic squamous cell carcinoma. Conglomerate left level 4 and 5 lymph nodes.
e,f   Metastatic squamous cell carcinoma. Bulky left pharyngeal carcinoma involving the epiglottis and pyriform sinus. Low-density, peripherally enhancing left jugular chain level 2/3 necrotic lymph node.

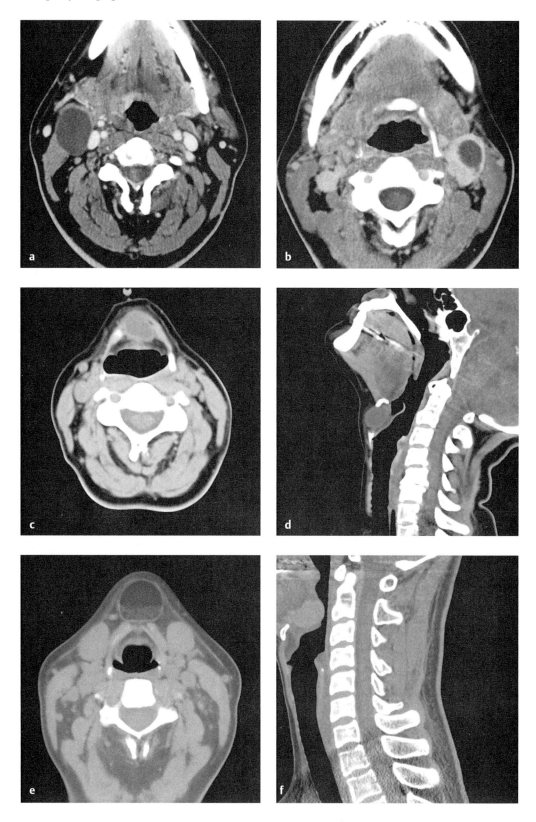

◆ Cervical Developmental Cysts and Masses

Branchial cleft cysts are found in the lateral neck and result from incomplete migration or obliteration of one of the four branchial clefts during embryologic development. Most are derived from the second branchial cleft, and these are located below the mandibular angle, bounded by the submandibular gland, the carotid artery, and the sternocleidomastoid muscle. Typically, the cyst is filled with mucoid material and asymptomatic unless superinfected. It is usually diagnosed in adolescence or young adulthood after a patient presents with lateral neck inflammation or palpable mass. First-branchial-cleft cysts are less common and appear as small cysts located near the external auditory canal or within the parotid gland. If the cyst is not infected, contrast-enhanced CT shows a round, well-circumscribed, thin-walled, nonenhancing mass. An infected cyst will have variably dense contents and an enhancing, irregular wall. Surgical excision is the definitive treatment.

Thyroglossal duct cysts arise from an epithelial tract that persists after the embryonic descent of thyroid tissue from the tongue base to the low paratracheal neck. Most are midline, between 2 and 4 cm in diameter, and closely apposed to the hyoid or strap muscles. Cysts located near the thyroid gland may be more lateral in position. Ultrasound shows a well-circumscribed unilocular or multilocular mass with variable echogenicity depending on the cyst's content. Contrast-enhanced CT findings include a thin-walled cyst, located in the midline at or below the level of the hyoid bone, with a peripheral rim of enhancement. Thick irregular walls, internal septations, or surrounding inflammatory changes indicate superinfection. Calcifications and soft tissue nodules suggest the possibility of thyroid carcinoma, which can sometimes develop in a thyroglossal duct cyst. Fat within an anterior midline neck cyst is diagnostic of a dermoid, another, less common, developmental anomaly. Surgical resection of the cyst and thyroglossal duct is necessary to prevent recurrence.

Lingual thyroid refers to a developmental anomaly in which the embryonic thyroid fails to migrate from its origin at the base of the tongue to its normal position in the lower neck. The diagnosis is usually made incidentally or in the course of investigating an apparently absent cervical thyroid gland. Usually asymptomatic, ectopic thyroid tissue can enlarge during upper respiratory tract infections, pregnancy, or puberty and can rarely cause dysphagia, dysphonia, dyspnea, or hemoptysis. Thyroid ultrasound confirms absence of thyroid tissue in its expected location. CT shows a hyperdense soft tissue mass at the base of the tongue and no thyroid gland in its expected position. Treatment depends on the patient's thyroid function at the time of presentation. Because patients often have some degree of hypothyroidism, surgical removal has the potential to render the patient profoundly hypothyroid (**Fig. 3.24**).

Fig. 3.24a–f
a,b Type 2 branchial cleft cysts. (**a**) Well-defined, round, 3-cm cystic mass with homogeneous fluid attenuation center and imperceptibly thin capsule. It displaces the carotid space posteromedially, the sternocleidomastoid posterolaterally, and the submandibular gland anteriorly. (**b**) Complicated, thick-walled, infected cyst.
c,d Thyroglossal duct cyst. 2-cm midline cyst with slightly indistinct enhancing margins located anterior to the epiglottis and interposed between the hyoid and thyroid cartilages. Minimal adjacent inflammatory fat stranding within the anterior epiglottic space.
e Dermoid cyst. Midline, thin-walled, fat-filled, cyst containing layering soft tissue attenuation granules.
f Lingual thyroid. Well-defined, high-attenuation mass at the base of the tongue (foramen cecum). Normal thyroid gland is absent from its characteristic location in the lower neck.

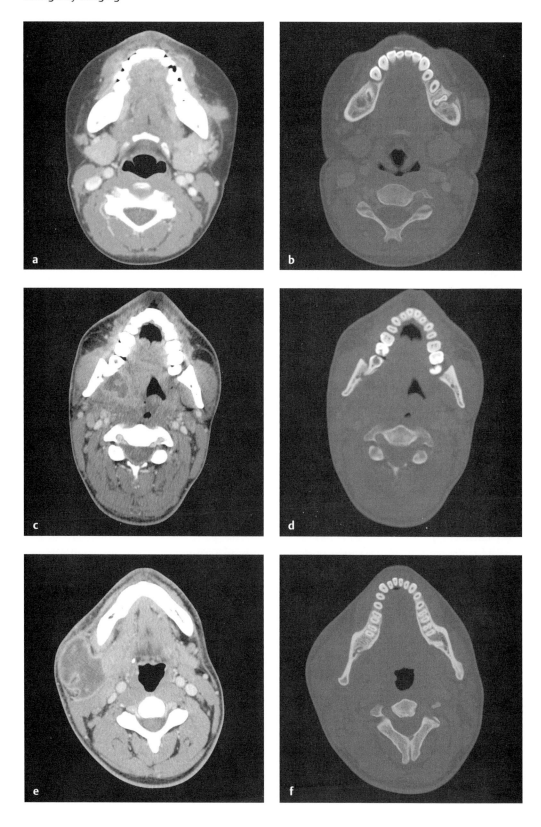

◆ Dental Disease and Odontogenic Abscess

Poor oral hygiene, diabetes, and smoking contribute to gingivitis, dental caries, and periodontal disease. Infection that begins in the space between the gum and tooth, or within a cavity that communicates with the dental pulp, can migrate to the tooth root, where it can form a periapical abscess and localized infection of the adjacent mandible or maxilla. Erosion through the cortex can result in buccal, masseteric, or sublingual fossa and submandibular space abscesses. Patients present with acute facial swelling, pain, dysphagia, and dysphonia.

In odontogenic abscess, CT shows periradicular lucency and often a small mandibular defect with an adjacent area of inflammatory change or peripherally enhancing fluid collection. Asymptomatic periodontal and dental disease is frequently identified on head and face CT obtained for other indications. Mandibular osteomyelitis is identified by erosion, cyst or sinus formation, and periosteal new bone. Periodontogenic abscesses are generally treated with tooth extraction, abscess drainage, and antibiotics (**Fig. 3.25**).

Fig. 3.25a–f
a,b   Buccal space abscess. Focal inflammatory stranding within the fat adjacent to a defect in the lateral mandibular cortex that communicates with an area of bone resorption surrounding the left third molar root. Periosteal new bone formation surrounds the mandible adjacent to the involved tooth.
c,d   Masticator space abscess. 1.5-cm well-defined, peripherally enhancing mass with low attenuation center located in the medial pterygoid muscle adjacent to the lower right third molar. The molar is horizontally oriented with periradicular osseous resorption, periosteal calcification, and a defect in the medial mandibular cortex.
e,f   Submandibular abscess. Large right submandibular space abscess. Small defect in the medial mandibular cortex adjacent to the right lower third molar root is contiguous with a portion of the abscess and indicates odontogenic origin.

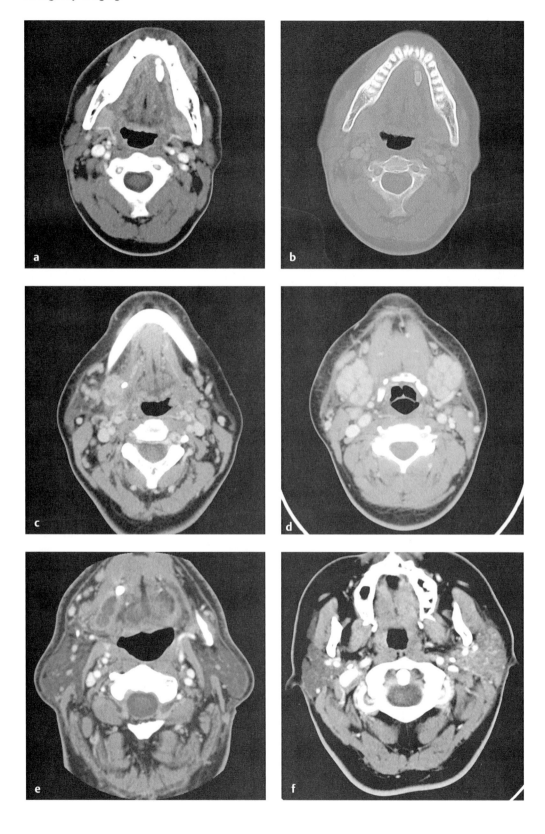

◆ Sialolithiasis, Sialodochitis, and Sialadenitis

Excepting mumps, sialolithiasis is the most common salivary gland disease. Alkaline and viscous secretions promote stone formation within the ducts or intraglandular tributaries, and obstruction by a stone can be complicated by bacterial infection of the duct (sialodochitis) or of the gland (sialadenitis). The submandibular gland is more frequently involved than the parotid gland, and sialolithiasis is more common in men than in women.

While sialadenitis is often due to ductal obstruction, viral infections (especially mumps), autoimmune diseases, and drugs that reduce salivary flow are other causes. Most patients present with pain and swelling of the gland made worse by eating (salivary colic). In some cases purulent material may drain from the salivary duct.

Ultrasound is sensitive for detection of calculi, but CT with contrast provides a more comprehensive evaluation of the gland and can identify any associated deep abscess. In uncomplicated sialolithiasis, one or more stones will be seen in the gland or corresponding duct. A distended duct indicates sialodochitis and is characterized by a distal obstructing stone, ductal wall enhancement, and variable periductal and periglandular inflammatory fat stranding. In acute sialadenitis, the gland is diffusely enlarged and enhances with intravenous contrast. In chronic sialolithiasis, the gland atrophies, often appearing small and infiltrated with fat (**Fig. 3.26**).

Fig. 3.26a–f
a–c Sialolithiasis. (**a,b**) Several sialoliths in the distal left submandibular duct. (**c**) Sialolith at the junction of the right submandibular gland and duct.
d Bilateral submandibular sialadenitis. The glands enhance symmetrically with adjacent subcutaneous fat stranding and platysma muscle thickening, more severe on the right.
e Sialodochitis. Right distal submandibular duct calculus with ductal dilatation and wall enhancement.
f Parotid sialadenitis. The left parotid gland is enlarged and enhances relative to the right parotid.

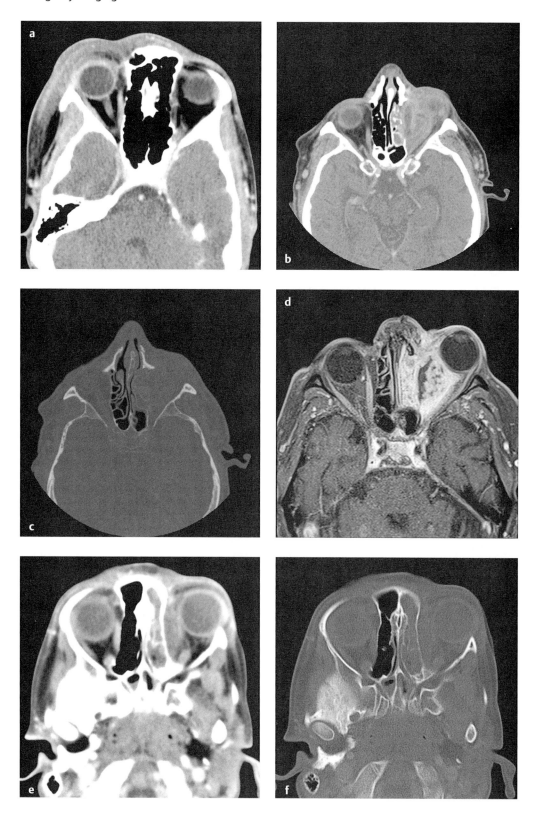

◆ Orbital Cellulitis and Abscess

Orbital cellulitis can be described as either preseptal or postseptal, depending on whether or not soft tissues deep to the orbital septum are involved. Preseptal cellulitis involves the eyelid and periorbital soft tissues and usually arises from a facial dermal infection. Postseptal cellulitis is often due to adjacent sinusitis and can involve the subperiosteal space, the extraconal space, and the orbital apex. Intraconal involvement is uncommon.

Patients with preseptal cellulitis have swelling and erythema of the eyelids, as well as chemosis. Ophthalmoplegia, proptosis, and deteriorating visual acuity in addition to periorbital swelling indicate postseptal involvement.

CT, usually obtained with contrast, evaluates the anatomic extent of disease, extension of any inflammatory changes posterior to the orbital septum, and any other orbital or intracranial complication. The most common finding is increased retroseptal fat edema or stranding, but subperiosteal abscess, cavernous sinus or superior ophthalmic vein thrombosis, meningitis, and intracranial abscess can complicate orbital cellulitis in severe, neglected, or refractory cases.

Inflammation confined to the eyelids and preseptal orbital tissues, as well as mild retroseptal inflammation, may be managed with antibiotics.

Orbital abscess can complicate frontal, maxillary, or ethmoid sinusitis. The most common location is along the medial orbital wall and is due to transosseous spread of bacteria from an adjacent ethmoid sinusitis. Symptoms are similar to those seen with orbital cellulitis and include swelling and erythema of the eyelids, chemosis, proptosis, painful ophthalmoplegia, and diminished visual acuity. Postseptal abscesses are almost always extraconal. Intraconal abscesses are rare and seen only in penetrating trauma, following ocular surgery, or in the setting of orbital malignancy.

Contrast-enhanced CT will show retrobulbar fat stranding, a defined intraorbital fluid collection with an enhancing rim, and adjacent sinus opacification and should be carefully evaluated to exclude involvement of the orbital apex or cavernous sinus. Orbital abscesses are treated with antibiotic therapy and, in some cases, surgical drainage (**Fig. 3.27**).

Fig. 3.27a–f
a Preseptal cellulitis. Soft tissue inflammation limited to the eyelids and adjacent skin and subcutaneous tissues. The retroseptal and intraconal fat is uninvolved.
b Fungal orbital abscess. Left ethmoid and medial orbital retroseptal, extraconal, enhancing mass containing areas of necrosis. Associated bone destruction and distortion of the posteromedial globe.
c–f Bacterial orbital abscess. Convex, marginally enhancing fluid collection interposed between the medial orbital wall and the medial rectus muscle. Left ethmoid sinusitis with complete opacification of the air cells and hyperostosis of the lamina papyracea.

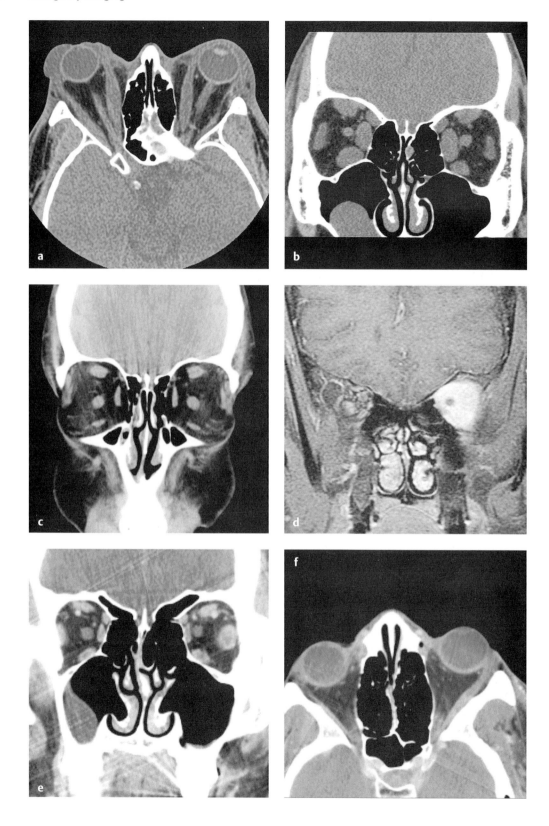

◆ Orbital Inflammatory Disease

Graves orbitopathy is the most frequent cause of proptosis in adults. It develops several years after the onset of thyroid disease and is considered to be an autoimmune phenomenon distinct from thyroid dysfunction. Lid retraction, proptosis, ophthalmoplegia, and chemosis reflect orbital fat hypertrophy and orbital muscle enlargement that sequentially involves the inferior, medial, superior, and lateral rectus muscles.

CT and MRI show symmetrically enlarged extraocular muscles with a spindle-like appearance; the muscle is thickest at the center and thinnest at the tendinous insertions. Inflammatory stranding, increased orbital fat, eyelid edema, stretching of the optic nerve, and tenting of the posterior globe may also be seen.

Treatment is primarily conservative, as many cases of Graves orbitopathy are self-limiting, spontaneously improving within 2 to 5 years. Eyelid-lengthening surgery can prevent corneal damage from exposure. In severe cases, orbital decompression with medial or lateral orbital fracture may be required.

Orbital pseudotumor, or idiopathic orbital inflammatory syndrome (IOI), is a nongranulomatous inflammatory disease with no known local or systemic cause.

After Graves orbitopathy, IOI is the second most common cause of proptosis and is associated with other inflammatory and autoimmune conditions including Wegener granulomatosis, fibrosing mediastinitis, autoimmune thyroiditis, and sclerosing cholangitis. Patients typically present with acute onset; painful, unilateral proptosis; and eyelid swelling. Diplopia and decreased visual acuity are sometimes associated. IOI often involves the extraocular muscles, but, in contrast to Graves orbitopathy, the distal tendinous attachments are usually affected and muscles are thickened along their entire extent. Isolated inflammation of the lateral rectus muscle favors IOI, as this is usually the last muscle involved in Graves disease.

CT or MR imaging appearances vary in IOI and include intra- or extraconal fat infiltration, a well-defined focal intraorbital mass (tumefactive type), or enlargement of one or several extraocular muscles (myositic type). The lacrimal gland, optic nerve sheath, sclera, and retrobulbar soft tissues can be involved.

Steroid therapy is the mainstay of treatment for IOI and results in rapid improvement. Recurrences are common and may be seen in up to 25% of patients (**Fig. 3.28**).

Fig. 3.28a–f
a,b Graves myositis. Bilateral proptosis. Enlarged inferior, medial, and superior rectus muscles. Sparing of the tendinous insertions results in a spindle-like appearance in longitudinal section. The lateral rectus is not involved. Marked preseptal soft tissue hypertrophy indicates severe chemosis.
c Graves orbitopathy with orbital fat hypertrophy. Marked orbital fat hypertrophy with normal extraocular muscles.
d Idiopathic orbital inflammation. Diffuse inflammatory infiltration with enhancement of the orbital apex soft tissues on fat-suppressed, postgadolinium, T1-weighted MRI.
e,f IOI with myositis. Isolated enlargement of lateral rectus with involvement of musculotendinous insertions. This appearance would be very unusual in Graves disease.

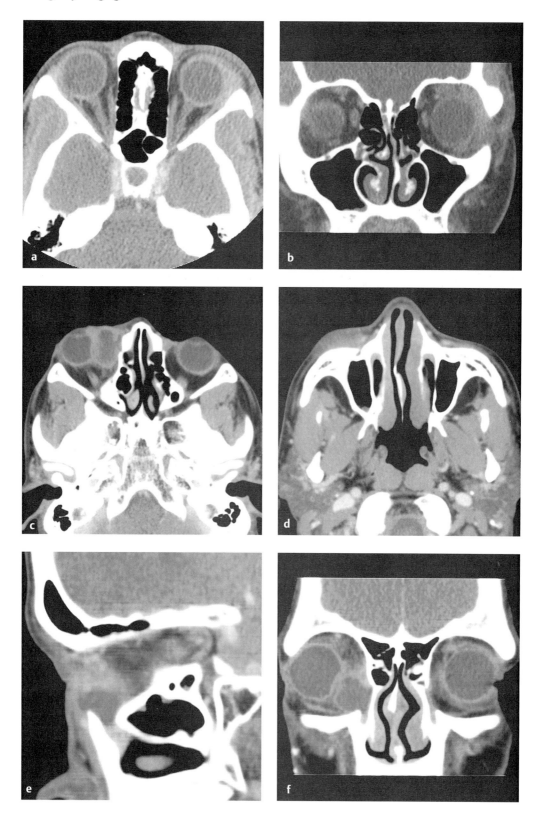

◆ Dacryoadenitis and Dacryocystitis

Acute dacryoadenitis is an uncommon inflammation of the lacrimal gland, often due to extension from adjacent conjunctivitis. Infectious etiologies may be viral, bacterial (usually gram positive), or fungal and noninfectious causes include Sogren syndrome, sarcoidosis, Graves disease, and idiopathic orbital inflammation. Patients present with rapid onset of unilateral chemosis, orbital pain, and superolateral orbital fullness. If severe, orbital mobility may be limited and the globe displaced inferomedially. CT shows enlargment of the lacrimal gland with variable adjacent inflammatory changes. The primary differential diagnosis is orbital cellulitis and lacrimal gland neoplasm. Management includes culture and antibiotics and most patients recover uneventfully.

Inflammation involving the nasolacrimal sac is most often due to ductal obstruction by a dacryolith, developmental stenosis in neonates, or acquired stenosis in adults. Etiologies include rhinitis, paranasal sinus mucocele, enlarged turbinates, septal deviation, nasolacrimal duct carcinoma, and foreign body. Patients present with a medial canthal inflammatory mass, with pain, erythema, and edema. Purulent discharge may be evident at the puncta.

Contrast-enhanced CT demonstrates the inflamed lacrimal apparatus, which appears as a peripherally enhancing cyst in the anteromedial orbit. CT also evaluates potential complications such as periorbital or orbital cellulitis, and identifies any predisposing anatomic variants or obstructing masses. Treatment is with antibiotics, or in some cases surgical drainage may be necessary (**Fig. 3.29**).

Fig. 3.29a–f
a,b Dacryoadenitis. The left lacrimal gland is enlarged in comparison to the right gland. Associated preseptal cellulitis.
c-f Dacryocystitis. Thick-walled, peripherally enhancing, inferomedial, anterior orbital mass that is contiguous with the nasolacrimal duct, displaces the globe laterally, and is associated with moderate preseptal/premalar cellulitis.

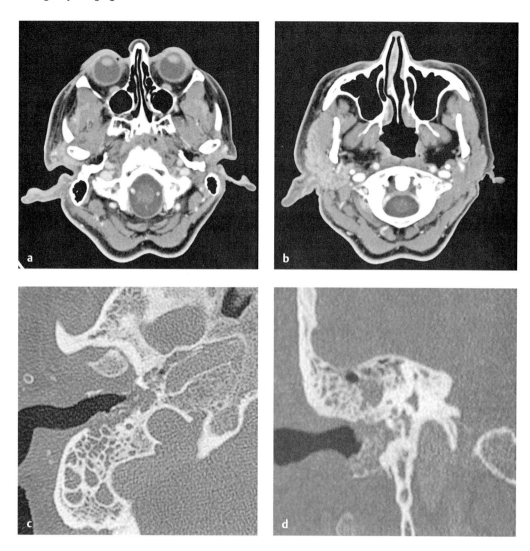

◆ Necrotizing External Otitis

Necrotizing external otitis is a severe invasive infection of the external auditory canal, usually caused by *Pseudomonas aeruginosa* in elderly patients with diabetes mellitus. In immunosuppressed and AIDS patients, *Aspergillus* is another cause. Cellulitis initially involving the external auditory canal can rapidly spread to surrounding superficial soft tissue, parotid gland, adjacent deep neck spaces, and the the skull base.

Otalgia, otorrhea, and temporomandibular joint pain are frequent symptoms. Soft tissue induration and granulation tissue within the external auditory canal should be evident on physical exam, and laboratory analysis typically detects an elevated erythrocyte sedimentation rate. Cranial neuropathies, venous sinus thrombosis, meningitis, or intracranial empyema indicate skull base or intracranial extension.

Contrast-enhanced CT identifies auricular and external auditory canal wall soft tissue thickening and may show bone erosion and adjacent abscess formation. Fluid is usually present in the middle ear and mastoid air cells. Squamous cell carcinoma can have a similar appearance but is more clinically indolent. Temporal bone osteomyelitis is indicated by opacified air cells, frank osseous erosion, and obliteration of the normal fat within the stylomastoid foramen. MRI is useful for evaluating the extent of soft tissue disease as well as any intracranial complications.

Treatment includes meticulous glucose control in diabetic patients and an extended course of systemic antibiotics (**Fig. 3.30**).

Fig. 3.30a–d
a–d   Necrotizing external otitis with associated parotitis and osseous erosion. (**a,b**) Right-sided dermal and subcutaneous auricular and external auditory canal soft tissue thickening and enhancement. Right parotid enlargement and enhancement. (**c,d**) The mastoid air cells and tympanic cavity are completely opacified. The posterior wall of the temporomandibular joint, anterior mastoid bone, and ossicles are eroded.

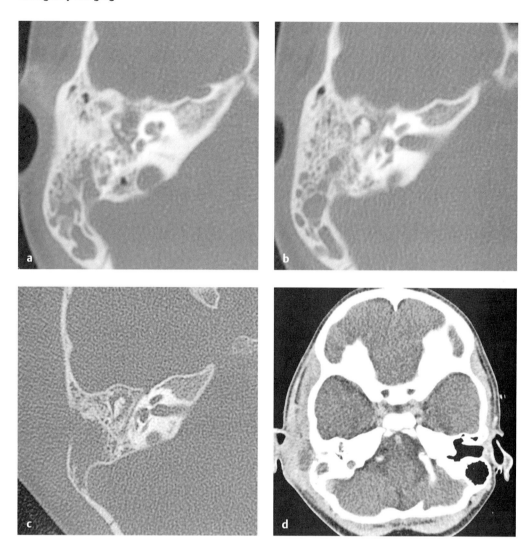

◆ Otitis Media and Mastoiditis

Otitis media is a common childhood infection that results from adenoid hypertrophy and consequent eustachian tube dysfunction. In this setting, fluid that accumulates in the tympanic cavity becomes secondarily infected, usually by *Streptococcus* or *Haemophilus influenzae*. In children, fever, retroauricular swelling, and erythema are common findings, but symptoms in infants and younger children are often nonspecific and include irritability, feeding difficulties, and ear pulling. Older children and adults more commonly present with pain, middle ear fluid, and a detectible conductive hearing loss.

CT is not usually necessary for diagnosis and management of otitis media, but if imaging is performed, it will always show middle ear and mastoid air cell opacification. In uncomplicated otomastoiditis, the ossicles and mastoid septa are intact, and fluid typically resolves with antibiotic therapy. Resistant or inadequately treated infections can be complicated by skull base osteomyelitis (coalescent mastoiditis or petrous apicitis) or periauricular soft tissue cellulitis/abscess.

Longstanding or past episodes of recurrent otitis media result in sclerotic, poorly pneumatized mastoids, and this finding is often incidentally identified on head CT obtained for other reasons. Cholesteatoma is an acquired middle-ear condition in which epithelial cells proliferate in the tympanic cavity as a result of chronic retraction of a portion of the tympanic membrane. Seen exclusively in patients with chronic otitis media, it can lead to ossicular erosion, hearing loss, or facial nerve compromise.

Coalescent mastoiditis is a consequence of mastoiditis in which the mastoid septa or cortex are dissolved by lytic inflammatory exudates. Prolonged fever, ear pain, otorrhea, and variable degrees of retroauricular swelling and erythema are typical. Direct extension of infection to deep cervical and intracranial structures in severe cases can lead to facial pain, cranial neuropathy, and focal neurologic or neuropsychiatric symptoms.

Thin-section CT optimally evaluates the mastoid septa and walls. Lateral mastoid wall erosion with penetration of the external mastoid cortex may give rise to a subperiosteal abscess. Involvement of the mastoid tip can result in formation of a high cervical ("Bezold") abscess as the infection spreads along the sternocleidomastoid muscle into the superficial neck. Erosion of the medial sigmoid sinus plate and subsequent intracranial extension can cause meningitis, epidural or cerebral abscess, or transverse/sigmoid venous sinus thrombosis. The latter can be associated with venous infarction (**Fig. 3.31**).

Fig. 3.31a–d
a,b Otitis media and mastoiditis. Fluid fills the tympanic cavities and mastoid air cells without erosion.
c,d Coalescent mastoiditis with Bezold abscess. The intramastoid septa and lateral wall of the mastoid bone are eroded. Extensive right periauricular cellulitis with loss of normal subcutaneous fat surrounds a small fluid collection lateral to the mastoid bone.

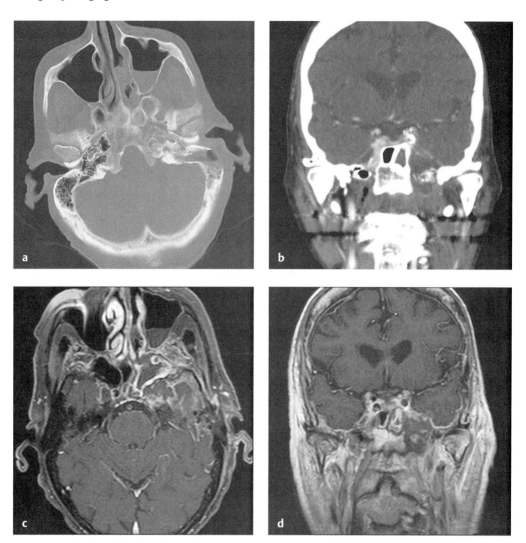

◆ Petrous Apicitis

Petrous apicitis, also known as apical petrositis, occurs when mastoiditis extends to the pneumatized petrous apex, and it has the potential to involve the adjacent cavernous sinus and central skull base. The combination of headache, abducens nerve palsy, and otorrhea is referred to as Gradenigo syndrome and is the most typical presentation of this disease. Patients with acute otalgia and a recent history of acute or chronic suppurative otitis media should be imaged using a thin-section temporal bone CT protocol or MRI to assess for petrous involvement, especially if cranial nerve deficits are present.

CT findings include petrous apex opacification with destruction of septa. Acute petrositis may appear as an expanding lesion with irregular margins, often with enhancement of the adjacent meninges and cavernous sinus. In contrast, chronic petrous apicitis, like chronic mastoiditis, may show only hypopneumatization and sclerosis on CT. MRI characteristics include hyperintensity on T2-weighted images (corresponding to fluid) in the air cells of the petrous apex with avid surrounding enhancement after gadolinium administration.

Because of the proximity of the petrous apex to critical neural structures, petrous apicitis frequently requires surgical drainage in order to prevent severe complications such as cranial neuropathy, cavernous sinus thrombosis, extradural empyema, meningitis or cerebritis, and brain abscess (**Fig. 3.32**).

Fig. 3.32a–d

a–d Petrous apicitis with extension to cavernous sinus, erosion of central skull base, and ipsilateral carotid artery thrombosis. (**a**) The air cells of the left petrous bone are opacified, as are the left mastoid air cells. The medial petrous bone is eroded and largely replaced by a low-attenuation, peripherally enhancing inflammatory mass. (**b**) The left cavernous sinus is expanded and the left carotid artery is thrombosed. (**c,d**) Postgadolinium T1-weighted MRI shows a peripherally enhancing abscess involving the left cavernous sinus, the Meckel cave, and the floor of the middle cranial fossa. The left supraclinoid internal carotid artery flow void is absent consistent with thrombosis. The adjacent sphenoid sinus is fluid-filled, with marked mucosal enhancement.

4
Spine

◆ Approach

The aim of spinal imaging in acute trauma is to detect fractures, evaluate their stability, and identify associated soft tissue injuries. Other emergent indications include atraumatic pain (usually in the setting of an underlying malignancy or predisposition to infection) and acute myelopathy or radiculopathy.

CT with multiplanar reconstructions is significantly more sensitive and specific for detection and exclusion of cervical spine fractures than plain radiography and is now considered the standard of care in acute trauma. Five specific clinical criteria—validated by the National Emergency X-ray Utilization Study (NEXUS) and widely used in emergency departments and trauma centers—permit the emergency physician to exclude cervical spine fracture without imaging:

- No midline tenderness
- No focal neurologic deficit
- Normal alertness
- No intoxication
- No painful distracting injuries

MRI is indicated for patients with neurological deficits, prolonged obtundation, or unstable spinal injuries. Flexion and extension radiographs are never indicated in the emergency setting, as muscle spasm can mask ligamentous instability and truly unstable injuries can be made worse.

Both the thoracic and lumbar spine are normally included on chest and abdomen CT in the setting of polytrauma, and as long as high-quality reformations are available, a separate dedicated spinal examination need not be performed. Plain radiographs are usually adequate to screen for thoracic and lumbar spine injuries in patients with low-energy mechanisms, with CT to follow if an abnormality is identified.

To avoid missing craniocervical dissociation injuries, which can be subtle, several measurements in the cervical spine are useful. The tip of the basion should be within 9.5 mm of the tip of the dens on CT (12 mm on lateral radiograph). The tip of the basion should be between 6 and 12 mm from a line drawn along the posterior cortex of C2 (the posterior axial line). This is referred to as the basion–axial interval. Injury to the transverse ligament, which affixes the dens to C1, increases the atlantodental interval, which should be less than 3 mm in adults and 5 mm in children on both CT and radiographs.

In the lower thoracic and lumbar spine, the interspinous distance and interpedicular distances on frontal radiographs and coronal CT increase by about 2 mm at each level from craniad to caudad. Isolated widening of either of these distances at a single spinal level should raise suspicion for fracture. Disk herniations should be identified when present and can be practically described as either (1) broad-based disk bulge, (2) central, paracentral, foraminal, or lateral protrusion, or (3) extruded or sequestered disk, in which disk material is separated from the body of the disk.

Anterior compression and burst fractures can be described by the ratio of the affected vertebral body height to the average height of the adjacent superior and inferior vertebral bodies; for example, if the adjacent vertebral body height average is 25 mm and the affected vertebra is 20 mm, it has a 20% loss of height. Canal compromise can similarly be expressed as a percentage of the expected canal diameter at the affected level.

Anatomic Checklist

Cervical Spine

- Prevertebral soft tissues
- Anterior spinal alignment
- Posterior spinal alignment
- Spinolaminar alignment
- Basion–dens interval (< 12 mm on radiograph, < 9.5 mm on CT)
- Basion–axial interval (< 12 mm on radiograph, 6–12 mm on CT)
- Atlantodental interval (< 3 mm)
- Occipital condyle–lateral mass relationship
- Dens–lateral mass relationship
- Facet articulations
- Vertebral bodies
- Vertebral artery canal
- Intervertebral disks and uncovertebral articulations
- Spinal canal
- Spinal cord and epidural soft tissues
- Neuroforamina

Thoracolumbar Spine

- Paraspinous soft tissues
- Anterior spinal alignment
- Posterior spinal alignment
- Intraspinous distance
- Interpedicular distance
- Vertebral bodies
- Intervertebral disks and facet articulations
- Transverse processes
- Spinal canal
- Spinal cord and epidural soft tissues
- Neuroforamina

◆ Imaging

Cervical Spine Radiographs

Indications: Pain, radiculopathy. Trauma significant enough to warrant imaging should be evaluated by CT.

- AP
- Lateral
- Odontoid
- Oblique

Thoracic Spine Radiographs

Indications: Minor trauma, some patients with pain.

- AP
- Lateral

Lumbar Spine Radiographs

Indications: Some patients with minor trauma and lower back pain. Generally not indicated for uncomplicated lower back pain in patients under 50 or without a history of underlying malignancy.

- AP
- Lateral
- Sacrum
- Oblique lumbar radiographs are rarely indicated

Spine CT

Indications: Trauma, radiculopathy.

Technique: 0.6-mm dataset with 2-mm axial, 2-mm sagittal, and 2-mm coronal reformations. Images localized to area of clinical concern. Postcontrast images can be obtained for osteomyelitis/diskitis or epidural abscess when MRI is contraindicated or not available.

Spine MRI

Indications: Neurologic deficit in trauma, radiculopathy, pain, and suspected ligamentous injury.

Sequences: Sagittal T1, sagittal T2, axial T1, axial T2.

Options: T1+gadolinium sequences can be obtained if there is concern for osteomyelitis/diskitis, epidural abscess, or tumor. Fat suppression techniques (STIR, T1 with fat saturation) are also commonly used.

◆ Clinical Presentations and Differential Diagnosis

Clinical Presentations and Appropriate Initial Studies

Cervical Trauma

- Cervical spine CT
- MRI for suspected spinal cord injury, ligamentous injury or epidural hematoma
    - Occipital condyle fracture
    - Atlantoaxial dissociation
    - Rotatory subluxation of C1 on C2
    - Dens fractures
    - Hangman fracture (C2)
    - Flexion injury
    - Extension injury
    - Unilateral or bilateral jumped facets

Thoracolumbar Trauma

- Thoracic or lumbar spine CT (or reconstructions/reformations from multidetector chest/abdomen CT)
- MRI for suspected spinal cord injury, ligamentous injury, or epidural hematoma.
    - Anterior compression fracture
    - Burst fracture
    - Chance-type fracture
    - Flexion-distraction injury
    - Fracture-dislocation

Pain

- No imaging study for acute back pain in patients under 40 without trauma or other comorbid conditions.

- MRI and CT can be considered for pain unresponsive to conservative measures or for patients with underlying malignancy or risk of infection.
    - Muscle spasm
    - Disk herniation
    - Degenerative disk disease
    - Primary or metastatic bone tumor
    - Spondylolysis/spondylolisthesis
    - Osteomyelitis diskitis

Myelopathy

- MRI with or without gadolinium. CT with contrast may be considered if MRI is contraindicated.
    - Acute or subacute cord compression
    - Pathologic fracture
    - Primary spine tumor
    - Osteomyelitis/diskitis
    - Epidural abscess
    - Multiple sclerosis/demyelination
    - Spinal cord ischemia
    - Infectious myelitis
    - Radiation myelitis
    - Spinal cord neoplasm

Radiculopathy

- MRI with or without gadolinium. CT with contrast may be considered if MRI is contraindicated.
    - Herniated disk
    - Degenerative disk/facet disease
    - Spinal canal/neuroforaminal stenosis
    - Schwannoma
    - Meningioma

Differential Diagnosis

Collapsed Vertebra

- Metastasis
- Multiple myeloma
- Lymphoma
- Osteoporosis
- Trauma
- Osteomyelitis/diskitis

Enlarged Vertebra

- Paget disease
- Aneurysmal bone cyst
- Hemangioma
- Giant cell tumor

Extradural Mass

- Extruded disk
- Metastasis
- Plasmacytoma
- Lymphoma
- Hematoma
- Abscess
- Meningioma

Intradural Mass

- Meningioma
- Metastasis

Intramedullary Mass

- Astrocytoma
- Ependymoma
- Hematoma
- Infarct

Intramedullary Signal Abnormality

- Demyelinating disease/transverse myelitis
- Contusion
- Neoplasm
- Ischemia

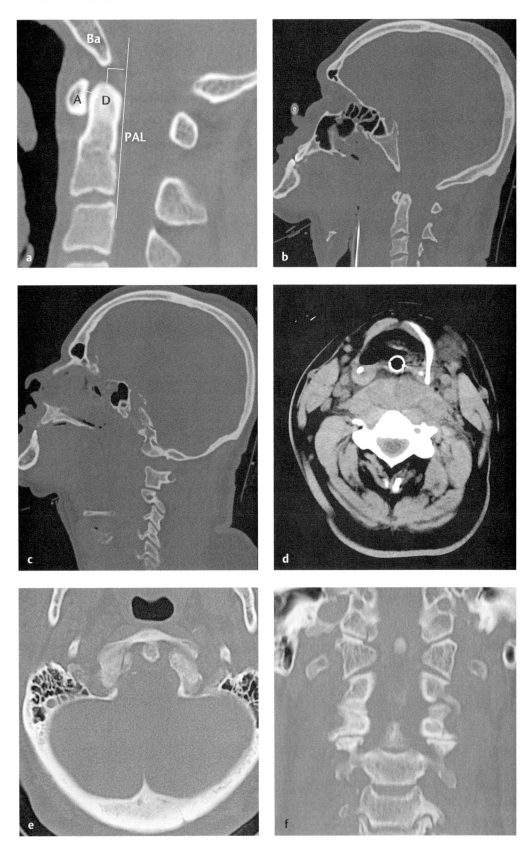

◆ Craniocervical Junction Injuries

Atlantooccipital dislocation (AOD) is a consequence of very high-energy trauma; usually diagnosed at autopsy rather than on imaging studies. In AOD, the skull is dislocated with respect to the lateral masses of C1, and this can be directly assessed on CT by evaluating the congruity of the atlantooccipital articulations. Displacement can be along either the transverse or craniocaudal axis and is usually associated with marked prevertebral soft tissue swelling.

Complete AOD (dislocation) is a fatal injury, but partial AOD (subluxation) may be compatible with life. To ensure detection of an unstable but potentially survivable injury, the atlantooccipital articulation should be specifically evaluated on any lateral radiograph or cervical spine CT obtained for trauma. The most useful measurements are the basion–dens interval, the basion–axial interval, and the atlantodental interval, which assesses integrity of the transverse C1 ligament.

Occipital condyle fractures, considered rare prior to the advent of CT, are diagnosed with increasing frequency. Depending on the mechanism of injury, several types of occipital condyle fracture have been identified.

- Type I: impaction fracture of the occipital condyle due to axial loading
- Type II: basilar skull fracture, usually due to direct impact, that extends to the occipital condyle
- Type III: avulsion injury at alar ligament attachment due to bending and rotation

In Type I and II injuries the alar ligaments and tectorial membrane are intact, and these fractures are generally stable. Because the alar ligament is disrupted in Type III fractures, they are potentially unstable. Type III fractures are more likely to be associated with lower cranial nerve deficits (**Fig. 4.1**).

Fig. 4.1a–f
a Normal craniocervical relationships. The basion–dens interval (Ba–D) should be < 9.5 mm, the atlantodental interval (A–D) should be ≤ 3 mm in adults and ≤ 5 mm in children, and the basion–posterior axial line (Ba–PAL) interval should be between 6 and 12 mm on a sagittal CT reconstruction. The occipital–C1 and C1–C2 articulations should be symmetric and congruent on coronal and parasagittal images.
b–d Atlanto-occipital dislocation. (**b**) NCCT. Abnormally widened basion–dens interval, basion–axial interval. (**c**) Anterior subluxation of the lateral mass of C1 with respect to the occipital condyle. (**d**) Marked prevertebral soft tissue swelling at the level of the hyoid bone. Extensive subarachnoid hemorrhage surrounds the upper cervical spinal cord.
e,f Type III occipital condyle fracture. Nondisplaced right occipital condyle fracture due to avulsion of the alar ligament.

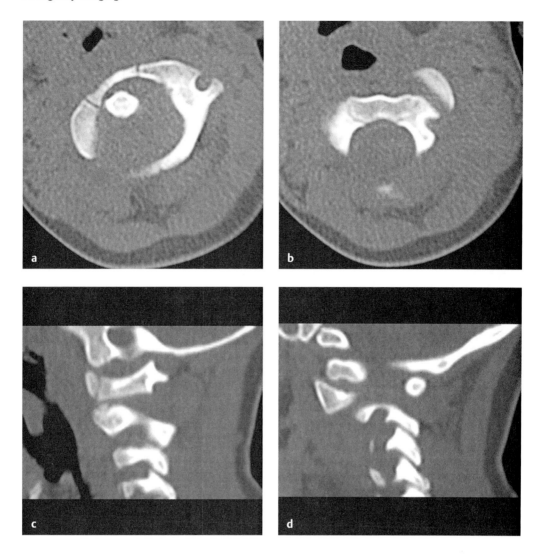

◆ Atlantoaxial Rotatory Subluxation

Atlantoaxial rotatory subluxation is a consequence of motor vehicle accidents and sports-related injuries in older adolescents and adults but may be nontraumatic in children. In trauma, disruption of the alar ligament, atlantoaxial joint capsule, and transverse ligament permits hyperrotation of C1 relative to C2 with widening of the atlantodental interval. Patients present with their head tilted to one side and rotated toward the opposite side.

AP or odontoid radiographs will show asymmetry of the lateral atlantodental intervals. CT is diagnostic and demonstrates rotation of the C1 ring with respect to the C2 lateral masses. If not clinically obvious, dynamic imaging with scanning before and after voluntary head turning can establish whether or not subluxation is fixed.

Fixed subluxation can be reduced by cervical traction followed by active range of motion (ROM) exercises. Rarely, C1–C2 fusion can be considered for persistently fixed and painful rotation (**Fig. 4.2**).

Fig. 4.2a–d
a–d Atlantoaxial rotatory subluxation in a child. (**a,b**) C1 is rotated to the right with respect to C2. The left C1 facet is subluxed anteriorly with respect to C2. (**c**) Normal right atlantoaxial articulation. (**d**) The left lateral mass of C1 is located anterior to the articulating surface of C2.

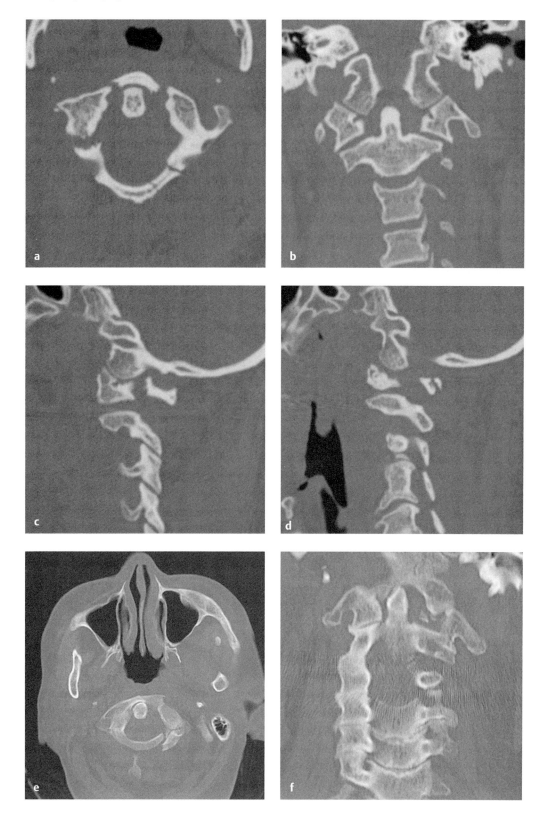

◆ C1 Burst (Jefferson) Fracture

Axial forces transmitted through the occipital condyles to the C1 lateral masses result in multipart fractures of the C1 ring with radial displacement of the fragments away from the C2 odontoid. A common injury mechanism is diving headfirst into shallow water. Because the fracture widens rather than narrows the spinal canal, patients often present with pain but without neurologic dysfunction. Associated spinal cord injury is usually absent unless there is a retropulsed fragment. Stability of this fracture depends on whether or not the transverse atlantal ligament is intact.

The "classical" Jefferson fracture is a four-part fracture with bilateral anterior and posterior arch fractures. Two- and three-part fractures are common variants reflecting eccentric loading and usually involve one lateral mass and the adjacent occipital condyle.

Coronal CT reformations will show displacement of the C1 lateral masses away from the odontoid. If the combined lateral atlantodental intervals are > 7 mm, transverse ligament rupture is possible. Sagittal CT reconstructions will show prevertebral soft tissue swelling as well as a widened atlantodental interval. The normal atlantodental interval is ≤ 3 mm in adults and ≤ 5 mm in children. An atlantodental interval >6 mm indicates definite transverse ligament disruption. Associated cervical spine fractures, especially of C2, should be excluded.

Multidetector CT more precisely delineates the C1 ring fractures, their extent of displacement, and any other synchronous fractures of the cervical spine. Minimally displaced fractures may be treated conservatively with hard collar immobilization. If the transverse atlantal ligament is disrupted, the injury will likely require halo placement or C1–C2 surgical fixation (**Fig. 4.3**).

Fig. 4.3a–f
a–d "Classical" Jefferson fracture. Unstable, four-part fracture involving the anterior and posterior arches of C1 with combined transverse atlantodental intervals of 15 mm and slight lateral displacement of the C1 lateral mass with respect to the body of C2.
e,f Lateral mass C1 fracture ("atypical" Jefferson fracture). Comminuted C1 left lateral mass fracture with three major fragments. The dens is normally related to the anterior arch of C1 indicating integrity of the atlantodental ligaments. This fracture is due to asymmetric axial loading.

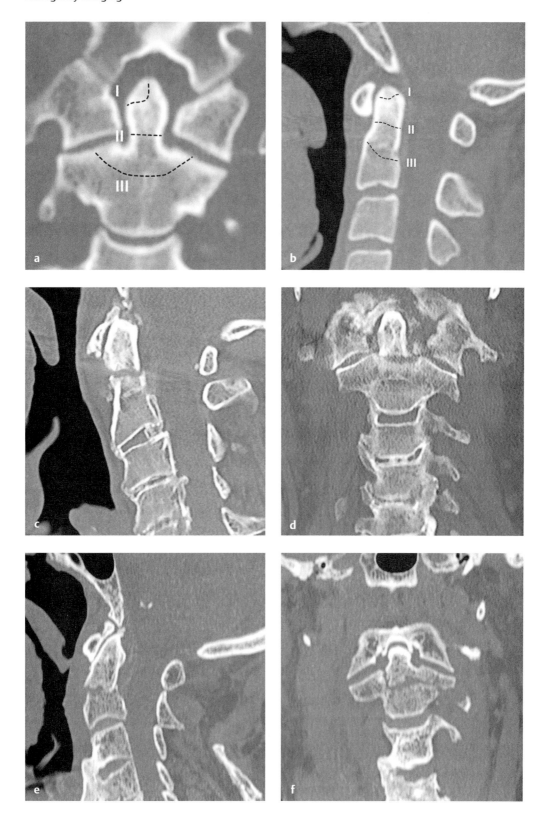

◆ Odontoid (Dens) Fracture

C2 fractures are common and are frequently seen in elderly patients who fall from standing or sitting. Hyperflexion, hyperextension, and lateral flexion mechanisms can all result in fractures that separate the odontoid from the vertebral body.

Type I fractures are avulsions of the odontoid tip at the attachment of the alar ligaments. These are rare but sometimes seen in patients with atlantooccipital dislocation. Type II fractures traverse the odontoid base.

Because the dens is mainly composed of dense cortical bone, they are prone to nonunion, and patients often require operative repair. Type III fractures separate a fragment that includes both the dens and a portion of the C2 body. Thanks to the larger area of cancellous bone-to-bone contact, type III fractures tend to heal with immobilization and do not usually require surgical fixation. Types II and III are also referred to as "high" and "low" dens fractures, respectively (**Fig. 4.4**).

Fig. 4.4a–f
a,b   Odontoid fracture classification. Type I fractures are odontoid tip avulsions at the attachment of the alar ligament. Type II fractures traverse the base of the dens. Type III fractures involve only the C2 body.
c,d   Type II odontoid fracture. Transverse fracture through the base of the odontoid with adjacent epidural and prevertebral hematoma.
e,f   Type III odontoid fracture. Transverse fracture through the upper body of C2 with minimal dorsal angulation of the odontoid fragment.

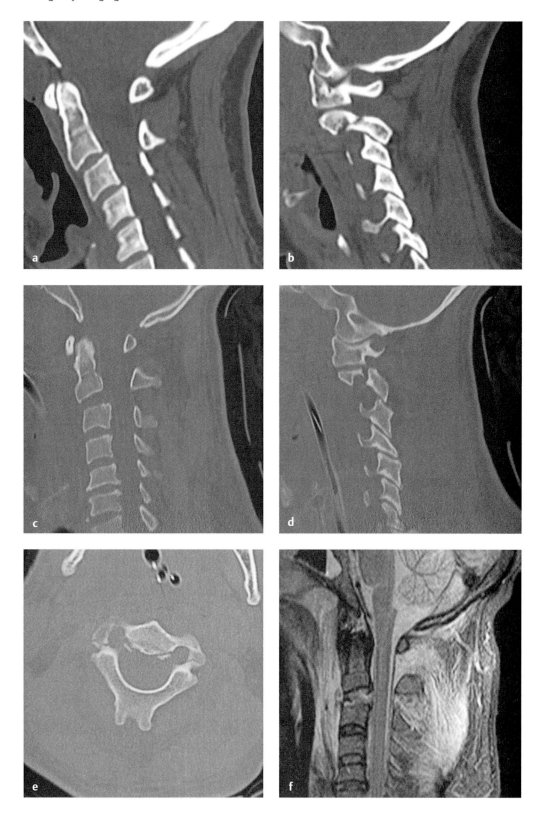

◆ Traumatic C2 Spondylolisthesis

Traumatic C2 spondylolisthesis results from the combined effects of axial loading and either hyperextension or hyperflexion. Both C2 pedicles fracture with varying degrees of angulation and anterolisthesis of C2 on C3. Historically referred to as a "hanged man's" fracture or "hangman" fracture because of its similarity to the injury caused by judicial hangings, traumatic C2 spondylolisthesis most frequently results from high-speed motor vehicle accidents. Neurologic sequelae are uncommon. Because the fracture tends to widen, rather than narrow, the spinal canal, the spinal cord and nerve roots are not usually damaged. The "atypical" hangman fracture is a variant in which the coronal fracture traverses the posterior C2 body, rather than the pedicles.

CT is necessary for accurate evaluation of displacement and angulation, which impact classification and treatment decisions, as well as identification of vertebral foraminal fractures and potential vascular injury. As in all cervical spine fractures, CTA should be considered to exclude vertebral or carotid artery injury.

Fractures that do not show disk widening, angulation, or subluxation are considered stable (Type I) (**Fig. 4.5**).

◆ Effendi/Levine and Edwards Classification

- Type I: Bilateral pedicle fractures with intact disk and ligaments. No angulation or translation
- Type II: C2/3 disk disruption with angulation but no translation
- Type III: C2/3 disk disruption with angulation, translation, and facet subluxation or dislocation

Type I fractures are stable, types II and III are unstable (**Fig. 4.6**).

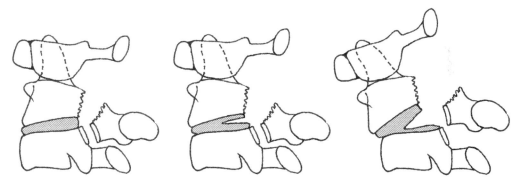

Fig. 4.6 Effendi/Levine and Edwards classification.

Fig. 4.5a–f
a,b Type I hangman fracture. Nondisplaced pedicle fractures with normal C2–C3 alignment and no disk space widening, translation, or angulation.
c–f Type III hangman fracture. (**c**) Anterior angulation and widening of C2–C3 disk space. (**d,e**) Bilateral pedicle fractures with C2–C3 facet subluxation. (**f**) T2-weighted MRI shows C2–C3 disk disruption and extensive prevertebral and nuchal ligament edema.

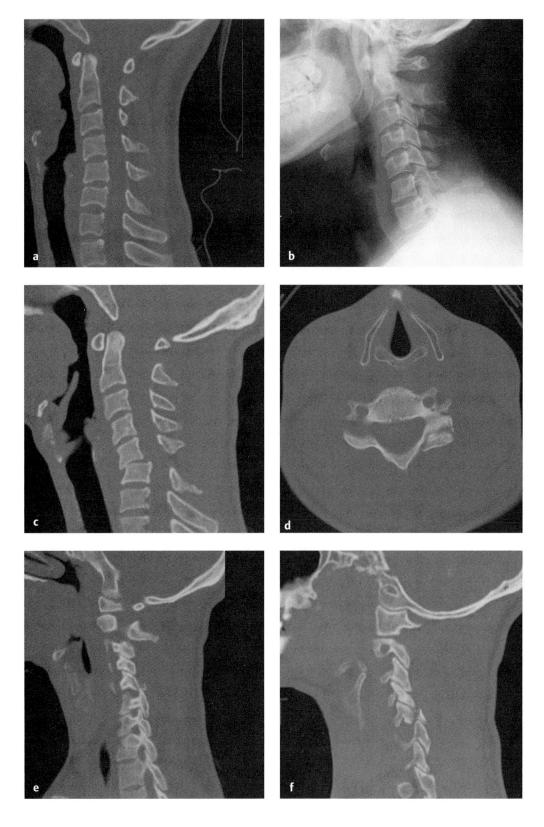

◆ Cervical Hyperflexion Injury 1

Cervical spine hyperflexion injuries result from whiplash mechanisms in which abrupt extension is followed by flexion or from axial loading forces acting upon a flexed neck. The latter are seen in head-on motor vehicle collisions and diving accidents. Hyperflexion injuries range, with increasing severity, from the stable hyperflexion sprain, in which only the posterior ligamentous complex is disrupted, to anterior vertebral subluxation, bilateral facet dislocation, and flexion "teardrop" or burst fractures.

Hyperflexion sprains may only show subtle spinous process distraction on lateral radiographs or sagittal CT reformations. If the injury is limited to the interspinous and nuchal ligaments, it is considered stable. Any degree of anterior vertebral subluxation, facet subluxation, or facet dislocation, however, indicates instability. MRI and/or delayed flexion and extension radiographs (after muscle spasm related to the acute injury has resolved) can be used to assess ligamentous injury and stability better.

The clay shoveler fracture is a horizontal fracture of a lower cervical spinous process originally described in workers who would abruptly contract their cervical muscles and flex the neck while shoveling heavy clay. The fracture may also result from direct impact and other complex mechanisms. Clay shoveler fractures are stable, as they do not involve the vertebral ring and are often incidentally discovered years after a forgotten injury.

Bilateral interfacet dislocation (BID) is a hyperflexion injury characterized by disruption of the anterior, middle, and posterior spinal ligaments. It is uncommon, extremely unstable, and associated with a high risk of spinal cord damage. On lateral cervical spine radiograph or sagittal CT reformation, the inferior articulating facet of the upper vertebra is displaced and locked anterior to the superior articulating facet of the lower vertebra. The upper vertebral body is anteriorly displaced by up to 50% relative to the lower one. Disk space and interspinous widening reflect the ligamentous nature of this injury. Small facet fractures may be seen (**Fig. 4.7**).

Fig. 4.7a–f
a Hyperflexion sprain. Slight kyphotic angulation at C5–C6 with splaying of the spinous processes indicates a posterior ligamentous complex injury.
b Clay shoveler fracture. Acute, transverse oblique, minimally displaced fractures limited to the spinous processes of C5 and C6.
c–f Bilateral interfacet dislocation. Focal kyphosis and anterolisthesis of C5 with respect to C6. The right inferior articulating facet of C5 is "perched" on the superior articulating facet of C6, resulting in an unpaired "naked" facet on the axial image. The left inferior articulating facet of C5, which should lie posterior to the C6 superior articulating facet, is dislocated anteriorly, resulting in the "reverse hamburger sign," in which the dorsal surface of the C5 facet contacts the anterior surface of the C6 facet.

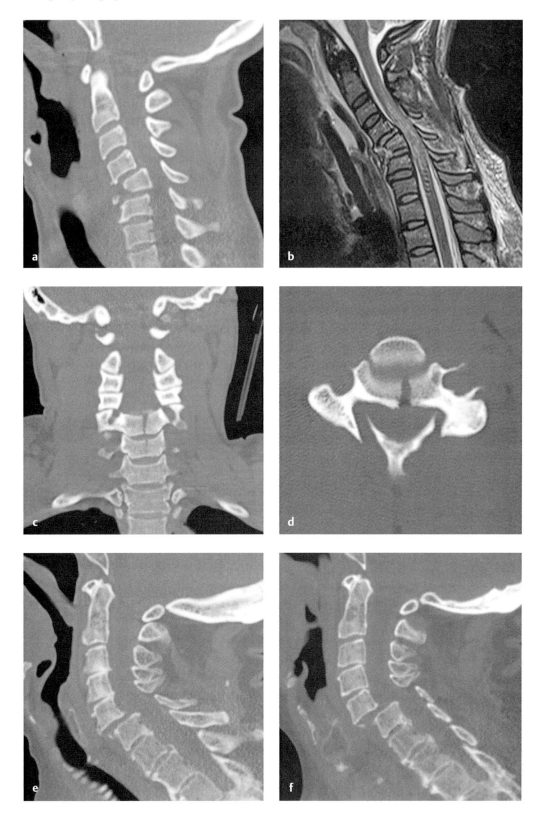

◆ Cervical Hyperflexion Injury 2

Hyperflexion teardrop fractures are the most devastating of the hyperflexion injuries and reflect severe axial loads with anterior and posterior ligamentous disruption, fracture of one or more vertebrae, and at least transient subluxation or vertebral body retropulsion. Anterior spinal cord injury is virtually always present, characterized by acute quadriplegia with loss of pain and temperature sensation but with variable preservation of the dorsal tracts that provide vibratory sense and proprioception.

CT with sagittal reformations shows a triangular "teardrop" fragment avulsed from the anterior inferior corner of a mid or lower vertebral body as well as focal kyphosis and posterior element distraction. The avulsed fragment frequently remains aligned with the anterior margins of the adjacent vertebrae, while the posterior fragment is displaced into the spinal canal. A typical burst fracture can occur if the injuring force is primarily axial; sagittal split, loss of vertebral height, dorsal fragment retropulsion, and laminar fracture are hallmarks.

Unilateral interfacet dislocation (UID) is a hyperflexion injury variant in which forced neck flexion is associated with simultaneous rotation, resulting in unilateral rather than bilateral facet dislocation. The diagnosis may be delayed, as patients often have either no neurologic deficit or isolated radiculopathy, and CT findings may be subtle. Dislocation can be dynamic, occurring at the moment of injury and reduced spontaneously prior to imaging. In this case a mildly widened facet joint may be the only clue to diagnosis.

Operative spinal fusion is necessary for hyperflexion teardrop fractures, burst fractures, and both types of interfacet dislocation in order to restore mechanical stability. Hyperflexion sprains and clay shoveler fractures can often be treated conservatively (**Fig. 4.8**).

Fig. 4.8a–f
a–d Hyperflexion teardrop fracture. Small anterior triangular fragment with posterior displacement of the C5 vertebral body and focal kyphotic angulation. T2-weighted sagittal MRI shows anterior prevertebral and nuchal ligament edema, fracture and marrow edema in C5, and spinal cord edema extending from C3 to C6. Coronal and axial images show typical sagittal split, which may be inapparent on lateral radiographs or sagittal reformations.
e,f Unilateral interfacet dislocation progressing to bilateral interfacet dislocation. Sagittal reformations show initial study with ~ 25% anterolisthesis of C5 with respect to C6; axial images (not shown) confirmed UID. Subsequent CT obtained after acute development of paraparesis show ~ 75% anterolisthesis and BID. Although UID is often considered relatively stable, it may be seen transiently in the presence of severe ligamentous disruption characteristic of BID.

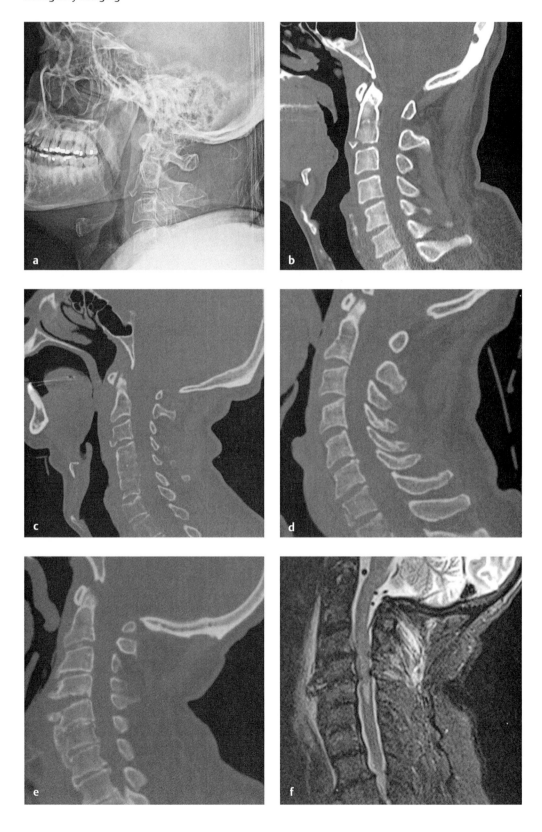

◆ Cervical Hyperextension Injuries

Like flexion injuries, cervical spine extension injuries can range from simple sprains to fracture-dislocations with significant neurologic deficit. The injury mechanism is sudden, severe hyperextension, usually due to impact to the head or lower face. In the less severe hyperextension sprain, prevertebral soft tissues are often swollen due to anterior longitudinal spinal ligament injury, but the middle and posterior vertebral columns remain intact and aligned.

Hyperextension with disruption of the anterior, middle, and posterior ligaments can result in severe spinal cord injury from transient dislocation at the time of impact. Prevertebral soft tissue swelling and subtle anterior disk space widening may be the only imaging evidence of this injury.

In hyperextension teardrop fractures, the anterior longitudinal ligament is avulsed and produces a teardrop fracture of the anteroinferior vertebral endplate. The fragment is characteristically (but not always) larger in the vertical than the horizontal dimension. In elderly patients this fracture usually occurs at C2 and is relatively stable. However, in younger patients, hyperextension injuries often involve the lower cervical spine and can be associated with acute central cervical cord syndrome: motor weakness below the level of the lesion that affects the upper extremities more severely than the lower extremities.

A triangular avulsed fragment is generally visible on lateral radiograph or sagittal CT reformation, with associated anterior disk space widening and prevertebral soft tissue swelling. Concomitant hyperextension injuries at other levels are not uncommon. In dislocation, MRI optimally evaluates ligamentous injury, intervertebral disk disruption, epidural hematoma, and spinal cord injury. On T2-weighted images, acute spinal ligament injury is seen as an interruption in the otherwise low-signal-intensity ligament surrounded by high-signal edema (**Fig. 4.9**).

Fig. 4.9a–d
a–d Hyperextension injuries with anterior ("teardrop") avulsion fractures in three patients. (**a,b**) C2 anterior inferior avulsed fragment with only minimal associated soft tissue swelling. (**c**) C3 avulsion in a patient with a partially fused cervical spine. Moderate prevertebral soft tissue swelling. (**d**) C5 avulsion fracture. The small triangular fragment is taller than it is wide (typical).
e,f Hyperextension injury without fracture. Isolated widening of anterior C4–C5 disk space. T2-weighted sagittal MRI shows extensive prevertebral soft tissue edema, dorsal nuchal ligament edema, canal stenosis from C3–C4 to C5–C6, and central cord high signal indicating acute injury.

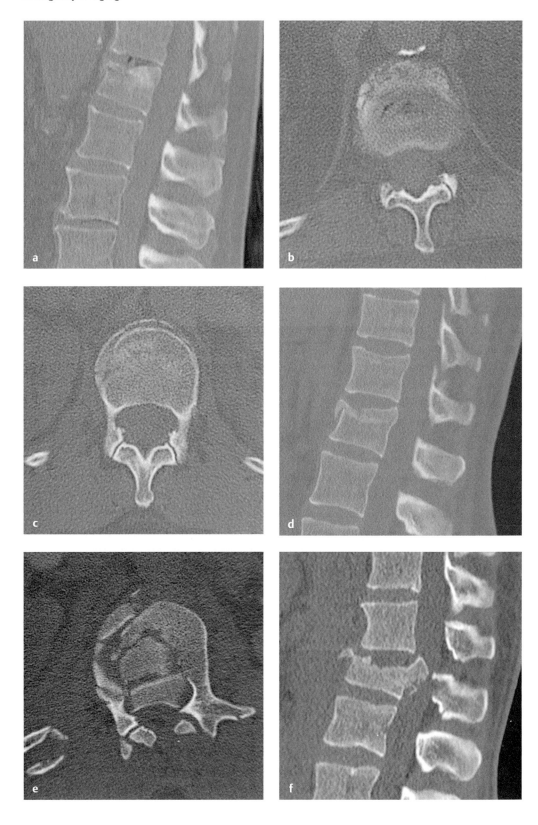

◆ Anterior Compression and Burst Fractures

Anterior compression fractures may result from acute axial loading injuries or can develop insidiously in vertebral bodies weakened by osteoporosis, metastatic disease, or infection. Most are considered stable but often require pain management and efforts to prevent further collapse. Alcohol, steroids, cytotoxic drugs, thyroid hormones, and heparin all predispose to osteoporosis and compression fractures. The presence of one anterior compression fracture increases the risk of subsequent fractures due to altered biomechanics of the kyphotic spine.

Compression fractures appear on lateral radiographs as vertebral body wedge deformities. Anterior height loss can be documented as the ratio of the ventral height of the involved vertebral body compared to the average of the heights of the two adjacent vertebrae. Fractures limited to the the anterior third of the vertebra are considered stable because of intact supporting spinal ligaments. On the normal AP radiograph, the vertebral pedicles should be intact, and the interpedicular and interspinous distances should gradually increase from craniad to caudad. Focal pedicle separation indicates a burst fracture with posterior element involvement. Focal interspinous widening suggests a posterior distraction injury.

On axial CT, the appearance of a double cortex at the anterior superior margin of the vertebra is characteristic. The contour of the spinal canal, the pedicles, lamina, and spinous processes should be otherwise normal.

Minimal burst fractures, in contrast to anterior compression fractures, involve the middle third of the vertebral body and are potentially unstable. In this case, the posterior vertebral body, which normally has a smooth arch that defines the anterior spinal canal wall, is flattened or disrupted.

Burst fractures are comminuted vertebral body fractures associated with significant anterior and middle vertebral height loss and are due to severe, acute axial load injuries. While they can occur at any spinal level, they are most frequently seen in the cervical spine and near the thoracolumbar junction. Burst fractures are distinguished from anterior compression fractures by involvement of both the anterior and middle thirds of the vertebral body (anterior and middle columns) and, not infrequently, posterior element disruption. The extent of middle column retropulsion, the relative size of the spinal canal, and the level of the involved vertebra determine the nature and degree of any associated neurologic compromise.

Axial images show a double cortex, significant vertebral height loss, and a retropulsed dorsal vertebral fragment. Sagittal reformations exclude the axially oriented fracture and spinal process distraction that are the hallmarks of the invariably unstable flexion distraction injury (**Fig. 4.10**).

Fig. 4.10a–f

a,b T12 anterior compression fracture. Anterior superior compression, sclerosis, and fragmentation with ~ 20% loss of anterior vertebral body height. No distortion of the posterior vertebral body wall.

c,d L1 minimal burst fracture. Anterior compression with "double cortex" sign. Flattening of the anterior spinal canal wall and slight posterior bulge of the upper vertebral body reflect middle vertebral column involvement and potential instability.

e,f L1 three-column burst fracture. Unstable, highly comminuted fracture involving all columns with severe canal narrowing, more than 50% height loss, and focal kyphosis. Adjacent rib fracture and paraspinous soft tissue hematoma.

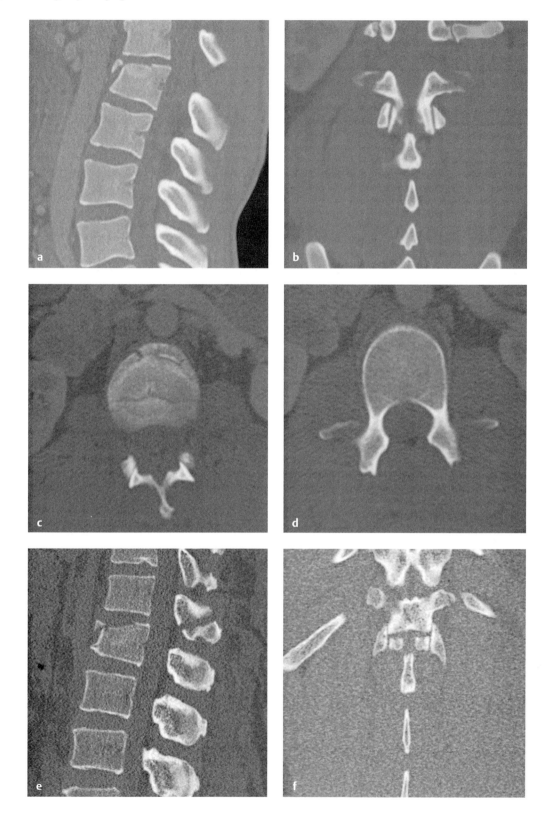

◆ Flexion-Distraction Injuries

The combination of flexion and distraction, as seen in lap-only seatbelt deceleration injuries, results in a horizontally oriented fracture through the vertebral body. Because flexion occurs about an axis at the anterior spinal margin, the anterior vertebral body is compressed and the posterior elements and spinous processes are distracted.

A common variant is the Chance fracture, in which flexion occurs about an axis located at the anterior abdominal wall and results in a horizontal fracture with less anterior vertebral height loss then in the typical flexion-distraction injury. Both fractures typically occur in the upper lumbar spine, are unstable, and always require surgical fixation.

AP and lateral radiographs can identify the horizontal fracture though the spinous process, laminae, or pedicles; distraction of the spinous processes; and any loss of anterior vertebral height. CT with coronal and sagittal reformations more sensitively evaluates the extent of injury, any potential disk disruption, and any spinal canal or cord involvement.

Flexion-distraction and Chance fractures are often associated with concurrent abdominal injury, particularly proximal intestinal and pancreatic contusion. Abdomen and pelvic CT with intravenous contrast should be always be obtained in this setting (**Fig. 4.11**).

Fig. 4.11a–f
a–d   Flexion-distraction injury at L1. L1 vertebral body fracture with anterior height loss and angulation, fractures through the anterior and middle third of the vertebral body, and distracted T12–L1 spinous processes. The inferior articulating facets of T12 do not articulate with the superior articulating facets of L1 on axial CT images ("naked facet").
e,f   Flexion-distraction injury with spinous process fracture. Anterior compression of L1 with horizontal fracture through the inferior articulating facets and spinous process of T12.

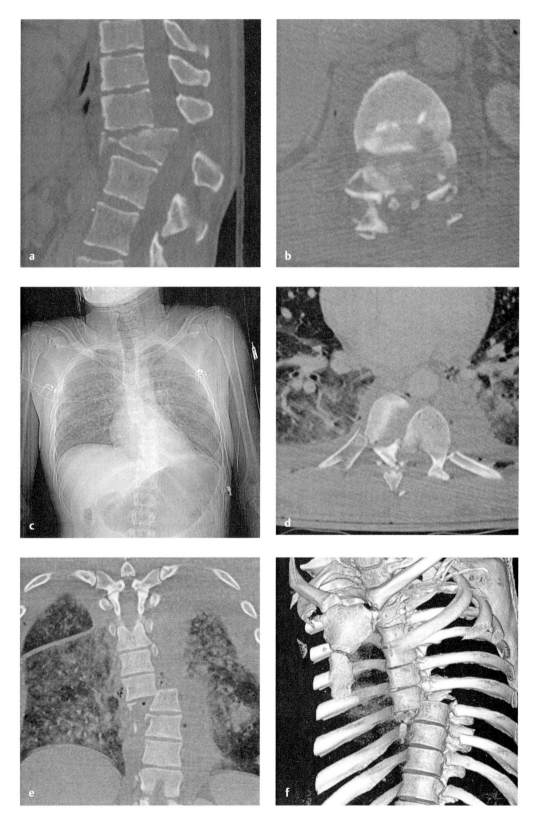

◆ Fracture-Dislocation

Spinal fracture-dislocation is the most severe type of thoracolumbar fracture and is invariably a grossly unstable injury, characterized by disruption of all three spinal columns and complete neurologic deficit below the affected level. It is due to severe, complex, shearing and rotational forces most commonly seen in motor vehicle collisions, impact from heavy objects, or falls. Surgical immobilization is almost always necessary to permit spinal stabilization and rehabilitation. Neurological deficits are usually immediate and permanent.

Fracture-dislocations can be detected on the initial supine AP radiograph obtained during resuscitation, and spinal continuity should always be carefully assessed. Most patients with an injury mechanism powerful enough to cause a spinal dislocation will undergo chest and abdominal CT, which readily identifies fracture-dislocations. Translation or rotation of the spine above and below the level of injury is diagnostic and best appreciated on sagittal, coronal, or 3D reformations. Axial findings include non-articulating ("naked") facets and visualization of two adjacent vertebrae on the same axial image ("double vertebra") (**Fig. 4.12**).

Fig. 4.12a–f
a,b Fracture-dislocation with anterior translation. T11 is anteriorly dislocated with respect to T12. Anterior T12 wedge deformity and wide splaying of the spinous processes indicates failure of anterior, middle, and posterior columns. The T11 and T12 vertebrae are both visible on the same axial image.
c–f Fracture-dislocation with anterior and transverse translation and rotation. CT scout image shows discontinuity of the mid-thoracic spine. The T7–T8 intervertebral disk space is completely disrupted, with anterior and transverse dislocation of T7 with respect to T8, large paraspinous hematoma, soft tissue gas, posterior pulmonary contusions, and a right pleural effusion/hematoma.

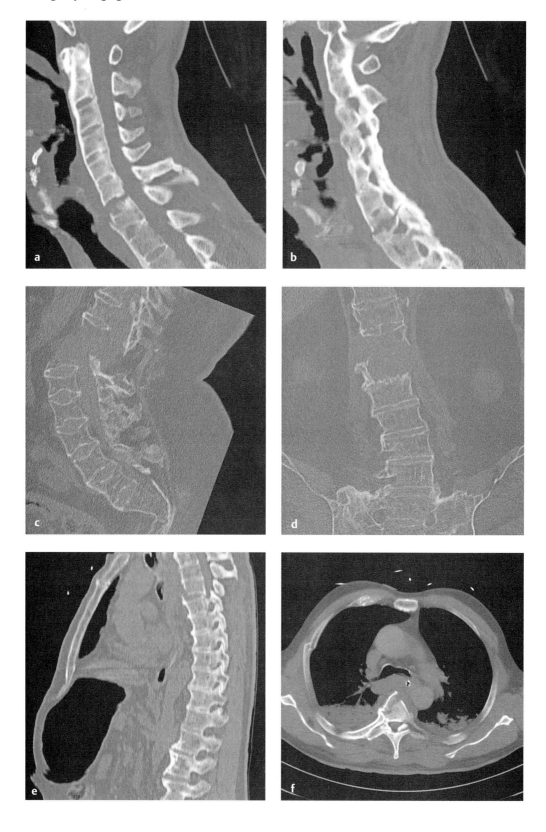

◆ Fused-Spine Fracture

The altered biomechanics in patients with rigid, fused spines, as seen in ankylosing spondylitis, diffuse idiopathic skeletal hyperostosis, osteogenesis imperfecta, and ossification of the posterior longitudinal ligament, result in a rigid, brittle spine. In these diseases, long segments of the spine are vulnerable to hyperextension or hyperflexion injuries, and most patients suffer complete spinal cord injury with para- or quadriplegia from the moment of injury.

Lateral spine radiographs or CT with sagittal reformation show a horizontal or oblique fracture through all spinal columns. Dislocation may not be obvious, particularly after immobilization, and failure to diagnose a fused-spine fracture in the neurologically intact patient can result in significant delayed neurologic decompensation. Surgical management aims to provide segmental internal fixation and stabilization. Unfortunately, recovery of neurologic function in patients with displaced fractures and cord injury is rare (**Fig. 4.13**).

Fig. 4.13a–f
a,b Fused-spine fracture in ankylosing spondylitis. Fracture through fused C6 and C7 vertebrae.
c,d Fused-spine fracture-dislocation in osteogenesis imperfecta. Fracture through the T12 vertebra with marked distraction and displacement.
e,f Upper thoracic hyperextension fracture-dislocation in patient with diffuse idiopathic skeletal hyperostosis (DISH). Associated paraspinous hematoma, pulmonary contusion, and rib fractures.

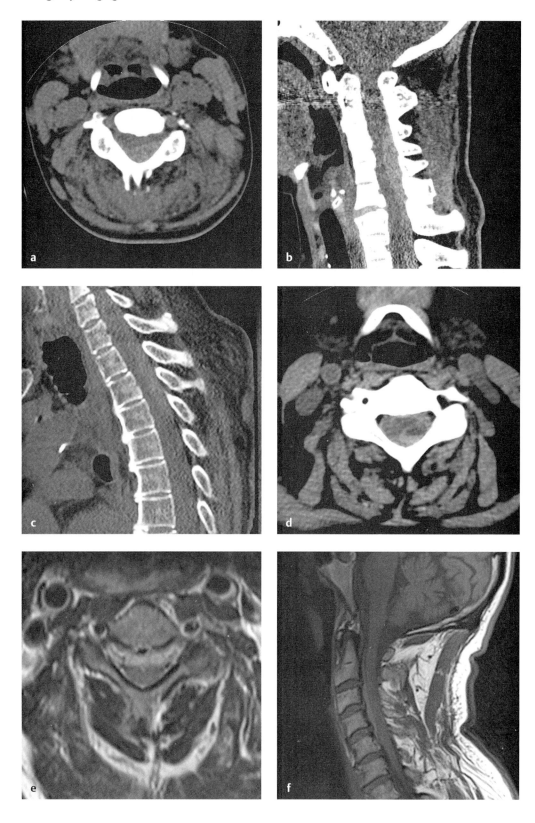

◆ Spinal Epidural Hematoma

Hemorrhage into the potential space between the dura and the adjacent bone may complicate spinal fracture or minor trauma such as a lumbar puncture or epidural anesthesia, or it may be spontaneous and atraumatic. Spontaneous epidural hematomas usually occur in patients with blood dyscrasias, coagulopathies, thrombocytopenia, neoplasms, or vascular malformations or in anticoagulated patients. Epidural hematoma often presents with severe localized back pain with radicular radiation that mimics disk herniation. Weakness, numbness, and lower motor neuron signs may also be present. In contrast to intracranial epidural hematomas, the source of bleeding is usually venous rather than arterial, and symptoms develop gradually as the hematoma enlarges over several days.

An acute spinal epidural hematoma appears on CT as a hyperdense mass in the spinal canal that extends over a few vertebral levels. MRI has a greater sensitivity in detecting small epidural hematomas. In the first 24 hours, the hematoma is typically isointense on T1-weighted and hyperintense on T2-weighted images. As time progresses, it becomes hyperintense on both T1 and T2.

Patients with significant or progressing neurologic deficits require surgical intervention, usually with laminectomy and clot evacuation. If the hematoma is small and deficits are minor or stable, patients can often be managed with observation and frequently achieve complete recovery (**Fig. 4.14**).

Fig. 4.14a–d
a,b   Spinal epidural hematoma in fused-spine hyperextension injury. High-attenuation dorsal, lentiform, intraspinous hematoma extending from C2–C3 to C6–C7. Widened C6–C7 disk space due to hyperextension injury and anterior ligamentous complex failure.
c,d   Atraumatic spinal epidural hematoma in an anticoagulated patient with syncope and acute weakness. Subtle, mixed-attenuation epidural collection dorsal to the lower cervical spinal cord on sagittal reformation. A blood-serum level within the hematoma is evident on the axial image dorsal and to the left of the cord.
e,f   Spontaneous cervical spinal epidural hematoma in patient with acute unilateral upper and lower extremity weakness (MRI). Sagittal T1-weighted image shows slightly hyperintense anterior epidural collection. Axial T2 weighted image shows hyperintense epidural collection compressing the thecal sac.

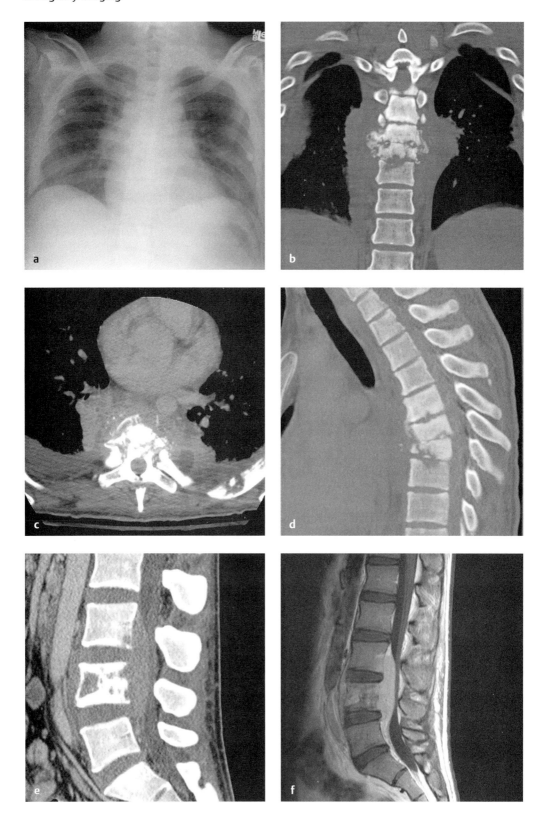

◆ Diskitis and Vertebral Osteomyelitis

Diskitis consists of infection of the intervertebral disk space and is virtually always associated with vertebral osteomyelitis. In children, diskitis/osteomyelitis is a consequence of hematogenous colonization of the intervertebral disk, which has a rich blood supply in the pediatric population. In older adults, it is often due to direct extension from a contiguous vertebral or paraspinous infection or is the result of direct inoculation during trauma or surgery. *Staphylococcus aureus* is the most commonly encountered pathogen, but *Streptococcus viridans* is more characteristic of infections in intravenous drug users and immunocompromised patients.

Neck and back pain, focal spinal tenderness, fever, and myelopathy are usual clinical findings.

The imaging hallmark of bacterial osteomyelitis/diskitis is destruction or edema involving two contiguous vertebral bodies and the interposed disk. Tuberculous osteomyelitis, in contrast to bacterial disease, tends to spare the disk and spread to adjacent vertebrae via the paraspinous soft tissues.

Early CT findings can be subtle and limited to mild loss of disk height and subtle endplate irregularity indistinguishable from degenerative change. As the disease progresses, vertebral collapse, paraspinal or epidural inflammatory changes, and abnormal paravertebral soft tissue or peripherally enhancing fluid collections can be seen. Plain radiographs are insensitive to early diskitis and may not indicate any abnormality for up to 4 weeks, but they are often the first study obtained for nonspecific back pain. CT or MRI should be pursued in patients with persistent pain or predisposing conditions.

MRI is the most sensitive modality for imaging suspected diskitis. T2-weighted images show increased signal in the disk and adjacent vertebral marrow. Findings on both T1- and T2-weighted sequences include vertebral collapse, vertebral body endplate destruction, and paraspinous soft tissue/fluid collections. Perivertebral soft tissue biopsy or fluid aspiration is necessary to identify a causative agent. Medical therapy consists of long-term antibiotic treatment. Surgery may be indicated for cord compression or débridement in the case of antibiotic therapy failure (**Fig. 4.15**).

Fig. 4.15a–f
a–d Diskitis osteomyelitis. Chest radiograph shows widened paraspinous soft tissues and apparently enlarged hila. CT with coronal and sagittal reconstructions show a large paraspinous soft tissue mass, obliteration of the T6–T7 intervertebral disk space, T5–T7 vertebral sclerosis, and end plate irregularity/erosion at T5–T6 and T7–T8. Focal midthoracic kyphosis is due to T5, T6, and T7 anterior collapse.
e,f Tuberculous osteomyelitis. Sagittal CT reformation and T1 postgadolinium MRI show L4 sclerosis and areas of vertebral destruction with a large adjacent prevertebral and epidural soft tissue mass. The L3–L4 and L4–L5 disk spaces are spared.

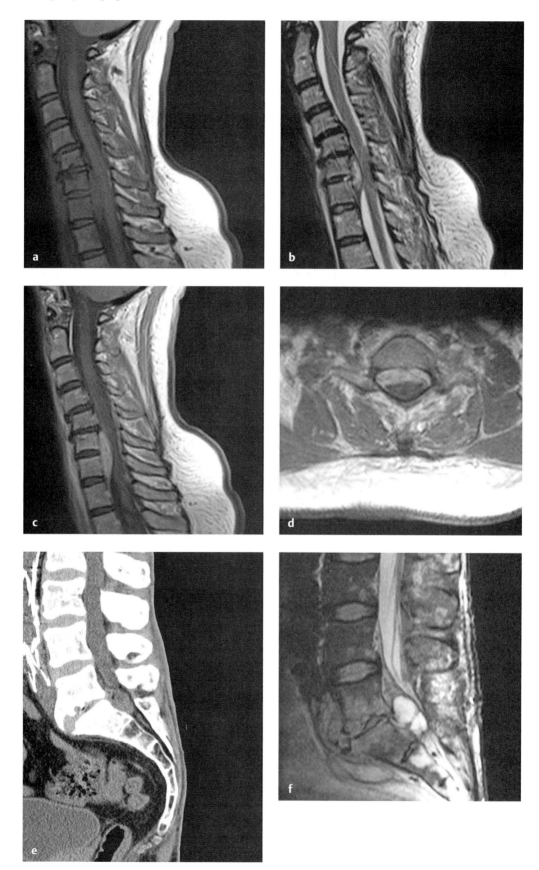

◆ Epidural Abscess

Spinal epidural abscess results from hematogenous seeding by an infection elsewhere in the body, direct inoculation during spinal surgery, contiguous spread from a retropharyngeal abscess that breaches the perivertebral fascia, or direct extension of a vertebral diskitis/osteomyelitis. It is usually caused by *Staphylococcus aureus,* and patients with diabetes mellitus, intravenous drug use, trauma, immunodeficiency, renal failure, spinal instrumentation, or malignancy are at increased risk. The clinical presentation is often subacute, with nonspecific back pain and later sensory symptoms, motor weakness, and bladder dysfunction. Delay in diagnosis or treatment may lead to paralysis or death.

Epidural abscesses cause neurologic deficits by compressing the spinal cord, cauda equina, or nerve roots or by vascular inflammation and occlusion. The most sensitive diagnostic test is MRI with gadolinium, although if MRI is unavailable in the emergency setting, spinal CT with contrast will usually identify an epidural mass and can detect most findings of osteomyelitis/diskitis. Epidural abscesses are intermediate to low in signal intensity on T1-weighted sequences and high in signal on T2 sequences, and they often show peripheral enhancement when mature. An epidural phlegmon appears as diffusely enhancing, thickened epidural soft tissue. Diffusion-weighted imaging will show the expected high signal (restricted diffusion) within the abscess. CT or conventional myelography may also be used to define an intraspinal extramedullary mass in patients who cannot undergo MRI. Management is by surgical drainage and concomitant antibiotic therapy in most patients (**Fig. 4.16**).

Fig. 4.16a–f
a–d Epidural abscess. Intermediate signal intensity, lentiform, anterior epidural mass dorsal to the C6 and C7 vertebral bodies that flattens the ventral spinal cord. (**a**) It is low in signal intensity on T1-weighted MRI, (**b**) high in signal intensity on T2-weighted image, and (**c,d**) enhances avidly on postgadolinium images.
e,f Epidural abscess due to adjacent L5/S1 *Mycobacterium avium intracellulare* osteomyelitis. Sagittal CT reformation shows L5/S1 disk space narrowing with sclerotic bone changes and an apparent soft tissue mass within the spinal canal posterior to S1. T1-weighted image with gadolinium shows enhancing prevertebral and epidural collections with areas of central low signal intensity.

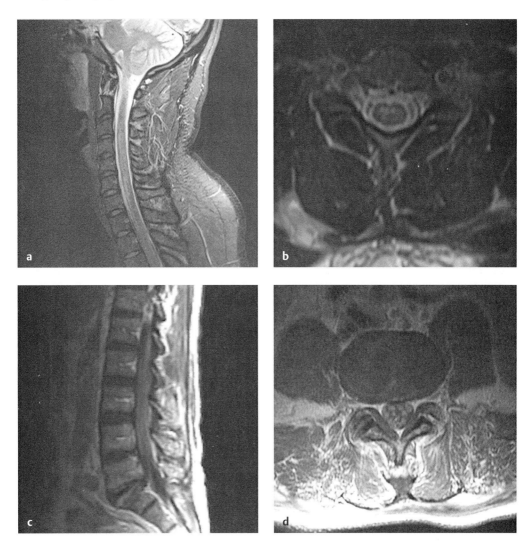

◆ Myelitis and Radiculitis

Myelitis is a primary inflammatory disease of the spinal cord that may be idiopathic, the consequence of viral or other infection, or a manifestation of multiple sclerosis, vasculitis, ischemia, radiation, or autoimmune disease. It usually extends over several segments, functionally transecting the cord. Weakness, sensory disturbance, and autonomic dysfunction develop rapidly, often reaching maximum severity within 10 days of symptom onset. Most patients have numbness and paresthesia in the legs and trunk and bandlike dysesthesia at the level of the lesion. Bladder dysfunction is common.

In almost all cases, T2 signal is increased on spinal MR imaging. Lesions usually are located in the central cord, involve greater than 60% of its cross-sectional area, and may show swelling or expansion of the cord.

Prognosis varies depending on etiology. Most patients will have good outcomes, but some experience persistent neurologic deficits. Treatment often includes steroids or other immunomodulatory therapies.

Radiculitis (spinal nerve root inflammation) presents with pain, weakness, or sensory loss in a nerve root distribution. Symptoms respect the sensory and motor territories of the root, an aspect that distinguishes radiculitis from cerebral infarct, myelitis, or peripheral neuropathy. Other symptoms include changes in reflexes and hyperesthesia, which can be mild to severe. Most single-level radiculopathies involve lumbosacral roots. Cervical roots are the second most commonly involved group, with thoracic radiculitis representing a minority of cases.

Radiculitis can be categorized as single-level disease or polyradiculitis and further divided into structural lesions such as disk herniation, spinal stenosis, tumors and leptomeningeal metastases, and nonstructural diseases including diabetes mellitus, HIV/AIDS, Lyme disease, and sarcoidosis.

MR is the most sensitive and specific modality for evaluation of radiculitis and will detect both structural lesions and abnormal radicular signal or enhancement due to inflammation. CT is useful in evaluating herniated disks, degenerative spinal changes, and canal and neuroforaminal stenosis at suspect levels (**Fig. 4.17**).

Fig. 4.17a–d
a,b Transverse myelitis in multiple sclerosis. Abnormally increased T2 signal within the anterior spinal cord at the level of T5–T6.
c,d HIV radiculitis. Diffuse thickening and enhancement of cauda equina roots on postgadolinium T1-weighted MRI.

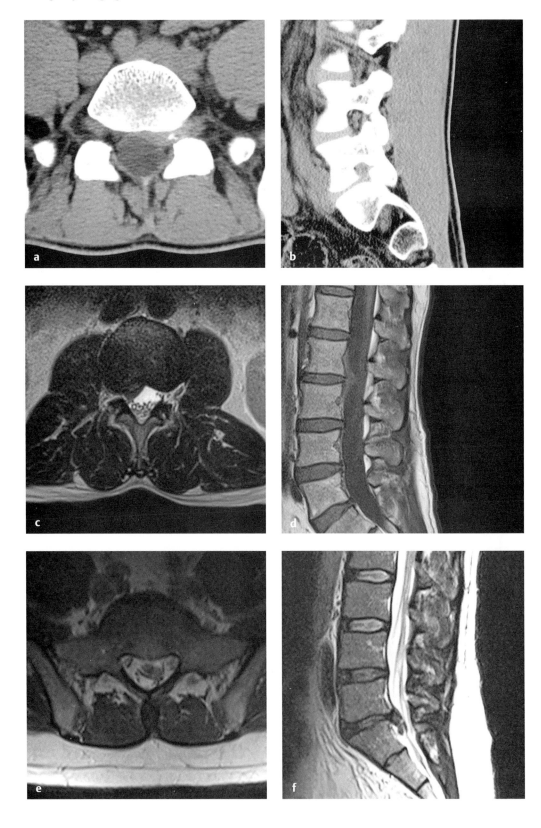

◆ Disk Herniation

Disk herniation is a general term that refers to displacement of the intervertebral disk material through a tear or weakening in the disk annulus. It may involve portions of the nucleus pulposus, vertebral endplate cartilage, and annulus fibrosis. If a herniation occurs through a focal tear or fissure in an otherwise intact annular shell, it is called a disk protrusion. Involvement of greater than half the circumference of an intervertebral disk is called a disk bulge. If a fragment is completely separated from the parent disk, it is described as an extrusion or sequestered fragment. Protrusions or extruded disks can be central, paracentral, subarticular (lateral recess), foraminal, or extraforaminal.

Radicular symptoms depend on the level and location of the herniated disk. For example, a paracentral protrusion at L4–L5 will compress the descending L5 nerve root, whereas a lateral protrusion will affect the already exited L4 nerve root. Patients may be entirely asymptomatic or present with an isolated dull ache or with pain and/or radiculopathy consisting of sensory disturbance and motor weakness. Concomitant paraspinal muscle spasm is often present.

MR imaging is optimal for delineating disk herniations, most of which occur at the L4–L5 or L5–S1 disk levels. Disk extrusions often appear hyperintense relative to the parent disk on T2 images. T1-weighted images accentuate the hypointense disk against the bright intraforaminal fat. Contrast is not generally necessary for evaluation unless there has been prior surgery, in which case it can be helpful in differentiating recurrent disk herniation from postoperative granulation tissue.

Prognosis is not dependent on the size or type of disk herniation, and many lesions will spontaneously regress. Spinal intervention should be based on clinical findings rather than imaging appearance (**Fig. 4.18**).

Fig. 4.18a–f
a,b L5–S1 Left lateral recess/foraminal disk protrusion. A broad protrusion involves the left paracentral spinal canal, lateral recess, and neuroforamen. A small dystrophic calcification is visible within the protruded disk material. On sagittal reformation, the L5–S1 neuroforaminal fat is completely obliterated with compression of the exiting L5 root. Contrast this appearance with that of the normal left L4–L5 and S1–S2 foramina, in which the exiting roots are surrounded by fat.
c,d Right lateral recess disk protrusion. T2-weighted MRI shows lateral recess compromise at the level of the cauda equina. The exiting L2 and descending L3 nerve roots would be potentially compromised. Low signal intensity within the L2–L3, L4–L5, and L5–S1 intervertebral disks is normally seen with aging and does not correlate with pain or neurological deficit.
e,f L5–S1 extruded (sequestered) disk. T2-weighted MRI shows a large fragment inferior to the L5–S1 disk level and anterior to the thecal sac dorsal to S1.

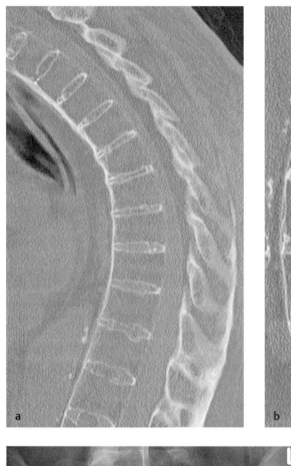

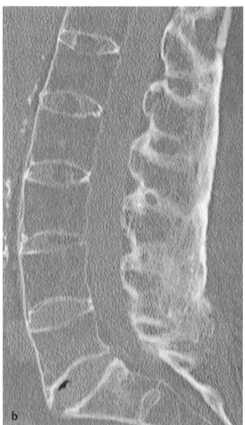

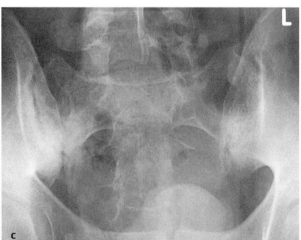

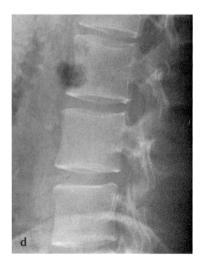

◆ Ankylosing Spondylitis

Ankylosing spondylitis (AS) is an inflammatory arthropathy that primarily involves the sacroiliac (SI) joints and the axial skeleton. The disease is more common in men and is associated with histocompatibility antigen B27. Patients describe the insidious onset of chronic low back pain that tends to be most pronounced on awakening and after periods of inactivity. Symptoms generally improve with movement and exercise. Because AS is a systemic inflammatory disease, fatigue, fever, and weight loss are common. The sacroiliac joints and lumbosacral spine are usually the first sites of disease, followed by progressive continuous craniad spinal involvement with ossification of the annulus fibrosis and ultimate osseous spinal fusion. Uveitis, aortitis, and (in men) prostatitis are nonarticular manifestations.

In early disease, the SI joints may appear widened due to subchondral erosions, but they later become sclerotic, become narrow, and eventually fuse. Erosions and sclerotic changes are typically seen in the most inferior portion of the iliac side of the SI joint. Fused SI joints may appear as a thin sclerotic line or may be completely obliterated on plain radiographs and CT. Early, and often very subtle, radiographic and CT findings of spinal disease include squaring of the vertebrae and sclerosis at the superior and inferior vertebral margins ("shiny corners"). Later syndesmophytic fusion produces a "bamboo spine" appearance that is virtually diagnostic. Peripheral joint involvement is also seen with uniform joint space narrowing, cystic or erosive changes, and subchondral sclerosis. The shoulder and hip joints are most frequently involved.

In patients with a compelling history, but without diagnostic radiographic findings, CT may be pursued as it is more sensitive for the detection of joint erosions and subchondral sclerosis. It is also indicated in the setting of trauma. Patients with any long-segment spinal fusion are at increased risk of spinal injury, particularly hyperextension fractures. Because fused-spine patients are at risk for multiple synchronous fractures with trauma, imaging of the entire spine is indicated for patients with ankylosing spondylitis in this setting (**Fig. 4.19**).

Fig. 4.19a–d
a,b Longstanding ankylosing spondylitis. Anterior fused syndesmophytes (bamboo spine), fused spinous processes, and thoracic kyphosis.
c,d Early ankylosing spondylitis. Right sacroiliac sclerosis with SI joint narrowing. The left SI joint appears fused. Lumbar vertebrae are squared with "shiny corners," indicating inflammation.

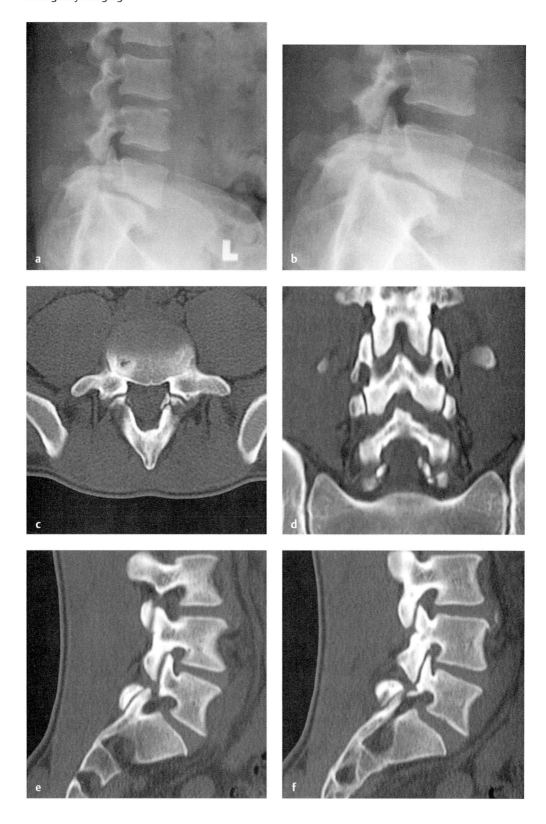

◆ Spondylolysis and Spondylolisthesis

Spondylolysis describes an osseous defect of the pars interarticularis of a lower lumbar vertebra, usually L4 or L5. It is frequently encountered in adolescents with back pain or incidentally discovered on lumbar radiographs or CT. Repetitive microtrauma in conjunction with congenital predisposition leads to bilateral stress fractures followed by bone separation and eventual spondylolisthesis: anterior translation of the involved vertebra with respect to the next lower one. Spondylolysis and spondylolisthesis may be asymptomatic but can also present with back pain, instability, and radiculopathy.

Lateral radiographs are usually adequate for identification of pars fractures. On oblique lumbar spine radiographs, the vertebrae have a "Scottie dog" appearance. On these studies, spondylolysis appears as a radiolucent line resembling a collar around the dog's neck. CT is more commonly obtained to confirm a suspicion of spondylolysis and directly shows the characteristic defect at the junction of the vertebral pedicle and the superior articulating facet of the intervertebral joint immediately below it.

The severity of spondylolisthesis, which is frequently associated with bilateral spondylolysis, is described in **Table 4.1** (**Fig. 4.20**).

Table 4.1   Severity of spondylolisthesis

Grade I	< 25%
Grade II	25–50%
Grade III	50–75%
Grade IV	75–100%
Spondyloptosis	> 100%

Fig. 4.20a–d
a,b   Spondylolysis with mild spondylolisthesis. Bilateral L5 pars interarticularis fractures with grade I anterolisthesis of L5 with respect to L4. L4–L5 endplate degenerative changes.
c–f   Spondylolysis. Bilateral L5 pars interarticularis defects without spondylolisthesis or L5–S1 neuroforaminal compromise.

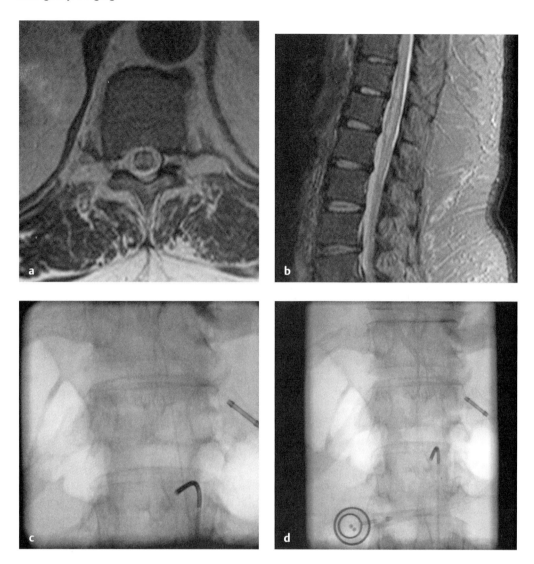

◆ Spinal Cord Infarct

Spinal cord infarction is an uncommon but potentially devastating disorder that results from acute spinal vascular compromise. Like cerebral infarction, spinal cord infarction may result from hypoxia and hypotension, cardiogenic thromboembolus, vasculitis, atherosclerosis, arteriovenous malformation, polycythemia, and hypercoagulability. Trauma, aortic pathology, hypertrophic degenerative diseases in the spine, and invasive procedures can also compromise spinal circulation in more specific territories.

Arterial infarcts, which are more common, tend to present with acute, severe back pain. Associated neurologic deficits vary depending on the vascular territory and spinal level involved but are usually characterized by bilateral extremity weakness, paresthesias, and inability to void. Most infarcts are due to anterior spinal artery occlusion and involve the central cord, commonly at lower thoracic levels. Infarcts of the dorsal cord, which is supplied by paired posterior spinal arterial territories, are rare.

Though insensitive to direct detection of spinal ischemia, CT is valuable for excluding other etiologies of acute myelopathy, such as spinal hematoma or vertebral fracture in acute trauma. Spinal MRI may be normal on initial examination, even in the setting of profound neurologic defects, but diffusion-weighted imaging can sometimes show early infarcts and should be included if possible. MRI can also identify other pathologies, including compressive or demyelinating lesions, vascular malformations, and infective myelitis.

Spinal arteriography can identify an occluded vessel, and selective thrombolysis can be effective in reversing or limiting neurologic deficit if undertaken early (**Fig. 4.21**).

Fig. 4.21a–d
a–d   Spinal cord infarct due to anterior spinal artery occlusion. (**a,b**) T2-weighted MRI shows abnormally increased signal throughout the central spinal cord at the level of the conus medullaris. (**c**) Spinal arteriogram shows filling of the hairpin loop of the artery of Adamkiewicz and embolic occlusion of the anterior spinal artery at the superior endplate of T12. (**d**) Postthrombolysis arteriogram shows improved distal flow, visible to the superior endplate of L1.

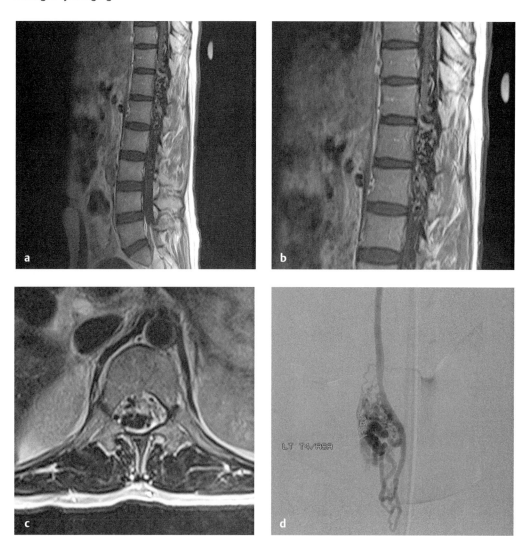

◆ Spinal Dural Arteriovenous Fistula

Spinal dural arteriovenous fistula (AVF) is the most common of the spinal cord vascular malformations, formed when a radiculomeningeal artery drains directly into a neighboring radicular vein, usually near the spinal nerve root. Increased arterial blood flow through the fistula recruits additional veins for drainage, which results in increased venous pressure, congestion, cord edema, and ischemia. The clinical syndrome of insidious and progressive lower cord myelopathy is called Foix-Alajouanine.

MRI is sensitive for detection of most larger dural AVFs and will show vascular flow voids in or enhancing vessels on the surface of the spinal cord. Diffuse multi-level hyperintensity on T2-weighed images indicates cord edema but does not directly correlate with the location of the fistula. Contrast-enhanced MRA, CT angiography, or CT myelography can all noninvasively diagnose and localize a fistula. Spinal catheter angiography permits optimal analysis of the fistula in anticipation of endovascular occlusion or surgical ligation (**Fig. 4.22**).

Fig. 4.22a–d
a–d   Spinal dural arteriovenous fistula. A tangle of vascular flow voids and enhancing vessels surrounds the conus medullaris and distal spinal cord. Axial T2-weighted images shows the AVF anterior to the distal cord. (**d**) Spinal angiogram with filling of the anterior spinal artery via an injection at T4. The anterior spinal artery is enlarged and fills a serpiginous cluster of vessels from above. Embolic coils have already been placed in a distal artery supplying the malformation.

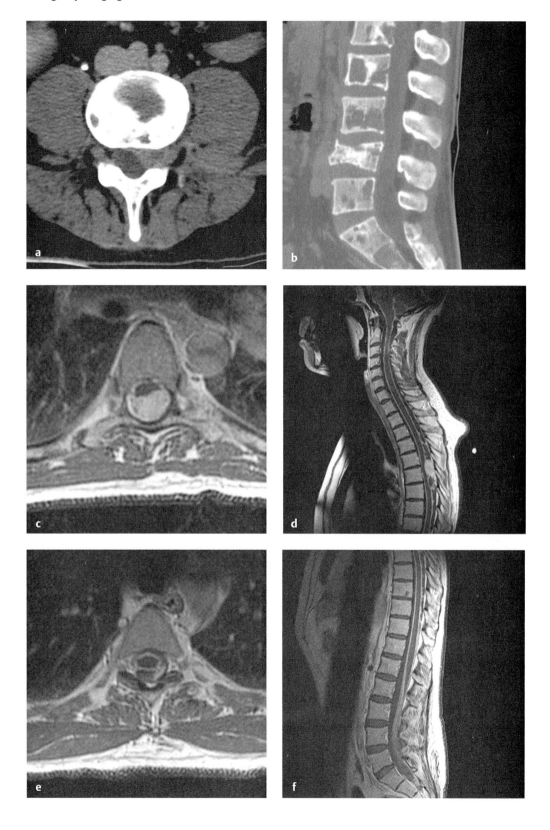

◆ Spinal Metastatic Disease

Tumor metastatic to the spine may be extradural, intradural-extramedullary, intramedullary, or a combination of these locations. Extradural metastases are most common, arise from the vertebrae and adjacent tissues, and are usually seen with primary tumors of the breast, prostate, uterus, and lung. Myeloma and lymphoma can also involve the vertebrae and mimic metastatic disease. Most metastases are found in the thoracic spine, but they can occur at any level. If the involved vertebra is fractured due to tumor replacement or insufficiency, the spinal cord can be compressed by a retropulsed bone fragment. Tumors within the spinal canal can also compress the cord.

Patients typically present with back pain, sensory, motor, or bowel/bladder dysfunction. In the patient with a known malignancy, the goal of emergent imaging is to identify any acute fractures, any destructive spinal lesion that is at risk for fracture, and any soft tissue compression of the spinal cord that might require urgent radiation therapy or surgical decompression.

While plain radiographs can detect pathologic fractures, spinal deformities, and grossly lytic or sclerotic lesions, they are insensitive to small lytic lesions and may not reveal any changes until up to half of a vertebral body is affected. Consequently CT and MRI are preferred for assessing extent of disease, the integrity of the vertebral column, and the paraspinal soft tissues. Osteolytic metastases appear as soft tissue attenuation lesions with irregular margins and cortical bone destruction. Osteoblastic metastases are sclerotic and irregular.

Intradural and intramedullary metastases are rare and usually due to intrathecal seeding of a primary CNS neoplasm such as medulloblastoma, ependymoma, or gliomas (drop metastases). T1 postcontrast MRI shows meningeal thickening and enhancement as well as surface nodules of the spinal cord and/or nerve roots (**Fig. 4.23**).

Fig. 4.23a–f
a–b Metastatic renal cell carcinoma. Multiple lytic and sclerotic lesions throughout the lumbar spine and sacrum. A left paracentral intraspinal soft tissue mass arises from the L4 vertebra, fills the left lateral recess and neuroforamen, and displaces the thecal sac to the right.
c–f Multiple intrathecal "drop" metastases from a malignant vestibular schwannoma. Postgadolinium T1-weighted MRI of the thoracic and lumbar spine shows a focal extramedullary mass that compresses the lower thoracic cord. Neoplastic involvement is indicated by diffuse thickening and enhancement of the entire thecal sac and lumbar nerve roots.

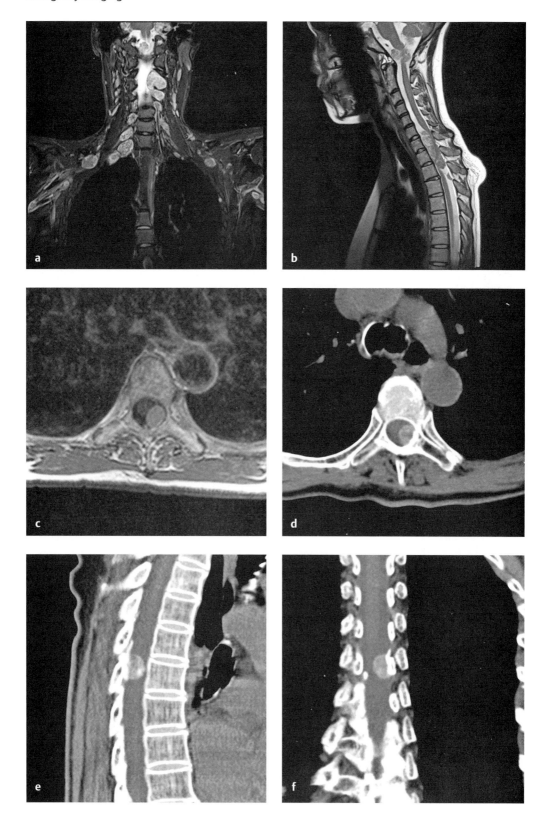

◆ Spinal Schwannoma and Meningioma

Schwannomas are slow-growing, usually benign, tumors that arise from peripheral nerves and spinal nerve roots. They are the most common intradural-extramedullary tumor of the spine. Most are solitary and sporadic, but multiple tumors can be seen in patients with neurofibromatosis type 2 and in familial schwannomatosis. Patients present with back or neck pain and motor or sensory symptoms localized to the involved spinal level.

Although these tumors are detectable on CT, MRI with gadolinium is far more sensitive and specific. Schwannomas are generally well circumscribed, are contiguous with the involved nerve roots, and enhance avidly with contrast. Rather than expand the spinal cord as ependymomas and astrocytomas do, schwannomas displace the cord, conus, or filum away from an eccentric, extramedullary mass. Schwannomas are more frequently associated with hemorrhage, intrinsic vascular changes, and intratumoral cyst formation than neurofibromas are, but they may be indistinguishable on CT or MRI.

Meningiomas are the second most common intradural-extramedullary spinal tumor. They arise from meningoepithelial cells present in the spinal cord leptomeninges. Although most are histologically benign, they can cause spinal cord compression. Like schwannomas, multiple meningiomas can be seen in patients with neurofibromatosis type 2. The thoracic spine is most frequent location, followed by the cervical and lumbar spine. Patients with cord compression typically present with motor deficits. Less common manifestations include sensory deficit, pain, and incontinence.

MRI and CT show a well-defined, extramedullary mass that displaces the cord or nerve roots. Meningiomas often have a broad dural attachment or enhancing dural tail, and may have a "marble under the rug" appearance. They are usually isointense to the spinal cord on T1- and T2-weighted images and enhance avidly and homogeneously. Because they grow slowly, meningiomas tend to remodel bone rather than erode it, and they commonly calcify.

Surgical resection is usually recommended for larger, symptomatic tumors. In contrast to intracranial meningiomas, spinal tumors are unlikely to recur after removal (**Fig. 4.24**).

Fig. 4.24a–f
a,b Multiple cervical nerve root schwannomas in a patient with neurofibromatosis type 2. T2-weighted MRI shows multiple heterogeneous, well-defined, rounded masses that arise from the exiting cervical nerve roots and brachial plexus cords. Intraspinal and foramen magnum masses compress and displace the cervical cord dorsally.
c–f Thoracic spinal meningioma. A well-defined, calcified, intradural, extramedullary mass dorsal to T6 displaces the spinal cord anteriorly and to the right. The mass enhances homogeneously on postgadolinium T1-weighted MRI.

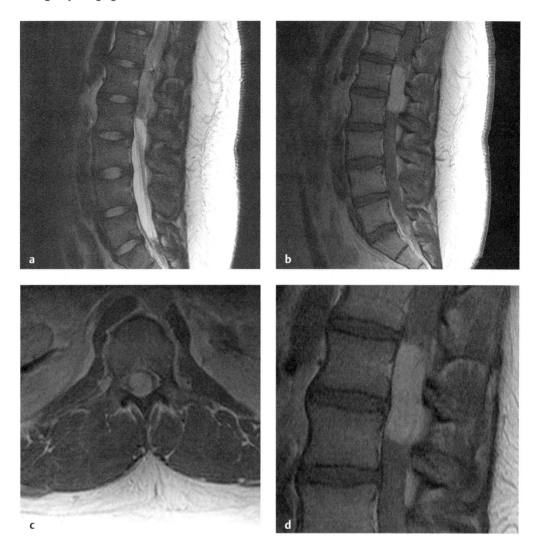

◆ Ependymoma

Ependymomas, the most common of the intramedullary spinal tumors, arise from the ependymal cells of the central cord and filum terminale. They can therefore occur anywhere within the bony spinal canal. Back pain with weakness and sensory changes are common. Ependymomas may gradually compress the cord as they grow, or may present acutely after intratumoral hemorrhage. They can also cause neurologic deficit as a result of superficial siderosis from repeated microhemorrhage. As with meningiomas and schwannomas, the incidence of spinal ependymomas is increased in patients with neurofibromatosis type 2.

They are slow-growing tumors, and at the time of diagnosis, CT or plain radiographs often show expansion and remodeling of the adjacent vertebrae. MRI is necessary for comprehensive evaluation of the tumor and associated findings such as adjacent cord edema, hemorrhage, spinal cord cysts, or syringohydromyelia. On T1-weighted images, ependymomas are isointense to the normal cord; they are hyperintense on T2 sequences and enhance intensely with gadolinium. All imaging modalities show symmetric cord expansion with variable microhemorrhage (hemosiderin staining).

Ependymomas have sharply defined borders. Associated cysts, while not uncommon in ependymoma, are more characteristic of spinal cord astrocytomas. The goal of surgery is complete excision, and this may be successfully achieved in over half of cases. In those patients, prognosis is good and recurrence is rare (**Fig. 4.25**).

Fig. 4.25a–d
a–d Ependymoma. (**a**) A distal intraspinal mass, slightly hyperintense to the normal cord, with focus of low intensity hemosiderin, arises from the proximal filum terminale and fills the spinal canal at L1–L2. (**b–d**) The mass enhances homogeneously on postgadolinium T1-weighted images and has well-defined margins.

5
Chest

◆ Approach and Analysis

Plain chest radiographs (chest X-rays, CXR) make up the bulk of imaging work in the emergency department. They are requested for virtually any suspected thoracic disease, to exclude (or detect) active tuberculosis in patients who will be admitted to hospital psychiatry units or to public shelters, and for screening in patients who will have urgent surgery. CT is reserved for patients with acute chest pain, hypoxia, and dyspnea in whom the chest radiograph does not provide a satisfactory diagnosis. The most common indications for CT are for investigation of possible pulmonary embolism, aortic dissection, and traumatic injury.

Anatomic Checklist

Radiographs

- Tubes and lines
- Trachea
- Heart
- Mediastinum and hila
- Central pulmonary vessels
- Lung parenchyma (including peripheral 1 cm)
- Bones
- Soft tissues

Computed Tomography

- Lower cervical soft tissues
- Trachea and airways
- Mediastinum and hila
- Aorta

Pulmonary Arteries and Veins

- Carotid, vertebral, and subclavian arteries
- Jugular, brachiocephalic veins, and superior vena cava

Heart, Coronary Arteries, and Pericardium

- Lungs
- Chest wall and diaphragm
- Upper abdomen

◆ Imaging and Anatomy

Radiography

Posteroanterior (PA) radiographs are obtained in full inspiration with the patient's chest against the detector and the arms positioned to rotate the scapulae away from the lungs. Anteroposterior (AP) portable radiographs, on the other hand, are obtained with the detector cassette behind the patient, the X-ray source about 6 ft (2 m) in front, the arms at the patient's sides, and the scapulae superimposed on the upper lungs. On AP radiographs the normal divergence of the X-ray beam and the increased distance between anterior thoracic structures and the detector leads to artifactual magnification of the cardiomediastinal silhouette and indistinct pulmonary vessels, particularly in larger patients. By contrast, because the X-ray source is behind the patient for PA radiographs, artifactual magnification of the heart is of less concern than on AP radiographs. Moreover, because the cassette for AP radiographs is against the patient's back, sometimes the skin can fold on itself against the cassette and produce a line similar to that seen with pneumothorax; this does not occur with PA radiographs. For these reasons, unless the patient cannot tolerate a PA radiograph, it is always preferred to a portable AP study.

Lateral radiographs are usually obtained with the right chest against the detector and the arms above or in front of the patient. The right hemidiaphragm appears continuous from front to back. The left hemidiaphragm blends into the cardiac shadow. Except for the rare patient with situs inversus, the gastric air bubble should be located immediately below the left hemidiaphragm.

Computed Tomography

Trauma

- Indications: Chest trauma (usually performed in conjunction with abdominal CT)
- Arterial phase: bolus track to aorta 150 HU
- Oral contrast: None
- IV contrast: 1.5 mL/kg at 4 mL/sec, followed by 20 mL saline at 4 mL/sec
- Images: 5-mm axial with 0.625-mm reconstruction and 1.25-mm coronal and sagittal reformations
- Approximate radiation dose: 1,200 mGy

"Routine"

- Indications: Evaluation of plain radiographic abnormalities, pulmonary nodules and masses, empyema
- IV contrast (optional): 1.5 mL/kg at 4 mL/sec, 40-second delay
- Images: 5-mm axial with 0.625-mm reconstruction and 1.25-mm coronal and sagittal reformations
- Approximate radiation dose: 320 mGy

Pulmonary Embolism

- Indications: Acute chest pain in setting of immobilization, hypercoagulable state, underlying malignancy, or other risk factors for pulmonary embolus

- Pulmonary arterial phase: bolus track to main pulmonary artery 150 HU
- IV contrast: 1.5 mL/kg at 4 mL/sec, followed by 20 mL saline at 4 mL/sec
- Images: 5-mm axial with 0.625-mm reconstruction and 1.25-mm coronal and sagittal reformations
- Approximate radiation dose: 650 mGy

Aortic Dissection

- Indications: Acute chest pain in setting of hypertension, connective tissue disorder, or other risk factors for arterial dissection or aortic rupture
- Arterial phase: bolus track to aorta 150 HU
- IV contrast: 1.5 mL/kg at 4 mL/sec, followed by 50 mL saline at 4 mL/sec
- Images: 5-mm axial with 0.625-mm reconstruction and 1.25-mm coronal and sagittal reformations
- Approximate radiation dose: 1,000 mGy

Anatomy

Knowledge of pulmonary segmental anatomy on radiographs and CT is necessary for accurate localization and description of pulmonary lesions (**Fig. 5.1**).

◆ Clinical Presentations and Differential Diagnosis

Clinical Presentations and Appropriate Initial Studies

Trauma

- CXR
- CT with contrast (arterial phase)
- Echocardiography to evaluate pericardial effusion and cardiac function
    - Aortic or other vascular injury
    - Hemothorax
    - Cardiac rupture
    - Hemopericardium
    - Pneumothorax
    - Pneumomediastinum
    - Pulmonary contusion or laceration

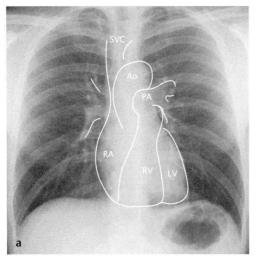

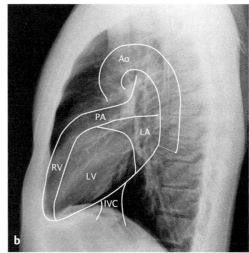

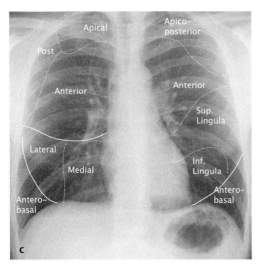

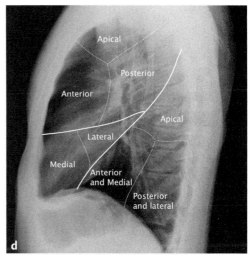

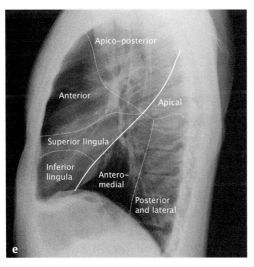

Fig. 5.1a–i

a,b Cardiomediastinal anatomy: radiograph. On the frontal view, the right heart border corresponds to the right atrium and superior vena cava/right atrial junction. The left heart border corresponds to the left ventricle. On the lateral view, the anterior border of the heart is made up of the right ventricle and pulmonary outflow tract, with the inferior and posterior margins formed by the left ventricle, inferior vena cava (IVC), and left atrium. The retrosternal space in adults should be free of soft tissue.

c–e Pulmonary segmental anatomy: radiograph. The lobar anatomy of the right and left lungs differs, with the right lung containing a middle lobe and the left upper lobe containing a roughly analogous lingular segment. On the lateral radiograph, the right (**d**) and left (**e**) lungs are superimposed upon each other. Localizing an intrapulmonary mass or lesion requires attention to both frontal and lateral views. (*Continued on page 210*)

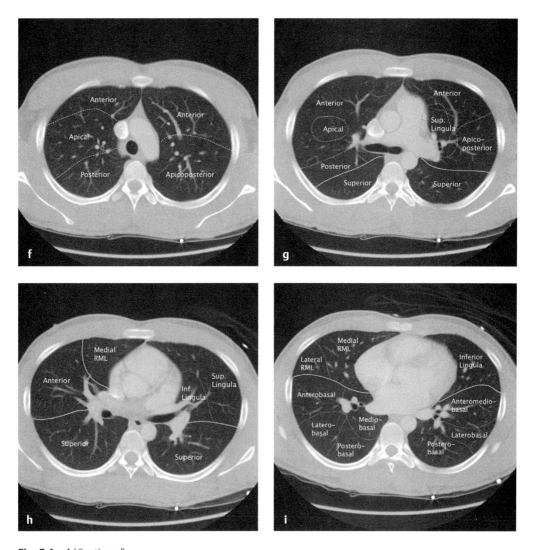

Fig. 5.1a–i (*Continued*)
f–i Pulmonary segmental anatomy: CT. Solid lines denote lobar divisions. Dotted lines indicate segmental borders. (**f**) Aortic arch; (**g**) pulmonary artery; (**h**) aortic root/left mainstem bronchus; (**i**) cardiac chambers.

– Aspiration
– Rib fractures (flail chest)
– Diaphragm injury
– Sternal fracture
– Clavicle dislocation
– Spine fracture or dislocation

Dyspnea

• CXR
• CT without contrast may be useful for further evaluating radiographic findings

• CT angiogram for exclusion of pulmonary embolism
    – Pneumothorax
    – Pleural effusion
    – Pneumonia
    – Aspiration
    – Reactive airways disease
    – Inhalational disease
    – Cardiogenic pulmonary edema
    – Noncardiogenic pulmonary edema
    – Acute respiratory distress syndrome
    – Pulmonary embolism

- Radiation pneumonitis (1–4 months posttreatment)
- Drug reaction

Chest Pain

- CXR
- Echocardiography to evaluate pericardial effusion and cardiac function
- CT angiogram for exclusion of pulmonary embolism
- CT angiogram for exclusion of aortic dissection or rupture
- Coronary CTA may be useful for assessing myocardial infarction risk in selected patients
  - Pneumonia
  - Pulmonary embolism/infarct
  - Myocardial ischemia
  - Aortic dissection or rupture
  - Pneumothorax
  - Pneumomediastinum
  - Neoplasm

Cough/Fever

- CXR
- CT without contrast may be useful for further evaluating radiographic findings
  - Pneumonia
  - Empyema
  - Septic pulmonary emboli

Differential Diagnosis

Pneumomediastinum

- Penetrating trauma
- Barotrauma (vomiting, Valsalva, asthma)
- Aspirated foreign body
- Esophageal tear
- Subdiaphragmatic free air

Anterior Mediastinal Mass

- Lymphoma
- Thymoma
- Substernal goiter
- Germ cell tumor

Middle Mediastinal Mass

- Lymphadenopathy
- Bronchogenic cyst
- Aortic or pulmonary artery aneurysm

Posterior Mediastinal Mass

- Neurogenic tumor
- Lymphoma
- Neurenteric cyst

Hilar Adenopathy

- Lymphoma
- Sarcoidosis
- Infection
- Metastatic disease

Pulmonary Edema

- Cardiogenic
- Fluid overload
- Head injury
- Acute respiratory distress syndrome (ARDS)
- Inhalational injury
- Transfusion reaction
- Drug-induced
- High altitude

Septal Lines/Interstitial Edema

- Left ventricular (LV) failure
- Mitral stenosis
- Pulmonary veno-occlusive disease
- Interstitial lung disease
- Lymphangitic carcinomatosis

Air Space Opacification

- Pulmonary edema
- Pneumonia
- Hemorrhage
- Adenocarcinoma (bronchioloalveolar cell)
- Sarcoidosis

Lobar Pneumonia

- *Streptococcus pneumoniae*
- *Klebsiella pneumoniae*
- *Staphylococcus aureus*
- Tuberculosis (primary)

Parenchymal Disease in HIV

- *Pneumocystis* pneumonia
- Tuberculosis
- Fungal infection
- Kaposi sarcoma

Interstitial Disease—Upper Lobe

- Tuberculosis
- Sarcoidosis
- Cystic fibrosis

Interstitial Disease—Lower Lobe

- Idiopathic pulmonary fibrosis
- Scleroderma
- Chronic aspiration
- Asbestos-related disease

Bronchiectasis

- Remote infection
- Cystic fibrosis
- Immunodeficiency
- Allergic bronchopulmonary aspergillosis

Solitary Pulmonary Nodule

- Granuloma (tuberculosis, histoplasmosis, coccidioidomycosis, cryptococcosis)
- Bronchogenic carcinoma
- Metastasis
- Adenocarcinoma
- Hamartoma
- Arteriovenous malformation

Multiple Pulmonary Nodules

- Metastases
- Septic emboli
- Granulomatous disease
- Rheumatoid arthritis
- Sarcoidosis

Miliary Nodules

- Tuberculosis
- Metastases
- Fungal disease
- Remote varicella pneumonia

Cavitary Nodules/Masses

- Tuberculosis
- Primary lung carcinoma
- Metastases (especially squamous cell carcinoma)
- Infected bulla
- Wegener granulomatosis
- Rheumatoid arthritis
- Septic emboli

Ground Glass Opacification (CT)

- Cardiogenic pulmonary edema
- Acute respiratory distress syndrome (ARDS)
- Atypical pneumonia
- Pulmonary hemorrhage

Perilymphatic Nodules (CT)

- Sarcoidosis
- Lymphangitic carcinomatosis
- Pneumoconiosis

Centrilobular Nodules (CT)

- Infectious bronchiolitis (*Mycobacterium avium intracellulare*, tuberculosis)
- Hypersensitivity pneumonitis
- Endobronchial tumor
- Respiratory bronchiolitis interstitial lung disease (RB-ILD)
- Pneumoconiosis

Pleural Effusion

- Trauma (hemothorax)
- Viral pleuritis (usually with otherwise normal chest radiograph)
- Congestive heart failure
- Hepatic failure
- Parapneumonic effusion
- Neoplastic effusion
- Pulmonary infarct
- Subphrenic abscess

Pleural Based Mass

- Metastasis
- Empyema
- Mesothelioma
- Fibrous tumor of pleura

Pneumothorax

- Spontaneous
- Iatrogenic
- Trauma
- Secondary to lung disease
- Secondary to pneumomediastinum or pneumoperitoneum

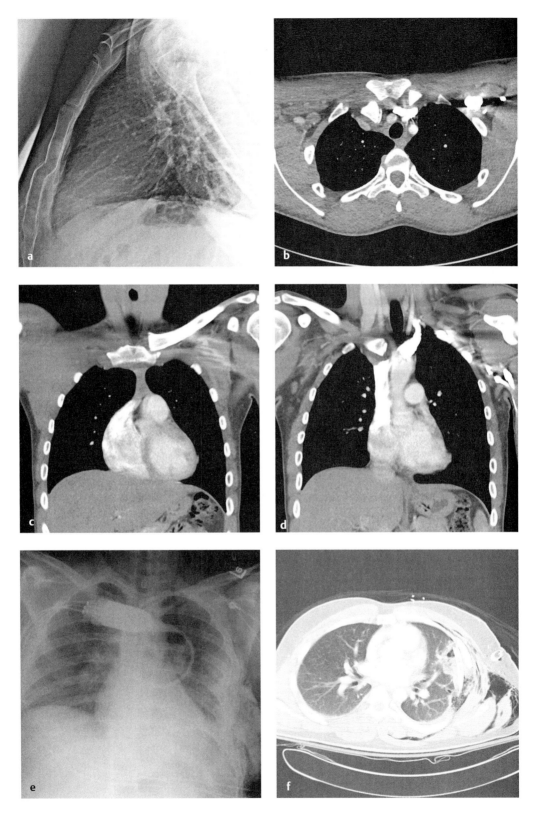

◆ Chest Wall Injuries

Sternal fractures are a marker of high-energy impact and are seen in approximately 8% of patients with blunt thoracic trauma. Retrosternal hematoma, myocardial contusion, coronary artery tear, aortic laceration, and tracheobronchial tear are potential associated injuries.

Sternal fractures are not visible on supine portable AP chest radiographs, but they can be detected with a true lateral view. In practice, they are usually diagnosed on CT and are most commonly located 2 cm below the sternomanubrial joint. Retrosternal hematoma may be the consequence of great vessel injury or hemorrhage from small vessels; identification of normal fat between a substernal hematoma and the aorta indicates that the hematoma is not due to aortic rupture.

Sternoclavicular dislocation consists of anterior or posterior displacement of the medial clavicle relative to the sternal manubrium. Posterior dislocation, in which the clavicular head is located dorsal to the manubrium, typically results from a blow to the dorsal shoulder or to the anteromedial clavicle and can be associated with serious morbidity; as the medial clavicular head is driven into the soft tissues of the thoracic inlet, it can impact or injure the trachea, esophagus, recurrent laryngeal nerve, or great vessels. Anterior disloca-

tion, resulting from a frontal blow to the ipsilateral shoulder, is more common and carries less risk of associated injury.

The sternoclavicular joint is difficult to assess on plain radiographs. CT permits accurate characterization of the dislocation and any hematoma or vascular impingement. Sternal dislocations are usually treated by closed reduction in the absence of associated mediastinal injuries.

The term *flail chest* refers to thoracic injury with five or more adjacent simple rib fractures or more than three segmental rib fractures; it can lead to impaired ventilation and respiratory failure in the trauma patient. The normal thorax increases in volume on inspiration. In flail chest, the affected side, lacking structural support, retracts inward under negative intrapleural pressure as the diaphragm contracts. On expiration, positive intrapleural pressure allows the free-floating segment of fractured ribs to bulge outward, referred to as paradoxical respiration. Flail chest is extremely painful, and patients display rapid shallow breathing. Hypoxia is usually a consequence of associated pulmonary contusion rather than simple hypoventilation. Management includes supplemental oxygen and analgesics and may require regional nerve blocks or epidural anesthesia in severe cases (**Fig. 5.2**).

Fig. 5.2a–f
a Sternal fracture. The upper portion of the sternal body is depressed by half its width at a point 4 cm distal to the sternal manubrial joint. No visible retrosternal hematoma.
b–d Sternoclavicular dislocation. (**b**) Axial. Posterior dislocation of the right medial clavicle, the head of which is interposed between the subclavian vein and the right carotid artery. No associated vascular hematoma or definite injury. (**c,d**) Coronal. The right medial clavicle is located posterior to the sternal manubrium. The left clavicle articulates normally.
e,f Flail chest. The left chest wall is deformed due to segmental left fifth–seventh rib fractures. A left pulmonary opacity corresponds to lung contusion. Noncontrast CT reveals depressed segmental rib fractures with adjacent anterior segment left upper lobe pulmonary contusion and laceration. Extensive soft tissue emphysema. Left thoracostomy tube.

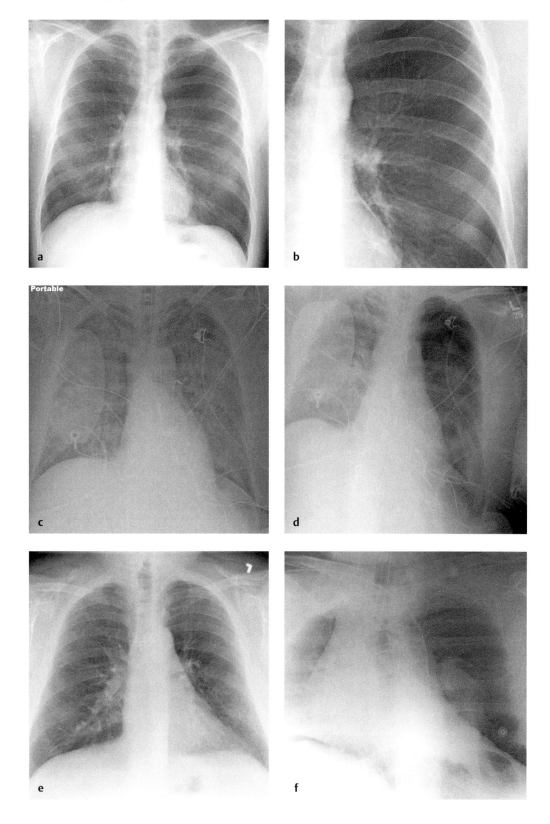

◆ Pneumothorax

Pneumothorax is the intrapleural accumulation of air due to a visceral pleural tear. It can be caused by barotrauma, rupture of a peripheral bleb or other pulmonary lesion, and blunt or penetrating chest trauma. Especially in traumatic pneumothorax, a one-way valve effect allows air to accumulate on inspiration that cannot exit the pleural space on expiration. As intrapleural pressure on the side of the pneumothorax exceeds atmospheric and contralateral intrathoracic pressure, the trapped air displaces and compresses the mediastinum, reducing cardiac output and systemic perfusion. Clinical signs include diminished breath sounds over the affected hemithorax, tachycardia hypotension, jugular venous distention, and contralateral tracheal shift.

Smoking is the most common risk factor for spontaneous pneumothorax, which is usually due to rupture of a subpleural bulla. Primary pneumothorax typically occurs in persons under the age of 35 and is not associated with lung disease. Secondary pneumothorax is associated with underlying lung disease, such as chronic obstructive pulmonary disease, asthma, cystic fibrosis, interstitial lung disease, and malignancy. Patients typically present with acute pleuritic chest pain and dyspnea, but many are only minimally symptomatic.

On upright PA radiographs, a fine, dense line that corresponds to the visceral pleura separates the lucent, air-filled lung from within the enlarged pleural space. Pulmonary vessels and other lung markings are not visible lateral to the visceral-pleural line. The heart and mediastinum are often normal in position but may be displaced to the opposite side in tension pneumothorax.

Supine, portable radiographs obtained in trauma patients often do not show pneumothoraces even when present, partly because air in the pleural space lies anterior, rather than lateral to the lung and the pleura is imaged en face rather than tangentially. Thoracic hyperlucency that extends over the upper abdomen is referred to as the "deep sulcus" sign and is a useful but indirect finding in acute trauma. Ultrasound can identify pneumothorax in the trauma setting, but findings are often subtle. Interrogation of the normal lung shows mobile dotlike echoes as the visceral pleura moves against the parietal pleura with respiration. In pneumothorax these mobile echoes are not seen.

Skin folds can simulate the appearance of a pneumothorax but are seen exclusively on portable AP chest radiographs. When the detecting plate is placed behind the patient, redundant skin can fold against the plate, causing an air–soft tissue interface external to the patient. A true pneumothorax will appear as a thin white line separating dark intrapleural air from dark air-filled lung. A skin fold (pseudopneumothorax) will appear as a dense edge against more lucent lung usually containing visible peripheral vessels.

In patients with hypoxia or vascular collapse, treatment should not be delayed while awaiting chest radiograph. A 14–16 gauge intravenous catheter can be inserted, either in the second anterior intercostal space in the midclavicular line or in the fifth intercostal space on the anterior axillary line, before a larger chest tube can be placed (**Fig. 5.3**).

Fig. 5.3a–f
a,b Tension pneumothorax. Left pneumothorax and pneumomediastinum. Rightward cardiac displacement.
c,d Deep sulcus sign on supine portable radiograph. (**c**) Initial study shows diffuse bilateral airspace opacity due to cardiogenic edema, intra-aortic balloon pump and external pacer/defibrillator pads. (**d**) Subsequent pneumothorax with abnormally deep and lucent left costophrenic sulcus compared with the right.
e,f Tension pneumothorax following laparascopic surgery. (**e**) Preoperative normal radiograph. (**f**) Large right pneumothorax with marked rightward mediastinal shift. Subdiaphragmatic air due to recent laparoscopy and gas insufflation.

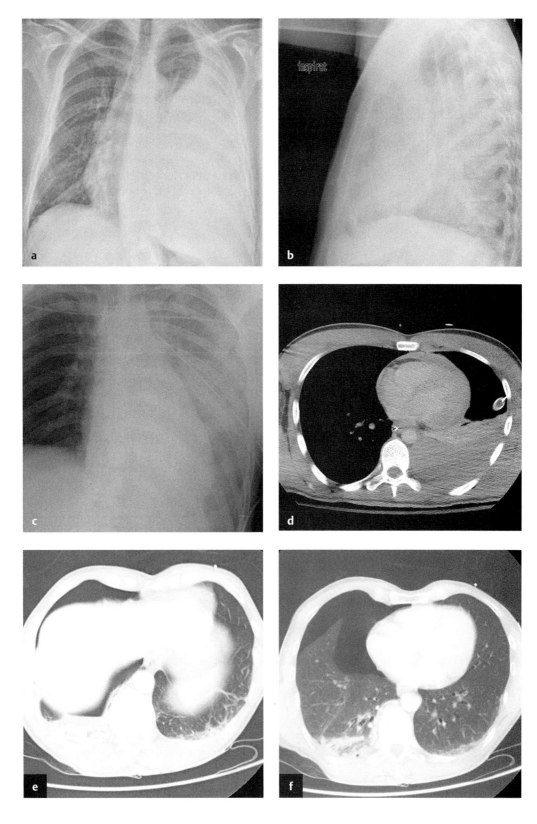

◆ Hemothorax

Injury to the chest wall, lung parenchyma, diaphragm, heart, or great vessels can result in intrapleural hemorrhage, most commonly from intercostal or internal mammary artery disruption. Hemothorax due to pulmonary parenchymal injury from stabbing or contusion is often small and self-limited because of the low pulmonary vascular pressure and usually subsides spontaneously or following placement of a pleural drain.

Massive hemothorax (> 1 liter) with clinical signs of shock and hypoperfusion is a surgical emergency due to potential heart and great vessel tamponade from the accumulated blood, acute hypovolemic shock, and hypoxia from lung collapse.

Supine chest radiographic findings are often subtle, depending on the volume of blood. Hazy increased density of the involved hemithorax with preserved vessel definition may be seen in smaller posterior hemothoraces. Large amounts of blood can fill the pleural space lateral to the lung and appear as a dense crescent-shaped collection. CT with arterial-phase contrast enhancement is diagnostic; acute blood products have an attenuation of 35–70 HU, and layering of intrapleural fluid with different densities due to combinations of clot, blood cells, and serum can be seen. In addition, CT optimally evaluates the integrity of the great vessels and identifies areas of arterial extravasation and other associated injuries.

Initial management is by placement of a chest tube, which permits evacuation of clot, reexpansion of the collapsed lung, and effective tamponade of low-pressure bleeding. Definitive surgical management depends on the nature of the injury and source of hemorrhage (**Fig. 5.4**).

Fig. 5.4a–f
a,b Hemothorax (stab wound). Massive left intrapleural fluid collection with compressed adjacent lung, contralateral mediastinal shift, and depression of the ipsilateral hemidiaphragm.
c,d Hemothorax (stab wound). Supine radiograph with hazy opacification of the left hemithorax and preservation of the right heart border. CT shows large left posterior blood collection, with lower lobe compressive atelectasis.
e,f Hemopneumothorax (bicyclist struck by car). Moderate right pneumothorax, small hemothorax with lower lobe compressive atelectasis.

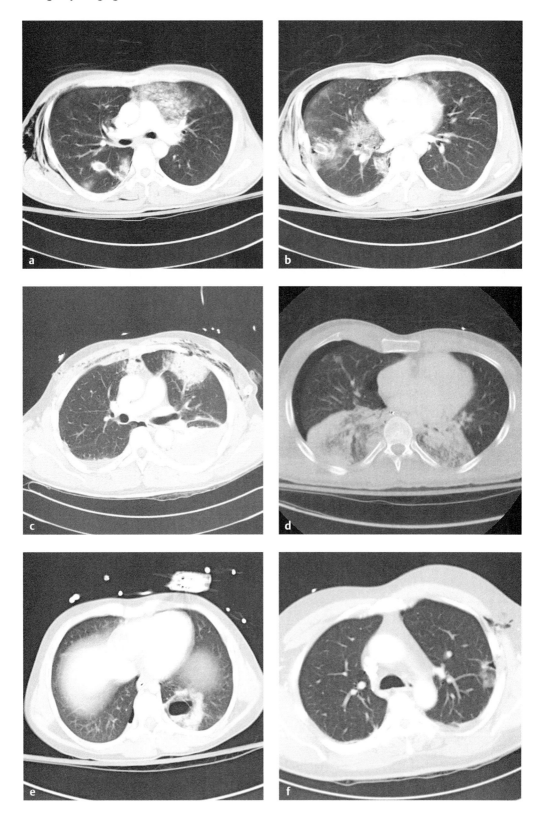

◆ Pulmonary Contusion and Laceration

Pulmonary contusion is a complication of blunt chest trauma and reflects focal parenchymal injury, edema, and interstitial and alveolar hemorrhage. Chest radiographic findings range from irregular nodular opacities to large areas of consolidation, but plain films are often nonspecific; aspiration pneumonitis can have a similar appearance and can also be seen in the trauma setting. On CT, pulmonary contusions appear as focal peripheral lung opacification adjacent to an area of impact. Posterior and lower lobes are more commonly affected. In contrast to lobar pneumonia, pulmonary contusions do not respect fissures and do not localize to a segment. They may be widespread, simulating ARDS or alveolar edema. In most cases, pulmonary contusion is apparent on the initial examination and does not worsen in severity. Radiographic clearing is rapid, and pulmonary contusions can resolve in as few as 72 hours.

Pulmonary laceration consists of a traumatic parenchymal disruption with subsequent formation of a hematoma or air-filled cavity (pneumatocele). The injury is typically due to shearing forces and is seen in blunt and penetrating injury. Lacerations are often obscured by concomitant pulmonary contusion, hemothorax, or pneumothorax and are easily missed on portable chest radiographs. Nearly all acute lacerations are detected with CT and appear as discrete round or oval air or fluid collections within an area of surrounding consolidation.

There are four types of pulmonary laceration. Type 1 (compression rupture injury) is most common and due to sudden compression of the chest wall with rupture of the inflated lung parenchyma. Type 2 (compression shear injury) results from compression of the lower chest with displacement of the lower lobe across the spine, causing a paravertebral cavity. Type 3 (rib penetration tear) is a small peripheral laceration adjacent to a rib fracture. Type 4 (adhesion tear) is the result of a preexisting pleuropulmonary scar (**Fig. 5.5**).

Fig. 5.5a–f
a,b Pulmonary contusion. Focal anterior segment left upper lobe airspace opacification (contusion). Small right pneumothorax. Right thoracostomy tube located in the major fissure. Extensive right axillary soft tissue emphysema.
c Lingular contusion. Left hemothorax.
d Bilateral lower lobe contusions. Right hemothorax. Subcutaneous emphysema.
e Compression shear pulmonary laceration (Type 2). Left lower lobe round paravertebral air collection within a larger area of air space opacity. Small right posterior hemopneumothorax.
f Rib penetration tear pulmonary laceration (Type 3). Small peripheral pneumatocele adjacent to rib fracture.

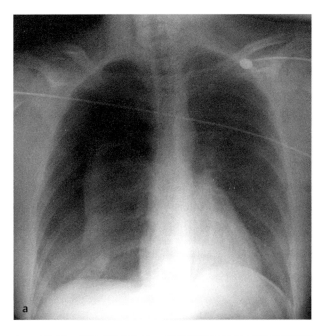

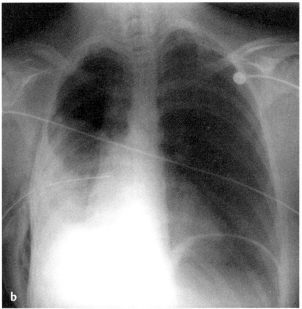

◆ Tracheobronchial Rupture

Tracheobronchial rupture is rarely encountered in clinical practice because most patients with this injury die from respiratory failure or exsanguination before arriving at the emergency department. Abrupt deceleration and intrathoracic shearing forces as well as compression of the airways between the sternum and thoracic spine in blunt trauma can disrupt the trachea or mainstem bronchus. Most injuries occur within 2.5 cm of the carina.

The most common imaging findings are pneumomediastinum and pneumothorax. Persistent pneumothorax after chest tube placement and suction is the hallmark of a major bronchial injury. With complete bronchial transection, the ipsilateral lung falls to the dependent (usually posterior) portion of the hemithorax; the "fallen lung" sign.

Chest CT can identify the exact site of the tear as a focal or a circumferential defect in the tracheal or bronchial wall. Other findings include airway wall contour deformity, extraluminal location of the endotracheal tube tip or herniation/overdistension of the balloon, pneumomediastinum, and deep cervical soft tissue emphysema (**Fig. 5.6**).

Fig. 5.6a,b
a,b Bronchial rupture. (**a**) The right lung is collapsed about the hilum and inferiorly positioned in the chest. Large right pneumothorax. (**b**) Persistent large pneumothorax following chest tube placement.

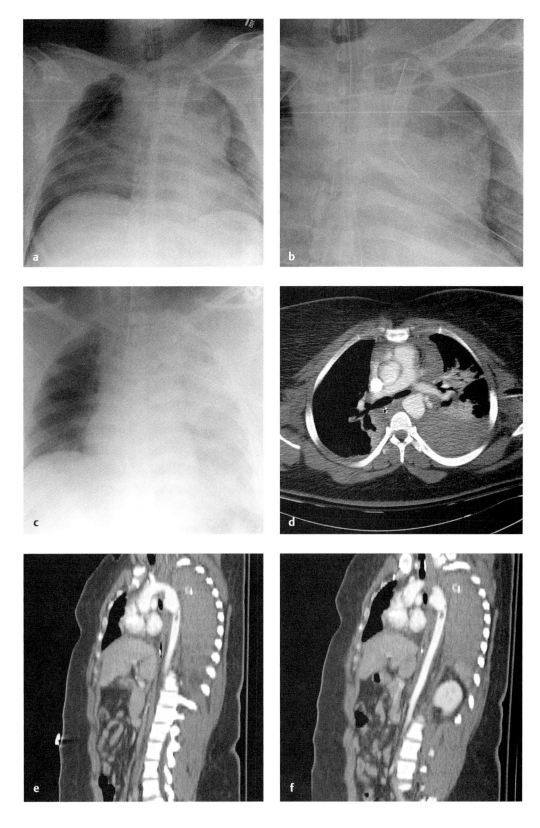

◆ Traumatic Aortic Injury

Thoracic aortic injury (TAI) is most commonly due to blunt trauma in high-speed motor vehicle accidents or falls. It can also result from stab or gunshot injuries to the chest. In most blunt impact mechanisms, the comparatively mobile heart and ascending aorta accelerate relative to the descending aorta, which is fixed to the spine. The aorta stretches or tears at a point just distal to the origin of the left subclavian artery. Other potential sites of injury are the proximal descending aorta, aortic root, and distal descending aorta. Patients with complete aortic transection, or laceration of all three layers of the vessel wall, exsanguinate before reaching the hospital. If a patient with TAI survives to reach the hospital, it is because the tear is likely transverse rather than longitudinal and the outer layer of the aorta (adventitia) remains intact.

Signs of a juxta-aortic hematoma on supine portable radiographs include mediastinal widening and indistinct margins, poor aortic contour definition, a widened paratracheal stripe, pleural effusion, caudal displacement of the right mainstem bronchus, and rightward displacement of an oro- or nasogastric tube. Many patients will have no mediastinal abnormality on portable chest radiograph. CT should be performed in patients with reported high-energy injury mechanism or who have upper rib, sternal, or scapular fractures on portable radiograph. A normal thoracic CT reliably excludes great vessel injury and can differentiate true aortic disruption from venous mediastinal hematoma by identifying direct findings of aortic injury: pseudoaneurysm, intimal flap, mural thrombus, arterial contrast extravasation, and focal change in aortic contour ("pseudocoarctation") (**Fig. 5.7**).

Fig. 5.7a–f
a,b   Traumatic aortic injury (11-story fall). Marked widening of the upper mediastinum with well-defined lateral border. Bilateral airspace opacities likely reflect pulmonary contusion. Left scapular body fracture.
c–f   Traumatic aortic injury. (**c**) Portable supine radiograph shows widened, ill-defined upper mediastinum. The left hemithorax is opacified. The orogastric tube is displaced to the right. (**d**) Postcontrast CT better defines a large left hemothorax and hemomediastinum. A small aortic pseudoaneurysm is visible adjacent to the left pulmonary artery. (**e,f**) Sagittal reformations show aortic intramural hematoma, intimal flap, and pseudocoarctation.

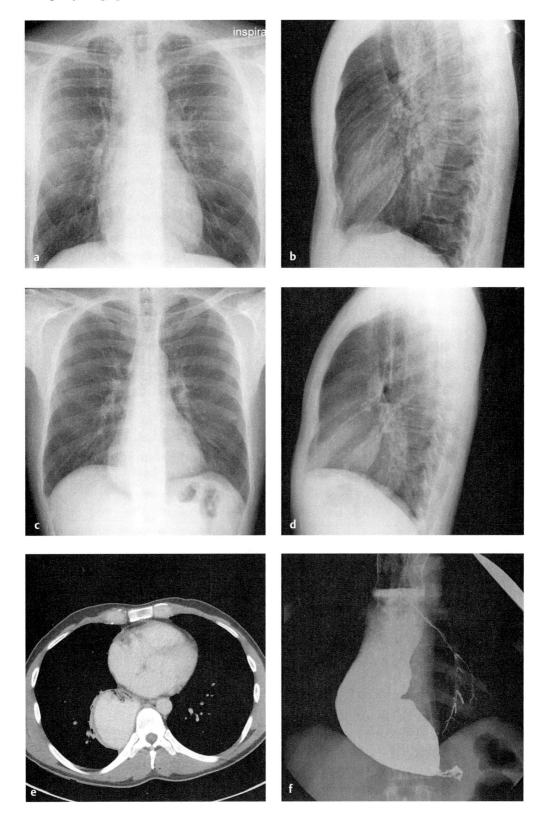

◆ Achalasia

Achalasia is a disorder of esophageal motility that results from failure of coordinated peristalsis and relaxation of the lower esophageal sphincter (LES) with swallowing. Degeneration of the Auerbach plexus leads to aperistalsis with consequent increased lower esophageal pressure and dilatation. Patients present with progressive dysphagia, vomiting, malodorous breath, aspiration, and weight loss. Complications of long-standing achalasia include esophageal carcinoma, aspiration pneumonia, esophagitis, and airway obstruction.

Barium esophagogram shows a dilated distal esophagus, aperistalsis, and failed LES relaxation, evidenced by a "bird's beak" appearance to the stenotic gastroesophageal junction. Plain chest radiographs are rarely diagnostic, but the food-filled distended esophagus or a mediastinal air-fluid level may be seen as well as a small or absent gastric air bubble. Esophagoscopy with manometry can be performed to document increased LES pressure and rule out complicating esophagitis or neoplasm.

Treatment aims to reduce lower esophageal sphincter pressure by surgical myotomy, dilations, or endoscopic injection of botulinum toxin (**Fig. 5.8**).

Fig. 5.8a–f Achalasia.
a,b The mediastinum is widened, with a double cardiac shadow along the right heart border. The esophagus is expanded and filled with granular material corresponding to retained food/fluid.
c–f Double cardiac shadow along the lower right heart border on frontal radiograph with retrocardiac density on lateral view. CT and esophagogram show gross esophageal dilatation proximal to stenosis ("bird beak") at the gastroesophageal junction. Incidental barium aspiration.

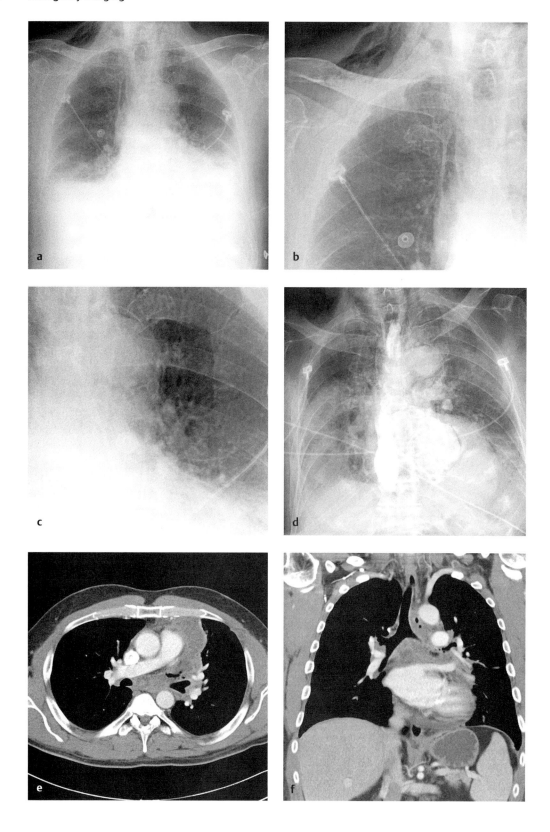

◆ Boerhaave Syndrome and Mediastinitis

Boerhaave syndrome entails complete esophageal rupture due to retching or vomiting. Perforation usually involves all layers of the distal posterior esophageal wall, and most patients are severely ill with acute-onset chest pain, dyspnea, blood-stained vomitus, and, in some cases, hypovolemic shock. Other signs and symptoms include tachycardia, fever, respiratory distress, and subcutaneous emphysema.

While a normal chest radiograph does not exclude small esophageal ruptures, pneumomediastinum and left-sided pleural effusion will be evident in most cases of Boerhaave syndrome. Esophagogram with water-soluble contrast material is diagnostic and will show contrast extravasation above the level of the diaphragm, often just proximal to the esophageal hiatus. CT, if performed, can demonstrate focal esophageal wall thickening, mediastinal fluid and edema, pneumomediastinum, and pleural effusion.

Treatment includes early surgical repair and drainage. The most severe complication is mediastinitis, which can be accompanied by septic shock and significant mortality.

Mediastinitis results from caudal extension of retropharyngeal or other deep cervical infection, hematogenous dissemination of distant infections, or, most commonly, direct inoculation into the mediastinal space due to surgery, trauma, or esophageal rupture. Acute mediastinitis is a surgical emergency with a high mortality. Chronic or slowly developing mediastinitis is less common but can be seen in tuberculosis, histoplasmosis, lung cancer, and sarcoidosis. The acute clinical presentation is nonspecific and includes fever, tachycardia, and chest pain. Dysphagia is commonly present, particularly in cases of esophageal rupture. When mediastinitis results from a descending head or neck infection, such as an odontogenic or deep neck infection, it is referred to as descending necrotizing mediastinitis.

Conventional radiography may show widening of the precervical and retropharyngeal soft tissues, sometimes with soft tissue gas, and mediastinal widening or mass. CT findings vary depending on the etiology but include extraluminal air, esophageal wall thickening, and mediastinal or lower cervical fluid collections. Treatment for mediastinitis consists of systemic antibiotic therapy and, if necessary, surgical débridement (**Fig. 5.9**).

Fig. 5.9a–f
a–d Esophageal rupture after vomiting. (**a–c**) Subcutaneous emphysema, pneumomediastinum, and left pleural effusion. (**d**) Gastrografin esophagogram shows extensive extravasation of contrast into the mediastinum and pleural space.
e,f Mediastinitis/mediastinal abscess. CT shows peritracheal, pericardiac, and subcarinal fluid collections containing multiple small air bubbles.

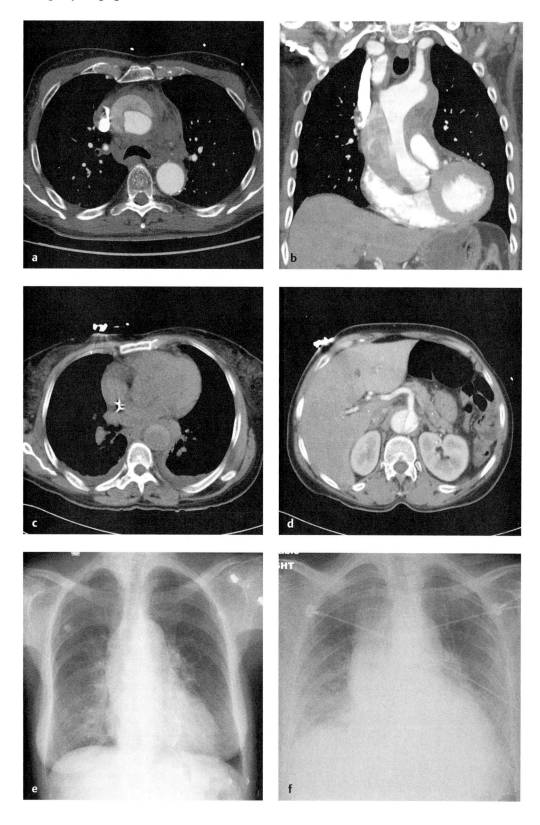

◆ Aortic Dissection and Nontraumatic Aortic Rupture

Aortic dissection is a consequence of spontaneous intimal disruption, usually due to a preexisting connective tissue disorder, hypertension, or vasculitis. Blood under arterial pressure enters and enlarges the potential space between the vascular intima and media and separates the two layers, proceeding proximally and distally from the initial tear. Potential consequences include carotid, subclavian, renal, and mesenteric artery occlusion as well as aortic rupture. Dissection may be preceded by aneurysmal dilation, and persons with an aortic diameter greater than 3 cm are at increased risk.

Thoracic aortic dissections are classified by their point of origin, and this determines treatment and prognosis. Stanford type A dissections begin in the ascending aorta and may or may not extend into the descending thoracic aorta. These dissections must be managed surgically due to their high rate of fatal complications, which include acute aortic regurgitation, rupture into the mediastinum or pleural space, and cardiac tamponade from rupture into the pericardium. Stanford type B dissections arise beyond the left subclavian artery origin, do not require surgery, and are managed by aggressive blood pressure control.

Patients present with sudden, severe chest pain that radiates to the back, sometimes described as ripping or tearing. Many are hypertensive at presentation, and renal, mesenteric, or cerebral ischemia may be associated if branch arteries are compromised. Nonenhanced CT is often performed prior to contrast administration, as it optimally evaluates acute intramural and extra-aortic hematoma, which is hyperdense compared with intraluminal blood. Contrast-enhanced CT in arterial phase provides excellent detail of the true and false lumens, any intraluminal thrombus, and local dilatation of the aorta. Conventional radiographs are often normal but can show aortic calcifications or aneurysm and, if compared with a prior examination, interval aortic enlargement or contour change.

Nontraumatic aortic rupture occurs in the setting of aortic dissection, aneurysm, coarctation, atherosclerosis, inflammation, mycotic disease, or erosion by an adjacent malignant tumor. Most such patients die from catastrophic blood loss before arriving at the emergency department. Those who survive to be evaluated may be dyspneic or hoarse and may have chest or upper back pain.

Mediastinal widening is the most common abnormality seen on portable radiographs. Other findings indicating aortic rupture include an indistinct aortic knob, widened paratracheal stripe, and depression of the left main bronchus. Thoracic CT identifies aortic intramural hematoma, mediastinal pleural hematoma, hemopericardium, and aortic abnormalities including dissection or pseudoaneurysm. Treatment requires urgent surgical intervention via open or endovascular repair (**Fig. 5.10**).

Fig. 5.10a–f
a,b Type A aortic dissection. Unopacified blood and thrombus fills the larger false lumen of a proximal aortic dissection with associated mediastinal hematoma.
c,d Type B aortic dissection. Acute hyperdense intramural hemorrhage surrounds the descending aorta on nonenhanced chest CT. CT angiogram at the level of the upper abdomen shows that the celiac trunk arises from the smaller true lumen. Nontraumatic aortic rupture.
e,f Ascending aortic (type A) dissection on plain radiographs. (**e**) Comparison radiograph from a prior admission shows baseline mild cardiomegaly. (**f**) Portable examination obtained in the emergency department for evaluation for acute chest pain shows interval enlargement of the cardiac contour with marked ascending aortic widening.

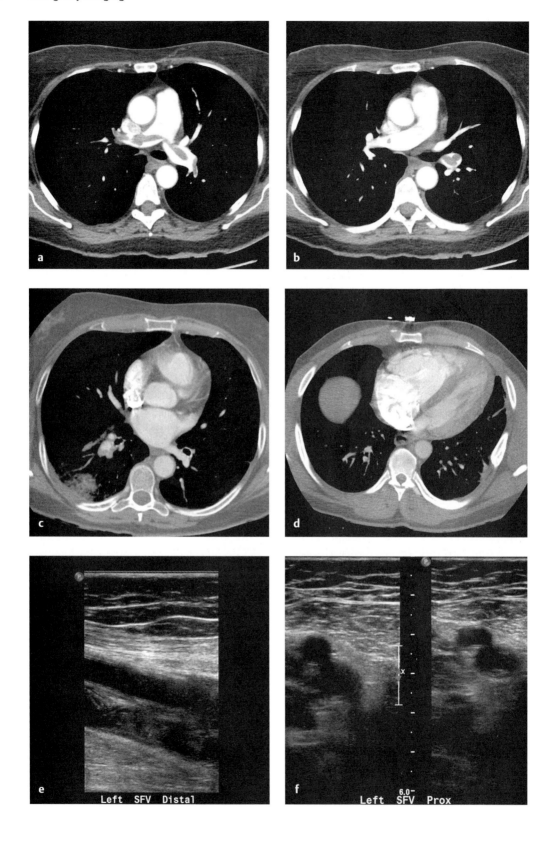

◆ Pulmonary Embolism and Deep Venous Thrombosis

Pulmonary embolism (PE) and deep venous thrombosis (DVT) are both manifestations of the same condition: venous thromboembolic disease. Pulmonary embolism consists of thrombus within the pulmonary arterial system that compromises lung perfusion. Risk factors include primary hypercoagulable syndrome, recent surgery, pregnancy, prolonged immobility, malignancy, and oral contraceptive use. Most emboli begin as thrombi in the deep veins of the leg and usually lodge in the segmental or subsegmental branches of the pulmonary arterial tree. Occasionally large emboli obstruct the central pulmonary arteries (saddle emboli). Patients with PE present with sudden onset of dyspnea, pleuritic chest pain, tachypnea, tachycardia, and hypoxemia.

A negative serum D-dimer effectively excludes pulmonary embolism in patients with low to moderate pretest probability, based on a collection of clinical findings known as the Wells criteria. Patients who are considered to be at high clinical risk, and those low to moderate risk who have an elevated D-dimer, should undergo CT angiography optimized for evaluation of the pulmonary vessels. When positive, CT shows central nonenhancing thrombus surrounded by contrast material. If right heart pressure is increased, the ventricular septum may appear straightened or bowed toward the left ventricle. Chest radiographs in patients with PE are typically normal or nonspecifically abnormal. Atelectasis, pleural effusions, or small peripheral opacities are commonly encountered, but they can be seen in many other conditions.

Lower-extremity DVT is a common disorder with predisposing factors that include immobilization, prior DVT, recent surgery, hypercoagulable syndromes, indwelling central venous catheter, increased estrogen state, and malignancy. Clinical findings include pain in the calf or thigh, unilateral leg edema, and warmth or tenderness. Ultrasound is most frequently used to differentiate DVT from other clinically similar entities such as cellulitis, ruptured Baker cyst, superficial thrombophlebitis, chronic thrombosis, and venous insufficiency, all of which can cause lower-extremity edema.

Noncompressibility of the affected vein is the single most reliable diagnostic finding. Other criteria include intraluminal thrombus visualization, vein enlargement, absent color flow signal, absent respiratory variation, and absent response to Valsalva maneuver.

DVT management includes low-molecular-weight heparin with appropriate analgesic pain control. Treatment of acute PE involves correction of hypoxemia with supplemental oxygen and immediate initiation of anticoagulation. Rarely, patients with hemodynamic compromise may require thrombolytic therapy or embolectomy (**Fig. 5.11**).

Fig. 5.11a–f
a,b Central "saddle" embolus. Large clot within the central pulmonary arteries.
c,d Segmental embolus. Lateral basal segment right lower lobe embolus with associated wedge-shaped peripheral opacity corresponding to a small pulmonary infarct. Increased right heart pressures due to large pulmonary embolus. The right ventricle is enlarged with straightening of the intraventricular septum.
e,f Superficial femoral vein thrombosis. Echogenic material fills and expands the superficial femoral vein. Transverse images without (left) and with (right) compression are identical.

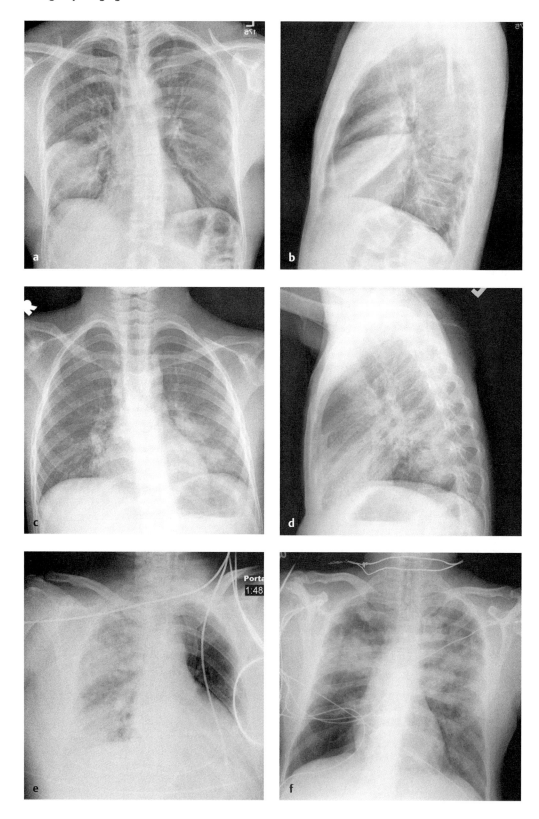

◆ Pneumonia

Pneumonia is an infection of the lung parenchyma caused by bacteria, viruses, or other microorganisms. Clinical manifestations include cough, fever, chills, and malaise. The elderly may present with confusion or other cognitive dysfunction.

Lobar pneumonias are characterized by opacification of a lobe or segment of a lobe with little or no associated volume loss, and commonly with an adjacent pleural effusion. They usually begin in the subpleural periphery and spread to adjacent alveoli via direct intra-alveolar connections (pores of Kohn and canals of Lambert). Because airways are not involved, they appear outlined as dark tubular structures within otherwise opacified lung parenchyma (air-bronchograms). Lobar pneumonias are typically confined by pleural surfaces, which permits localization on radiographs. Common causative organisms include *Streptococcus pneumoniae*, *Haemophilus influenzae*, and *Klebsiella pneumoniae*.

Bronchopneumonia (lobular pneumonia) involves the airspaces of the lung in patches around the bronchi or bronchioles. This pathological pattern is associated with *Staphylococcus aureus, Streptococcus pneumoniae, Pseudomonas*, tuberculosis, and *Enterobacter*. On CT, the "tree-in-bud" sign, in which tiny soft tissue density nodules at the ends of bronchioles appear as a budding tree, indicates infective bronchiolitis.

Bronchopneumonia is typical of postprimary, or reactivation, tuberculosis. The nidus of primary infection, usually in the apex, ruptures into a bronchus and spreads through the tracheobronchial tree to other regions of the lung. Resulting parenchymal destruction and residual scarring may result in cavity formation.

Because many different organisms can produce radiographic findings of bronchopneumonia, sputum and blood cultures may be necessary for precise diagnosis and management. Initial empirical treatment is often directed by clinical parameters such as severity of illness, immunologic status, and whether the infection was community- or hospital-acquired.

Aspiration pneumonia is the consequence of a direct chemical insult to the lung parenchyma by an aspirated solid or liquid material. The clinical presentation depends on the chronicity as well as the volume and pH of the aspirated contents. Several populations at risk include alcoholics, those undergoing general anesthesia, prolonged hospitalization, and mechanical ventilation. Aspiration pneumonia preferentially involves the posterior segments of the upper lobes and superior segments of the lower lobes, which are dependent regions, particularly in the supine patient (**Fig. 5.12**).

Fig. 5.12a–f
a,b Lobar pneumonia. Dense homogeneous consolidation of the right middle lobe lateral segment and portions of the medial segment.
c,d Bronchopneumonia. Heterogeneous airspace opacity predominantly involving the left lower lobe. The lingula is not involved, as the left heart border is sharply visible on the frontal radiograph.
e,f Aspiration pneumonia in two different patients. (**e**) Right upper and lower lobe consolidation. (**f**) Bilateral upper lobe/superior segment lower lobe heterogeneous consolidation.

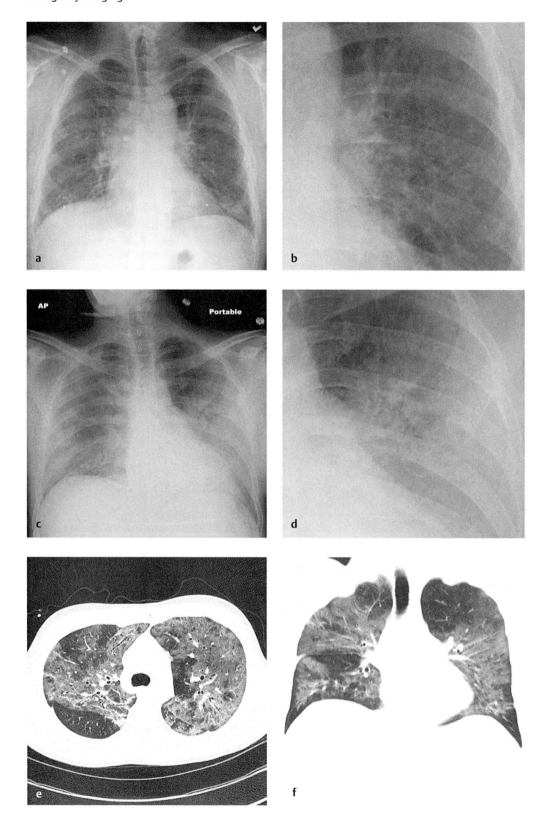

◆ Interstitial Pneumonia

Interstitial pneumonias characteristically involve the pulmonary interstitium with relatively little alveolar exudate. They are often associated with atypical pathogens such as *Mycoplasma, Chlamydia, Pneumocystis,* and viruses such as RSV, influenza, parainfluenza, and adenovirus. Symptom onset is insidious, and patients often complain of headache, myalgias, low-grade fever, and a nonproductive cough.

Radiographic features are normal or nonspecific in early pneumonia. Inflammatory cells migrate into and thicken the pulmonary alveolar walls, producing the characteristic reticular or reticulonodular pattern with diffuse or patchy airspace involvement. CT may show multifocal ground-glass opacities with bilateral, predominantly basilar linear or reticular opacities. Imaging findings are often symmetric. In chronic or recurrent interstitial pneumonia, traction bronchiectasis, consolidation, and honeycombing may be seen.

Pneumocystis pneumonia (PCP) is an atypical pulmonary infection caused by *Pneumocystis jiroveci,* previously known as *Pneumocystis carinii.* This pneumonia is restricted to immunocompromised populations such as those with HIV/AIDS, organ transplant recipients, or those on long-term steroid therapy. It is the most common opportunistic infection seen in patients with HIV and is one of the AIDS-defining illnesses, usually associated with a CD4 count below 200 cells/mm^3. Patients present with the gradual onset of malaise, dyspnea, weight loss, or a nonproductive cough.

Radiographic findings include diffuse perihilar opacities and fine reticular interstitial markings. Chest CT is more sensitive than radiography and shows ground-glass opacities in the perihilar or mid lung zones. A "crazy paving" pattern may also be seen, in which thickened interlobular septa overlie areas of ground glass density. Upper lobe pneumatoceles are common and predispose patients to spontaneous pneumothorax. Pleural effusions and hilar lymphadenopathy are sometimes present but are not common features.

Patients are treated with trimethoprim-sulfamethoxazole (TMP-SMX). If there is moderate to severe hypoxia, corticosteroids are often added. Prophylaxis with TMP-SMX for patients with CD4 counts less than 200 cells/mm^3 has helped decrease the incidence of PCP (**Fig. 5.13**).

Fig. 5.13a–f
a,b Influenza (H1N1) pneumonia. (**a**) Indistinct central vessels. (**b**) Subtle peribronchiolar thickening.
c–f Pneumocystis pneumonia. Plain radiographs show hazy opacities that obscure central vascular definition, granular opacities, and air bronchograms. CT shows heterogeneous ground-glass opacities that involve all lobes, superimposed air bronchograms, and interstitial thickening.

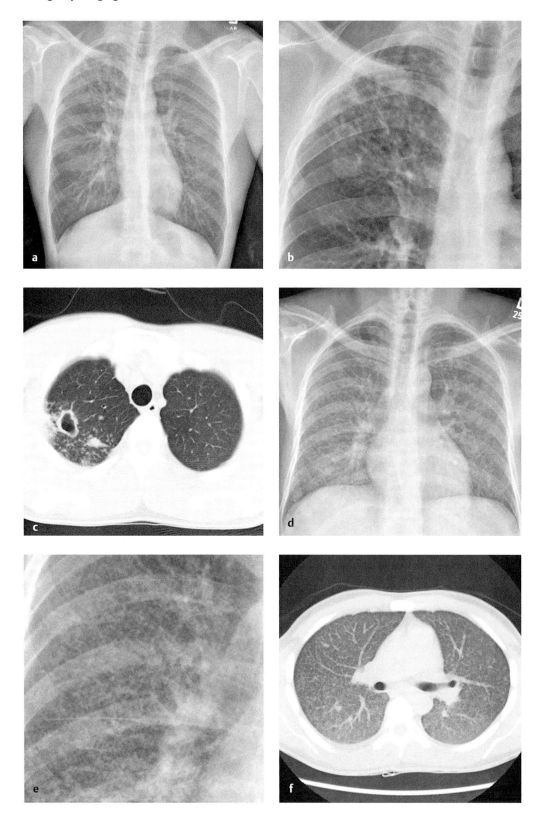

◆ Tuberculosis

Primary pulmonary tuberculosis (TB) results from the inhalation of mucus droplets containing tubercle bacilli exhaled by another infected person. The inhaled bacilli can cause a primary pneumonia or form a granuloma, often with associated ipsilateral hilar adenopathy (Gohn complex). Primary tuberculosis is often clinically and radiographically occult or can manifest as a nonspecific pneumonia. After a primary infection, the bacilli can die, they can remain dormant, or the infection can progress.

Postprimary TB results from reactivation of dormant bacilli or reinfection of a previously exposed patient. The risk of reactivation is highest within the first 2 years of initial infection, and rates are highest in children, the elderly, and patients whose immune systems are compromised by HIV or chronic diseases such as diabetes or renal failure. Patients with postprimary TB typically present with subacute fever, malaise, weight loss, fatigue, and night sweats. Most will also complain of a productive cough, with some reporting hemoptysis, pleuritic chest pain, and dyspnea. Reactivation should be considered in any HIV-positive patient with respiratory symptoms even if the chest radiograph is normal.

Radiographic findings include focal or confluent opacities in the apical and posterior segments of the upper lobes and the superior segments of the lower lobes. Cavitary disease is usually located in the upper lobes and reflects caseous necrosis in consolidated lung. Cavities are typically thick-walled with smooth inner contours and may contain air-fluid levels.

CT better defines areas of consolidation and detects associated findings such as cavitation, calcification, scarring, atelectasis, hilar adenopathy, and unilateral pleural effusion. Complications include vascular erosion, rupture into pleural space (bronchopleural fistula), tuberculous empyema, chest wall involvement, miliary disease, and endobronchial spread. The "tree-in-bud" sign—tiny, centrilobular, soft tissue–density nodules at the ends of branches arising from a single bronchiolar stalk—indicates infective bronchiolitis. It is commonly seen in endobronchial tuberculosis but is not diagnostic, as many other infectious and inflammatory conditions can cause it.

Miliary tuberculosis is due to hematogenous spread of tuberculosis to the lung from other organs. It is more frequently seen in immunocompromised patients. Fungal infections, varicella zoster, sarcoidosis, and some metastatic neoplasms can have similar appearances (**Fig. 5.14**).

Fig. 5.14a–f
a–c Postprimary endobronchial tuberculosis. Right upper lobe coarse nodular opacities with focal cavity visible below the clavicle. CT shows multiple tiny nodules and "tree-in-bud" upper lobe peribronchiolar opacities consistent with an infectious bronchiolitis/bronchopneumonia, as well as a 2-cm cavity with thick, irregular wall.
d–f Miliary tuberculosis. Innumerable 1–2-mm nodules distributed throughout the entire lung parenchyma.

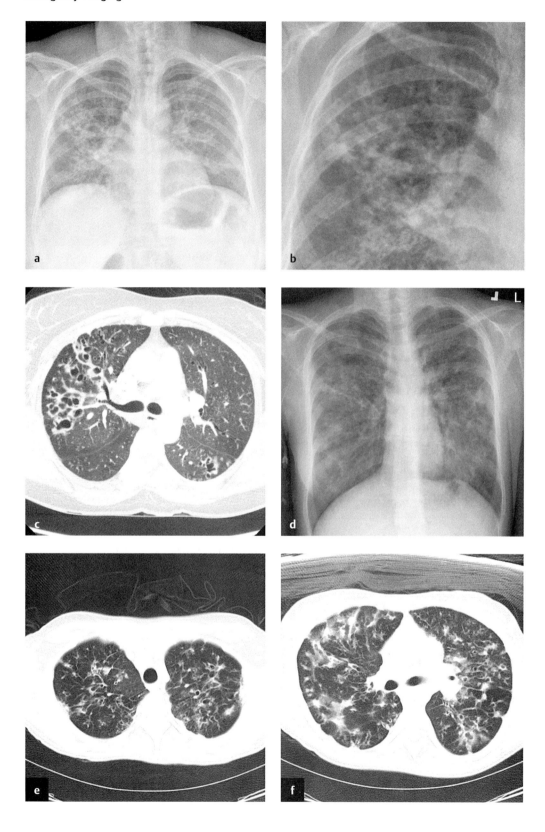

◆ Bronchiectasis and Cystic Fibrosis

Bronchiectasis—focal or generalized bronchial dilatation—is seen in various conditions, including cystic fibrosis, granulomatous diseases, necrotizing bacterial pneumonias, bronchogenic carcinoma, rheumatoid arthritis, systemic lupus erythematosus, and postradiotherapy. These can be categorized as postinfective etiologies, which are most common; congenital disorders; bronchiectasis secondary to bronchial obstruction; and fibrosis with loss of lung volume, among others. The clinical presentation is variable but includes recurrent chest infection, excessive sputum production, and hemoptysis.

Bronchiectasis is classified into four subtypes based on their macroscopic morphology, and these roughly correspond to clinical severity. (1) Cylindrical bronchiectasis is characterized by parallel, thick line markings radiating from the hilum, which are uniform in caliber without tapering. These are often referred to as "tram tracks" and represent enlarged segmental bronchi that have been widened by chronic disease. (2) Traction bronchiectasis results from traction by the surrounding fibrotic lung on the airway. (3) Cystic bronchiectasis is a severe form in which the bronchi show focal areas of cystic dilatation, sometimes containing air-fluid levels. (4) Varicose bronchiectasis is relatively uncommon and consists of bronchi with a beaded appearance due to alternating dilatation and narrowing.

Chest radiographs in patients with bronchiectasis are usually abnormal, with conspicuous or coarse bronchovascular markings, tram-track opacities, and air-fluid levels. CT better delineates the typical bronchial wall thickening, mucus plugging, and air-trapping that characterize the disease.

Treatment focuses on promoting sputum clearance, addressing the underlying disease, and management of intercurrent infections.

Cystic fibrosis (CF) is a disease of exocrine gland function that predisposes patients to recurrent respiratory infections and pancreatic enzyme insufficiency. Pulmonary disease is due to production of thick mucoid secretions that compromise the normal evacuation of tracheobronchial tree contaminants by epithelial cilia. Chronic colonization with pathogens such as *Staphylococcus aureus* leads to mucus plugging, inflammation, atelectasis, and scarring. These processes lead to a pattern of hyperinflation with coarse interstitial and airspace opacities that preferentially involve the upper lobes. Bronchiectasis appears as "tram-tracking" and reflects enlarged segmental bronchi widened by chronic infection and scarring.

Complications include spontaneous pneumothorax, chronic bacterial infection, and pulmonary arterial hypertension (**Fig. 5.15**).

Fig. 5.15a–f
a–c Bronchiectasis. Coarse bronchovascular markings with dilated, tubular air bronchograms; obscured central pulmonary vessels. CT better delineates multiple severely dilated, thick-walled bronchi and bronchioles, preferentially involving the right upper and middle lobes but also present in the left lower lobe and lingula.
d–f Cystic fibrosis. The lungs are hyperinflated with coarse bronchovascular markings. CT shows extensive moderate bronchiectasis with adjacent scarring and parenchymal opacity.

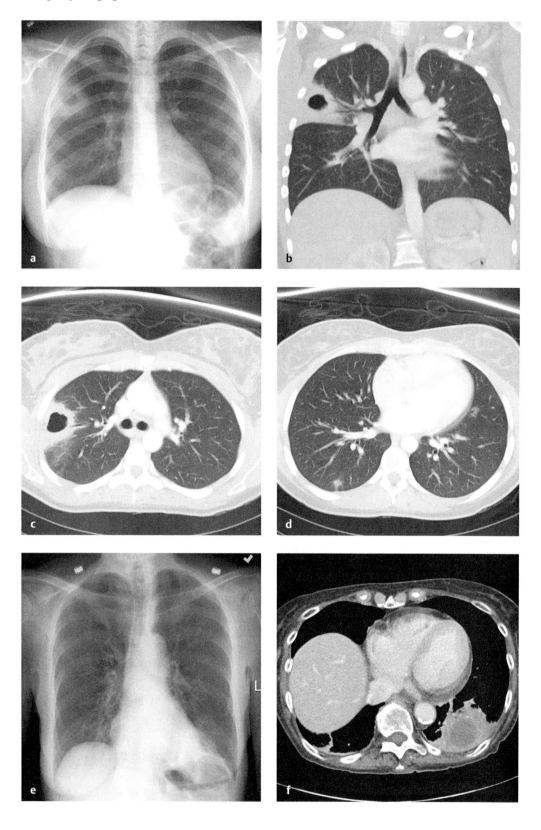

◆ Septic Pulmonary Embolism and Lung Abscess

Septic pulmonary emboli are infected thrombi that embolize into the pulmonary arterial system and cause focal pneumonitis, lung necrosis, and cavitation. *Staphylococcus aureus* is the most common pathogen, and intravenous drug users are at particular risk. Potential sources include infected cardiac valves in patients with endocarditis, indwelling catheters, prosthetic heart valves, pacemaker wires, osteomyelitis, or abscesses elsewhere in the body. The clinical presentation is often insidious, with signs and symptoms of fever, dyspnea, pleuritic chest pain, cough, or hemoptysis.

Chest radiographs may show ill-defined opacities, frank parenchymal consolidation, or peripheral, well-demarcated, rounded or wedge-shaped nodules. The latter often rapidly cavitate, in contrast to metastases and noninfected thrombotic emboli. CT shows multiple peripheral or subpleural nodules with or without necrotic centers and wedge-shaped peripheral infarcts. The "vessel" sign corresponds to a visible feeding artery leading to a pulmonary nodule. Empyema may complicate septic emboli in case of rupture through the visceral pleura.

Lemierre syndrome, in which a septic jugular thrombophlebitis complicates a pharyngeal infection, is commonly associated with septic emboli and secondary pneumonia.

Lung abscess is a localized, walled-off collection of pus within the lung parenchyma. It is most commonly due to aspiration pneumonia or septic pulmonary embolus. Less common causes include penetrating trauma, fungal or parasitic infections, and secondarily infected primary or metastatic neoplasm. Acute findings include fever, cough, shortness of breath, and pleuritic chest pain. Chronic abscesses may present with constitutional symptoms such as weight loss and fatigue.

Lung abscesses that complicate aspiration pneumonia tend to occur on the right side and often involve the superior segments of the lower lobes and the posterior segments of the upper lobes. An upper lobe cavity should suggest reactivation tuberculosis. Diagnosis is often made by chest radiograph; an abscess will appear as a mass if completely fluid-filled, or as a rounded lucency within an area of consolidation that may contain an air-fluid level. An abscess cavity is characteristically round on all projections. This finding helps to differentiate peripheral abscesses from empyemas, which are ovoid or lentiform. On CT, a lung abscess typically demonstrates a thick, well-demarcated wall with an irregular luminal surface and surrounding parenchymal consolidation.

Management consists of prolonged antibiotics, sometimes with bronchoscopic drainage. Lung abscesses are usually treated aggressively because of the potential for life-threatening complications such as hemoptysis and empyema (**Fig. 5.16**).

Fig. 5.16a–f
a–d Septic pulmonary emboli. Right upper lobe consolidation with central cavity. Smaller right lower lobe and lingular nodules reflect smaller, non-cavitary emboli. Posterobasal segment left lower lobe lung abscess.
e,f Posterobasal segment left lower lobe lung abscess. (**e**) Frontal radiograph shows left posterior costophrenic angle/retrocardiac soft tissue mass with obscured posterior hemidiaphragm. (**f**) Computer-enhanced CT reveals a well-defined low posterior segment low-attenuation fluid collection with surrounding enhancing rim and compressed lung.

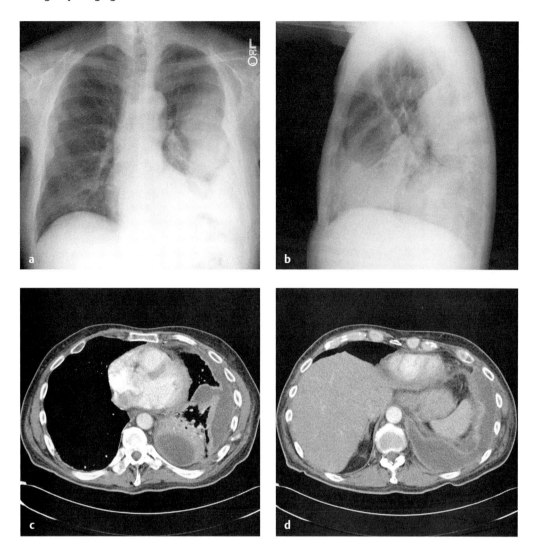

◆ Empyema

An empyema is a purulent intrapleural collection. Most often a complication of bacterial pneumonia, empyema can also result from chest or abdominal trauma, esophageal perforation, extension from a peripheral lung abscess, tuberculosis, osteomyelitis, or a secondarily infected chylo-, hemo-, or hydrothorax. Clinical presentation may mimic pulmonary infection, with pleuritic chest pain, cough, and fever. Patients may also present with weight loss, anemia, and night sweats. Decreased breath sounds, dullness to percussion, and a friction rub may be appreciated on physical exam.

On plain radiographs, empyemas are evident as pleural-based ovoid or lentiform densities. If an air-fluid level is present, it can appear to contact the chest wall. These findings help to differentiate an empyema from a peripherally located lung abscess, which can also contain an air-fluid level but is more characteristically round in all projections. On CT, the "split pleura" sign is formed by the separation of thickened, enhancing layers of visceral and parietal pleura, a feature that differentiates it from a simple pleural effusion. Loculations are often present within the empyema and may complicate attempts at catheter drainage. Empyemas have smooth walls and displace the surrounding parenchyma. In contrast, lung abscesses have thick, irregular walls and tend to destroy adjacent lung.

Empyema necessitans refers to an empyema that involves the thoracic wall and spontaneously drains through the skin. It is sometimes seen in tuberculosis and infected malignancies.

Most empyemas are managed by antibiotic treatment and percutaneous drainage. Open drainage may be necessary for persistent disease or chest wall involvement. In this case, the pleural cavity is marsupialized to the chest wall (Eloesser flap) (**Fig. 5.17**).

Fig. 5.17a–d
a–d Empyema. (**a,b**) Well-defined, lobulated pleural-based mass surrounding the left lower lobe with obscured diaphragm and heart border. (**c,d**) Postcontrast CT shows lobulated, thick-walled, pleural fluid collection with enhancing margins corresponding to visceral and parietal pleura.

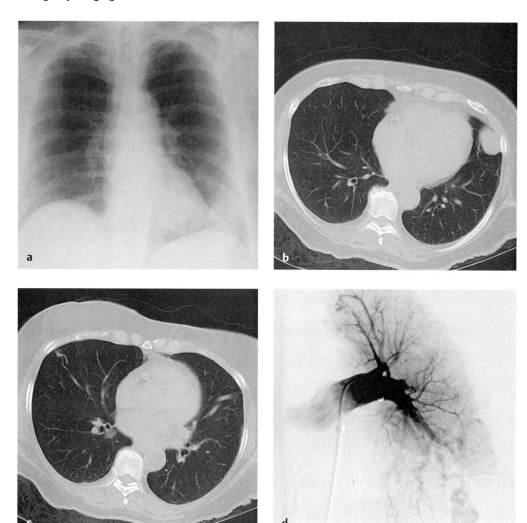

◆ Pulmonary Arteriovenous Malformation

Pulmonary arteriovenous malformations (AVMs) are uncommon pulmonary vascular abnormalities in which an abnormal communication between the pulmonary arteries and pulmonary veins bypasses the pulmonary capillary bed. Patients with multiple pulmonary AVMs typically have the autosomal dominant disease hereditary hemorrhagic telangiectasia (HHT), also known as Rendu-Osler-Weber syndrome. Although this condition is congenital, most patients remain asymptomatic until adult life. Pulmonary AVMs may also be acquired in cirrhosis with portal hypertension and in some chronic pulmonary infections, such as schistosomiasis, actinomycosis, or tuberculosis.

Signs and symptoms of HHT are due either to hemorrhage from vascular malformations or right-to-left intrapulmonary shunting that compromises the lung's normal function as a bacterial filter of the venous circulation. These include anemia from gastrointestinal hemorrhage, epistaxis from nasal mucosal telangiectasias, polycythemia or high-output cardiac failure from right-to-left pulmonary shunting, or seizure from cerebral abscesses.

On chest radiographs, a pulmonary AVM appears as a lobulated nodule with an enlarged feeding artery and draining vein or as a round or ovoid mass with uniform opacity, usually in the lower lobes. Most patients present with unilateral disease, and malformations tend to be small, typically 1 to 5 cm in diameter. Chest CT demonstrates smaller AVMs and more precisely delineates vascular supply.

Treatment includes transcatheter coil ablation or surgical resection, and prognosis for the solitary, nonsyndromic AVM is good (**Fig. 5.18**).

Fig. 5.18a–d
a–d Multiple pulmonary arteriovenous malformations in patient with hereditary hemorrhagic telangiectasia. (**a,b**) Radiograph and axial CT show a well-defined round lingular mass. (**c**) Axial CT shows lingular and right middle lobe paired dilated feeding pulmonary arteries and draining veins to the lingular mass and to a smaller right middle lobe AVM. (**d**) Pulmonary arteriogram preparatory to AVM embolization shows serpiginous lingular opacity corresponding to enlarged vessels.

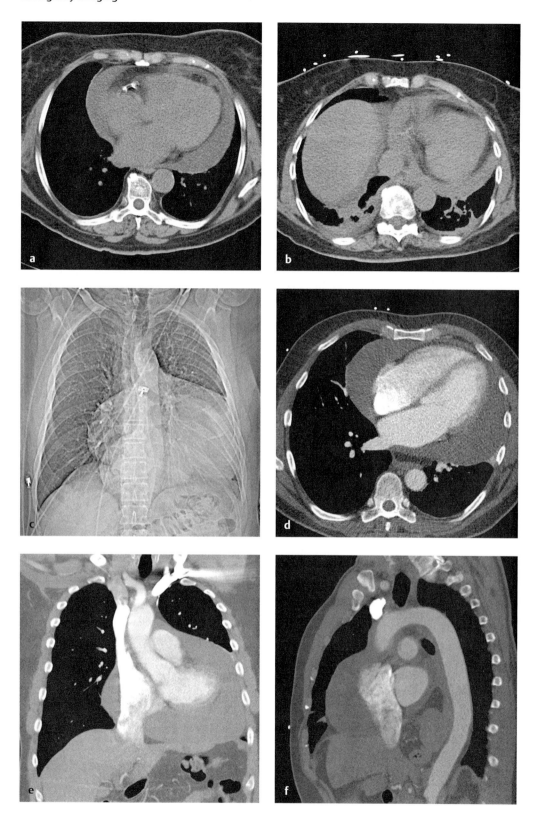

◆ Pericardial Effusion

The potential space between the parietal and visceral layers of the pericardium normally contains less than 50 mL of serous fluid. A pericardial effusion can be either serous, exudative, or hemorrhagic and consists of accumulation of fluid below the pericardium. Common causes of serous effusion include heart failure, pericarditis, nephrotic syndrome, and myxedema. Serous effusions can also be idiopathic or infectious or arise secondary to malignancy. Hemopericardium is caused by penetrating and blunt chest trauma, aortic dissection or aneurysm rupture, or myocardial infarction. Patients with pericardial effusion present with chest pain or discomfort, light-headedness, syncope, or palpitations.

In patients with large pericardial effusions, chest radiographs show apparent global cardiomegaly with a "water bottle" shape. Dilated cardiomyopathy can have a similar appearance. Echocardiography can immediately distinguish pericardial effusion from true cardiac chamber enlargement; it is frequently used at the bedside to estimate the volume of any effusion and assess its hemodynamic impact. If a rapidly developing effusion exceeds 150 mL, the patient is at risk for cardiac tamponade, a life-threatening impairment of cardiac filling and contractility. Clinical signs include tachycardia, muffled heart sounds, and distended neck veins. Effusions that develop over time are often compensated and can be very large (up to 1 L) without causing tamponade.

Chest CT, typically performed in chest trauma and acute severe chest pain, accurately identifies and characterizes pericardial effusion. A simple or serous effusion will measure between 0 to 15 HU. Greater density indicates hemorrhage, empyema, or a malignant pericardial effusion. CT often also identifies the underlying condition responsible for the pericardial effusion (**Fig. 5.19**).

Fig. 5.19a–f
a Serous pericardial effusion. Moderate effusion hypodense to intracardiac blood (11 HU).
b Hemorrhagic pericardial effusion. Large pericardial effusion isodense to nonenhanced liver and intracardiac blood (40 HU).
c–f Traumatic effusion (serous) following motor vehicle accident. CT localizer shows marked apparent cardiac enlargement and large fluid-filled hiatus hernia. CT shows normal cardiac dimensions with massive nonhemorrhagic pericardial effusion (15 HU).

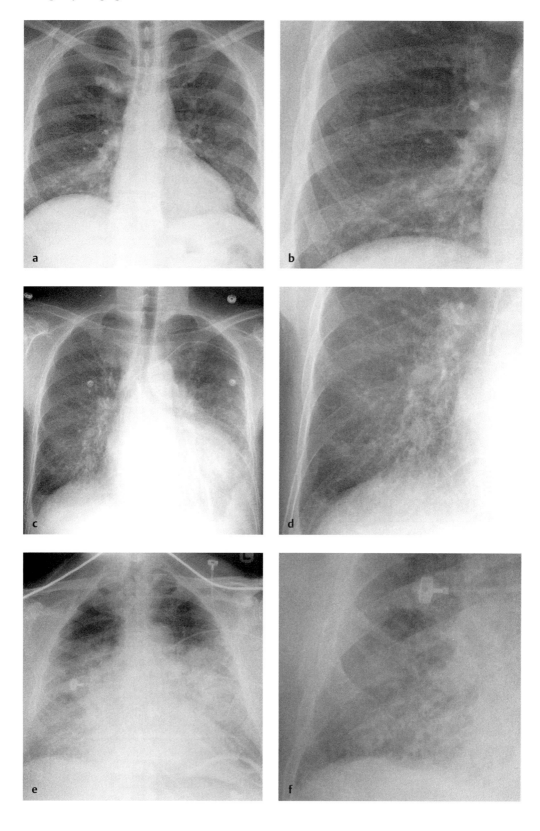

◆ Pulmonary Edema

Cardiogenic pulmonary edema develops when elevated pulmonary venous pressure leads to fluid accumulation in the extra-vascular lung parenchyma. It can be due to left heart failure or global fluid overload, as in renal disease or aggressive intravenous fluid therapy. Pulmonary edema is more likely to be of cardiac origin if the heart is dilated or other findings of left ventricular dysfunction are present. Clinical manifestations of pulmonary edema include dyspnea, tachypnea, hypoxia, wheezing, diaphoresis, and, in severe cases, blood-tinged, frothy sputum.

Cardiogenic pulmonary edema progresses from mild to severe through three stages: pulmonary venous hypertension, interstitial edema, and alveolar edema. Pulmonary venous hypertension is identi-fied by enlargement of upper-lobe pulmonary vessels to a point at which upper-lobe vessels appear equal or larger in size compared with lower-lobe vessels (cephalization). This is a reliable sign only on very high-quality radiographs.

As fluid accumulates in the pulmonary interstitium, central pulmonary vessels become increasingly indistinct, and pulmonary septal lines ("Kerley lines") appear in the peripheral 1 cm of the lung, which is normally free of markings on radiographs. Pleural effusions may also be present at this stage. As hydrostatic pressure increases further, interstitial fluid leaks into the alveoli and appears on radiographs as ill-defined ~ 2–3-mm nodules in the central and lower lungs. These may become confluent over time. Alveolar edema is relatively uncommon and often reflects an acute rapid cardiac decompensation, as seen in patients who suffer massive myocardial infarction or valve rupture. Conditions that can have a similar appearance include pneumonia, noncardiogenic edema (capillary leak, ARDS), pulmonary hemorrhage, and pulmonary alveolar proteinosis. In most of these conditions the heart size is normal.

Acute respiratory distress syndrome (ARDS) is a noncardiogenic pulmonary edema characterized by alveolar damage and lung capillary endothelial injury due to either direct lung injury or systemic illnesses. Sepsis, aspiration, pneumonia, acute pancreatitis, massive transfusion, severe trauma, and salicylate or cocaine overdose are associated conditions. The clinical presentation usually includes tachycardia, tachypnea, dyspnea, and hypoxemia.

Radiographically, ARDS is characterized by bilateral central alveolar opacities with sparing of the lung bases and costophrenic angles. Cardiogenic pulmonary edema, in contrast, tends to be most severe at the lung bases. Pulmonary venous cephalization and peripheral interstitial markings are usually absent, as these reflect increased hydrostatic pressure rather than pure capillary leak. Symptoms in ARDS may precede plain radiographic findings by up to 12 hours. After 24 hours of continued insult, multifocal opacities coalesce to form dense air-space consolidations with air bronchograms. The imaging features of ARDS tend to persist for days to weeks, whereas those related to cardiogenic pulmonary edema tend to resolve quickly with medical management. ARDS is associated with a 50% mortality, and many survivors are left with chronic pulmonary fibrosis (**Fig. 5.20**).

Fig. 5.20a–f
a,b Normal pulmonary vascularity. Central vessels are sharply defined. The peripheral 1 cm of the lung parenchyma should appear free of markings.
c,d Interstitial pulmonary edema. The heart is enlarged with indistinct central vessels and fine linear peripheral lung markings extending to the pleural surface (Kerley lines).
e,f Alveolar pulmonary edema. The heart is enlarged with completely obscured central vessels. peripheral nodular (~ 2-mm) opacities correspond to fluid-filled alveoli. The appearance of the pulmonary parenchyma is identical to that of pulmonary edema related to ARDS.

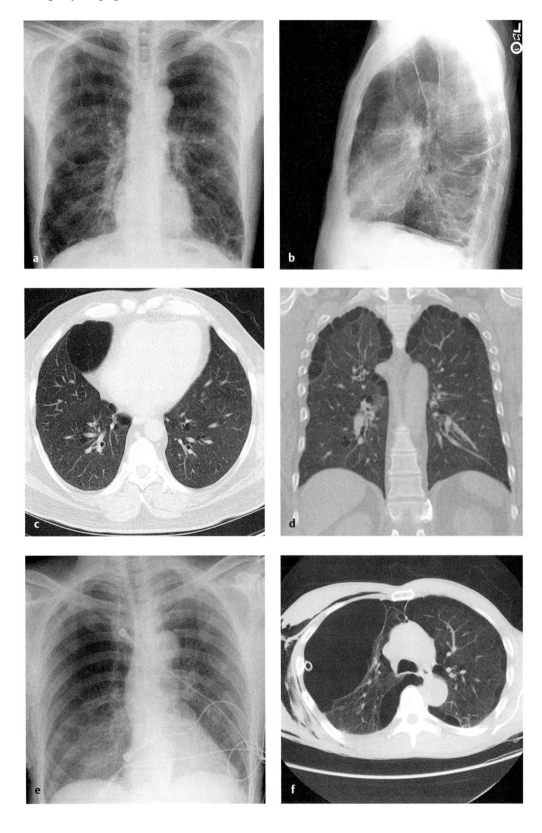

◆ Emphysema

Emphysema—destruction of the alveolar walls without fibrosis—leads to irreversible enlargement of pulmonary airspace distal to the terminal bronchioles. It can be due to several conditions including chronic obstructive pulmonary disease (COPD), alpha-1-antitrypsin deficiency, intravenous injection of methylphenidate (also known as Ritalin lung), and idiopathic giant bullous emphysema (vanishing lung syndrome). It may also be classified into the morphologic subtypes centrolobular emphysema, panlobular emphysema, and paraseptal emphysema.

Clinical features include tachypnea, chest wall hyperinflation, pursed-lip breathing, reduced breath sounds, and a notable absence of cyanosis. Patients are often referred to as "pink puffers," in contrast to those with chronic bronchitis, who are frequently cyanotic ("blue bloaters").

Conventional radiographs show flattened diaphragms, an increased anteroposterior diameter of the chest, and hyperlucent lungs with attenuated vascular markings. The cardiac silhouette often appears small in the setting of a hyperexpanded chest. Thin-walled cysts (bullae) are common at the apices, and very large ones may be occasionally mistaken for pneumothorax, but in the latter case, a visceral pleural white line should be visible. CT imaging is often used to determine the exact type and extent of emphysematous disease in the lung, as it has a high specificity for diagnosis. It is helpful in detecting early centrolobular emphysematous disease in COPD and differentiating it from other processes such as air trapping and bronchiectasis, which can be difficult to distinguish on plain radiographs (**Fig. 5.21**).

Fig. 5.21a–f
a,b Emphysema. Flattened diaphragm and increased anteroposterior thoracic dimension (hyperinflation), extensive bullous change, and fine linear scarring throughout the lung.
c,d Paraseptal emphysema. Multiple subpleural cysts with large right juxtacardiac bulla.
e,f Large right upper lobe bulla simulating pneumothorax. CT obtained after chest tube placement for presumed pneumothorax shows thoracostomy tube in a large right apical bulla, extensive emphysema with smaller subpleural bullae, subcutaneous air, and small postprocedure pneumothorax visible immediately behind the sternum.

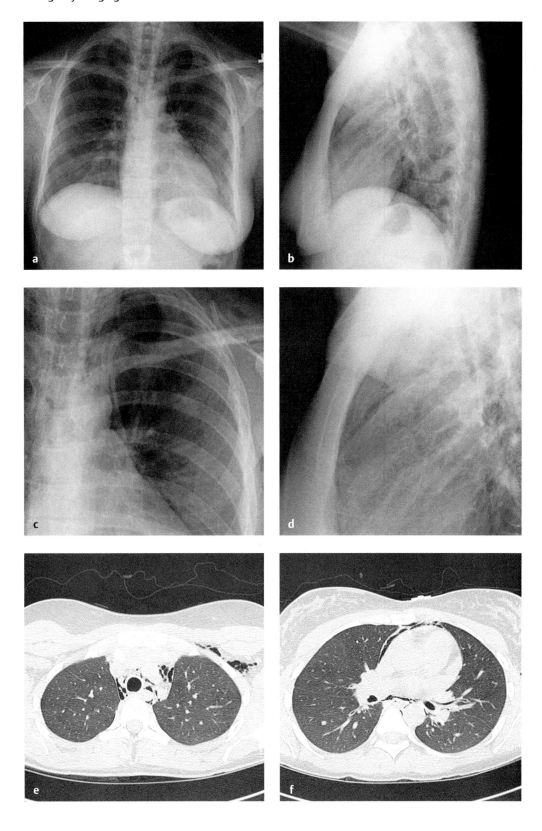

◆ Pneumomediastinum

Pneumomediastinum can be due to barotrauma or to disruption of the esophagus, trachea, or proximal airways. Barotrauma—disruption of the alveoli secondary to abruptly increased intrathoracic pressure—is seen in asthma exacerbation, croup, parturition, emesis, forceful fits of coughing, crack cocaine use, or as a complication of pneumonia, emphysema, or pulmonary fibrosis. Air escaping from the alveoli tracks along bronchovascular interstitial sheaths into the mediastinum. Patients typically experience chest pain, dyspnea, and fever, but they may be completely asymptomatic. A Hamman crunch (a crunching sound heard over the heart on auscultation of the chest) may be elicited on physical exam. Rarely, a tension pneumomediastinum may develop, in which venous return is impaired, compromising systemic perfusion.

Penetrating injuries to the trachea or esophagus, as well as esophageal rupture from retching or vomiting, can also result in pneumomediastinum.

Radiolucent streaks, bubbles, or collections of free air along the margins of the heart, in the retrosternal space, or surrounding the trachea are typical. Gas may outline the aorta or other great vessels, producing a "ring around the artery" sign. Air often dissects into the lower neck, resulting in subcutaneous emphysema. The "continuous diaphragm" sign refers to free air that accumulates superior to the diaphragm and inferior to the pericardium, causing the full length of the diaphragm to become visible. On lateral projection, pneumomediastinum is often visible behind the sternum and, in infants and young children, may outline the inferior and medial thymic margins. This finding is known as the "thymic wing" sign. Chest CT is more sensitive for detection of small amounts of mediastinal air and may be useful in identifying the cause, particularly in traumatic injury. It is generally not necessary for evaluation of spontaneous pneumomediastinum or obvious barotrauma.

Treatment depends on the clinical status of the patient and the underlying cause; almost all cases of spontaneous and many cases of traumatic pneumomediastinum resolve fairly quickly without specific intervention. In the setting of cardiorespiratory compromise, surgical intervention may be necessary (**Fig. 5.22**).

Fig. 5.22a–f
a–f Pneumomediastinum after cocaine use. (**a–d**) A thin collection of air surrounds the pericardium, upper mediastinal vessels, and trachea. (**e,f**) CT shows air confined to the mediastinum as well as subcutaneous air in the left axillary soft tissues.

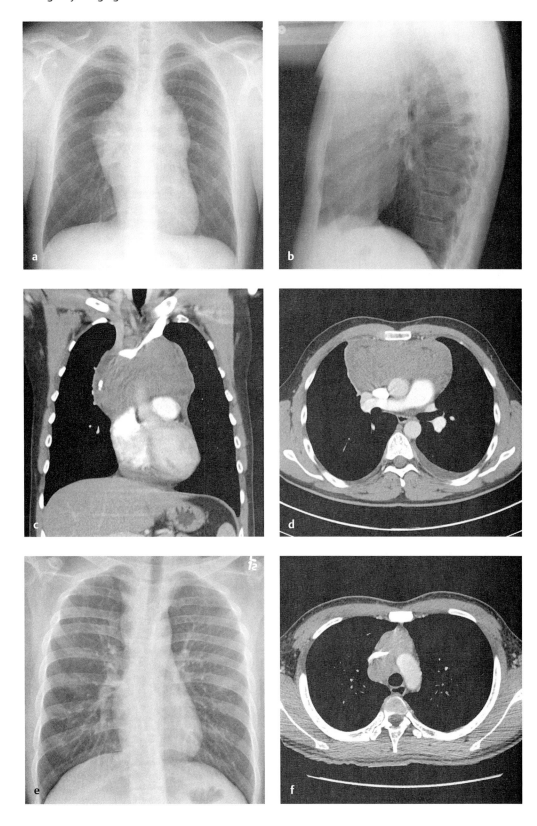

◆ Lymphoma

Lymphomas are a heterogenous group of malignancies that occur in different nodal and extranodal sites. In the chest, lymphoma can arise in the mediastinum, lung, pleura, or chest wall. Hodgkin disease (HD) arises primarily in lymph nodes and is further subdivided into nodular sclerosis HD, mixed-cellularity HD, lymphocyte-rich HD, and lymphocyte-depleted HD. It mainly affects younger individuals. In contrast, non-Hodgkin lymphomas (NHL) affect older patients and comprise a more diverse group of neoplasias reflecting clonal proliferations of B cells, T cells, or natural killer cells arrested in various stages of development. While the site of nodal involvement within the thorax may be suggestive, it is not sufficiently specific to differentiate the entities.

In the chest, Hodgkin disease frequently involves the anterior mediastinal nodes, while NHL tends to present in the subcarinal, paraesophageal, and internal mammary nodes. Pulmonary parenchymal involvement and mediastinal lymphadenopathy are more common in Hodgkin disease, but primary pulmonary lymphoma, which presents without significant evidence of nodal disease, is usually restricted to NHL.

Chest radiographs often show mediastinal widening with enlargement of the paratracheal lymph nodes. The right tracheal wall is normally outlined by air on both sides and appears as a 1–2-mm vertical stripe in the upper mediastinum. Paratracheal adenopathy widens or obliterates this normal structure. Single- or multiple-lung nodules with or without cavitation and less well-defined focal opacities with air bronchograms are sometimes seen. Subtypes with a predilection for the mediastinum include nodular sclerosis HD, lymphoblastic lymphoma, and diffuse large B-cell type. Further investigation with CT permits localization of abnormal lymph nodes and disease staging. Pleural effusions and thoracic wall disease are both more common in NHL (**Fig. 5.23**).

Fig. 5.23a–f
a–d Hodgkin lymphoma. A large, homogeneous anterior mediastinal mass fills the retrosternal space and obscures the superior cardiac margins and great vessels. Because the mass is confined to the anterior mediastinum and does not abut the trachea, the right paratracheal stripe remains well defined on the frontal radiograph.
e,f T-cell lymphoma in AIDS. Homogeneous superior mediastinal mass with marked right paratracheal soft tissue leading to obliteration of the right paratracheal stripe on the frontal radiograph.

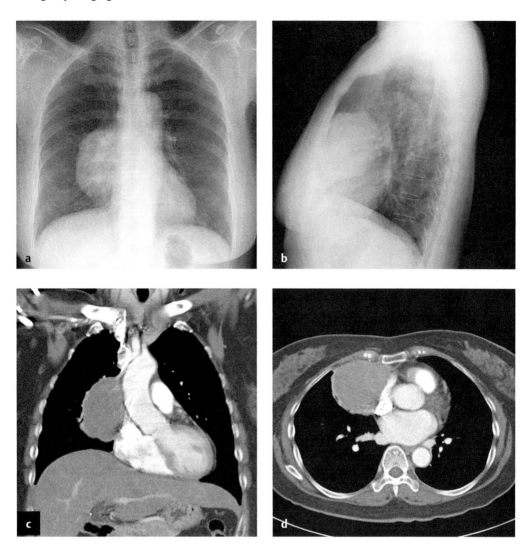

◆ Thymoma

Thymoma, the most common primary neoplasm of the anterior mediastinum, originates from the epithelial cells of the thymus. Most are slow-growing, solid, encapsulated tumors although some can be cystic, hemorrhagic, or necrotic. They can invade adjacent structures, but they rarely metastasize.

Many conditions have been associated with thymomas, but some of the most common are myasthenia gravis, pure red cell dysplasia, and hypogammaglobulinemia. Thymomas are rare in children and tend to occur in patients over 40 without gender predilection. Clinical presentations include venous obstruction, dysphagia, and stridor due to mass effect in the anterior mediastinum. Prognosis depends on histological subtype, surgical staging, and completeness of resection.

On plain radiographs, thymoma is visible as a well-defined anterior mediastinal or juxtacardiac soft tissue density. The mass usually projects into one of the hemithoraces. If the thymoma occurs on the right, the ascending aortic arch may be obscured. Conversely, if the thymoma extends to the left, the left cardiac border is obscured while the aortic knob is accentuated behind the tumor. Amorphous calcifications may be present. CT scan with contrast demonstrates a soft tissue attenuation mass usually located adjacent to the heart or between the sternum and great vessels (**Fig. 5.24**).

Fig. 5.24a–d Thymoma. Smoothly marginated mass arising from the right anterior mediastinum that abuts the ascending aorta and right atrium.

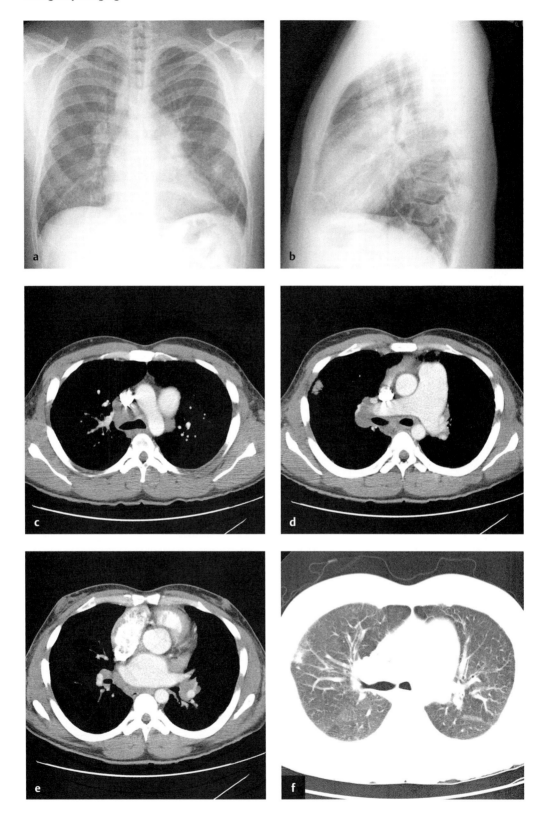

◆ Sarcoidosis

Sarcoidosis is an idiopathic, systemic granulomatous disease that involves the lung in over 90% of cases. Most patients are between the ages of 20 and 40, and there is a slight female predominance, especially among African-American women. Bilateral hilar and right paratracheal lymphadenopathy are the most common and recognizable radiographic findings. Differential considerations should include lymphoma and primary tuberculosis. Increased interstitial markings and interstitial fibrosis may also be present, particularly in the mid- and upper lung fields.

Contrast-enhanced CT can identify peribronchovascular thickening with characteristic mediastinal and hilar lymphadenopathy. Traction bronchiectasis and honeycombing are seen in long-standing pulmonary disease.

Treatment consists primarily of corticosteroids for significant exacerbations or for symptomatic disease. The likelihood of resolution depends on stage of disease at the time of diagnosis. Complications include pulmonary fibrosis, pulmonary arterial hypertension, and aspergillomas (**Fig. 5.25**).

- Stage 0: normal chest radiograph
- Stage I: hilar or mediastinal nodal enlargement only
- Stage II: nodal enlargement and parenchymal disease
- Stage III: parenchymal disease only
- Stage IV: end-stage lung disease (pulmonary fibrosis)

Fig. 5.25a–e   Sarcoidosis. Bilateral hilar and right paratracheal adenopathy. Mild peribronchovascular thickening with scattered peripheral interstitial nodules.

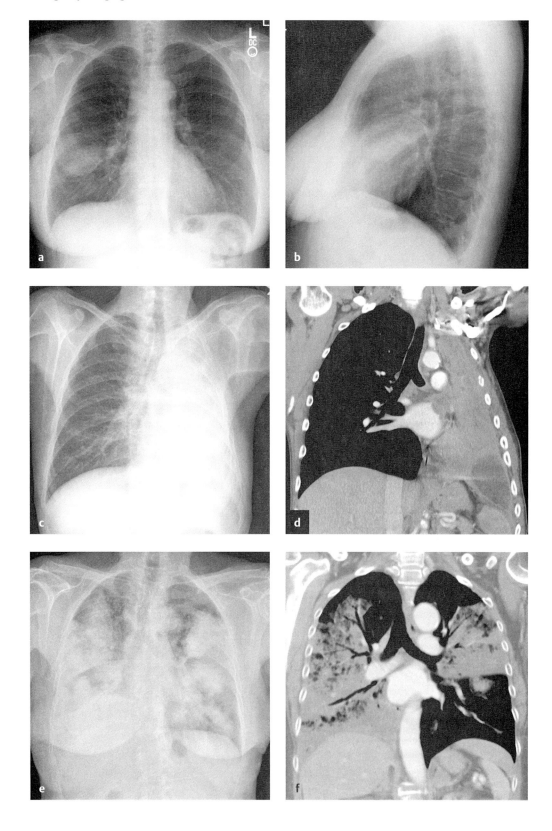

◆ Bronchogenic Carcinoma

Bronchogenic carcinoma is the most common cause of cancer death in both men and women. The primary risk factor is cigarette smoking, which is implicated in most cases. Patients may be asymptomatic or have chronic cough and dyspnea. Pneumonia, hemoptysis, pleuritic chest pain, and lymphadenopathy are other common presentations. Paraneoplastic syndromes seen with bronchogenic carcinoma include syndrome of inappropriate antidiuretic hormone (SIADH), Cushing syndrome, carcinoid syndrome, or hypercalcemia secondary to parathyroid hormone–related protein (PTHrP).

Primary lung malignancies comprise four main histologic subtypes, which are broadly divided into non–small-cell lung cancer (NSCLC) and small-cell carcinoma. NSCLC includes squamous cell carcinoma, adenocarcinoma, and large-cell carcinoma. Each subtype differs in terms of its clinical presentation, radiographic appearance, demographic, treatment, and prognosis.

Several features should raise suspicion for lung cancer on plain film: a lung parenchymal nodule or mass, hilar enlargement, widened mediastinum, or lobar or segmental collapse. Lung nodules appear as round or irregular foci of increased density and measure less than 3 cm. Their CT characteristics can be further described as ground glass, subsolid, or solid. An obstructing endobronchial mass can cause distal atelectasis or pneumonia. When this occurs in the right upper lobe, the concave, atelectatic upper lobe and convex right hilar mass form an edge resembling a reversed "s" (the Golden s sign).

Invasive mucinous adenocarcinoma is the most common subtype of adenocarcinoma of the lung. Characterized by glandular differentiation and mucin production, this variant, formerly termed mucinous bronchioloalveolar cell (BAC) carcinoma, arises from pneumocytes in the walls of the pulmonary alveoli. Patients with these mucoid-producing tumors present with chronic productive cough.

On chest radiograph, invasive mucinous adenocarcinoma may appear as a solid nodule, a partly solid mass, or a lobar or sublobar area of consolidation. This latter is referred to a lobar replacement pattern and appears as ground-glass opacification with air bronchograms and multiple internal cystic lucencies, more commonly seen in advanced disease. Mucin fills alveoli and small bronchi, producing consolidation that has lower attenuation than either pneumonia or atelectasis. Enhancing arterial branches are accentuated against this background of low-density consolidation and produce the "CT angiogram" sign, which is frequently seen in invasive mucinous adenocarcinoma (**Fig. 5.26**).

Fig. 5.26a–f
a,b Bronchogenic carcinoma in patient presenting with cerebral metastasis. Large mass located in the right middle lobe.
c,d Squamous cell carcinoma with left lung atelectasis. Occlusion of the left mainstem bronchus by neoplasm. Complete left lung atelectasis, posterolateral thoracic wall invasion with rib destruction, and loculated pleural fluid collection. The mediastinum is markedly displaced into the left hemithorax.
e,f Invasive mucinous adenocarcinoma. Multifocal air space opacities with prominent air bronchograms correspond to alveolar filling with neoplastic cells and mucoid material.

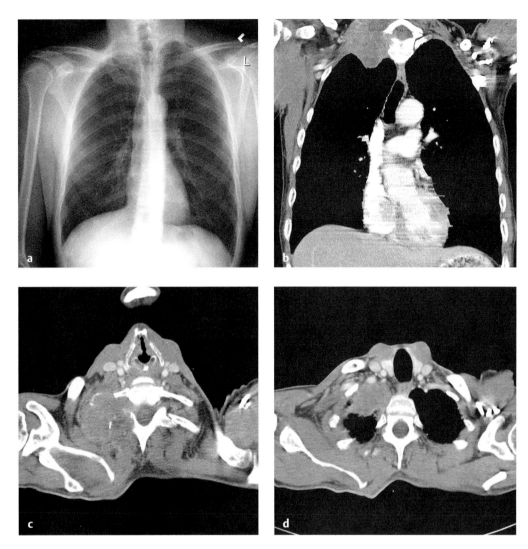

◆ Pancoast Tumor

Pancoast syndrome consists of shoulder pain, radicular pain in the C8-to-T2 distribution, and (variably) an ipsilateral Horner syndrome due to primary bronchogenic carcinoma of the lung apex.

Plain radiographs may show an apical mass or pleural thickening, and lordotic views may be helpful for confirmation or clarification. Local rib erosion or extension into the supraclavicular fossa may be present. CT will confirm a radiographic suspicion and identify any bony involvement but is poor at comprehensively evaluating the extent of soft tissue invasion. MRI, while not necessary for emergent diagnosis, is more accurate for documenting or excluding brachial plexus involvement, which is one feature that determines operability.

Treatment depends on the degree of soft tissue extension and invasion of the brachial plexus and subclavian vessels. Radiotherapy may be used to downstage the tumor in advance of resection, but, as with all lung carcinomas, the overall prognosis is poor (**Fig. 5.27**).

Fig. 5.27a–d Pancoast tumor. Radiograph shows very subtle asymmetry of the lung apices, with increased soft tissue density at the right superior sulcus. CT clearly defines a heterogeneous mass that has eroded an upper thoracic vertebra and extends well into the soft tissues of the lower neck.

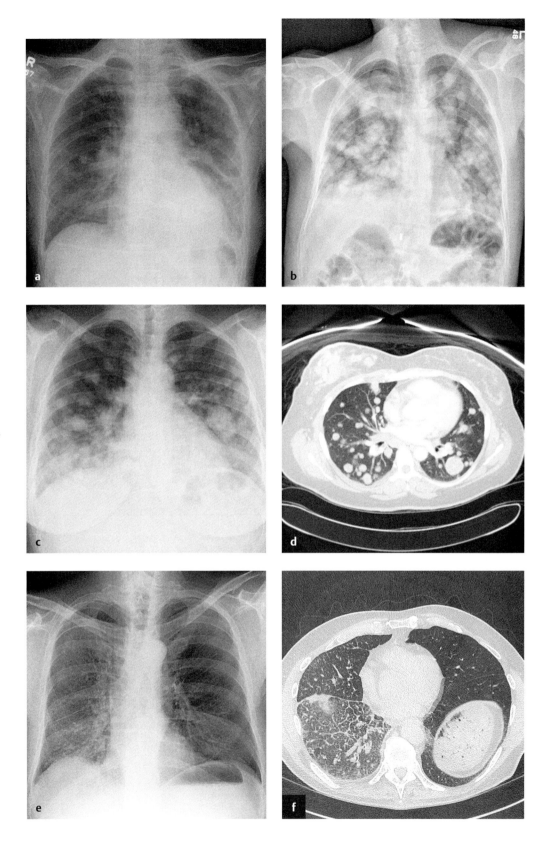

◆ Pulmonary Metastases

Because of its rich systemic venous exposure, the lung is a common site of metastatic disease. Most pulmonary metastases arise from common tumors such as breast, colon, prostate, bronchial, and renal carcinomas. Less common primary tumors that metastasize to the lungs include choriocarcinoma, Ewing sarcoma, osteosarcoma, melanoma, and testicular tumors. Pulmonary metastases per se are usually asymptomatic, and patients present with constitutional disease or symptoms related to the underlying primary malignancy. Hemoptysis and pneumothorax may result from bronchial or pleural invasion.

Metastases are often detected incidentally on chest radiographs obtained for various indications. Nodules vary in size from 5 to 15 mm and are usually multiple. In most patients, nodules less than 5 mm are not dense enough to be appreciated on plain radiographs, and visible nodules smaller than this are likely calcified granulomas, particularly if unchanged from prior radiographs. Nodules smaller than 2 cm are usually smooth and round, whereas larger nodules can be lobulated. Occasionally pulmonary metastases become confluent and form a single multinodular mass. Squamous cell tumors, especially those origi-

nating in the head and neck, may cavitate, and this finding, when present, is more common in the upper lobes. Multiple cavitating masses, however, are more typical of nonmalignant conditions such as Wegener granulomatosis, septic pulmonary emboli, and sarcoidosis.

Lymphangitic carcinomatosis is defined as tumor infiltration of the pulmonary lymphatics; most sources are lung, breast, and colon adenocarcinomas. Radiographs and CT show interstitial thickening, Kerley lines, and sometimes hilar adenopathy, which can be unilateral, focal, or bilateral. The possibility of lymphangitic carcinomatosis causing an interstitial edema pattern should be considered in those patents who have an underlying malignancy.

CT has a higher resolution and may be used to reveal smaller nodules than would be detected by plain radiography. In addition, CT may demonstrate a prominent pulmonary vessel supplying the metastasis, which is termed the "feeding vessel" sign. Malignant melanoma, osteosarcoma, and renal cell and thyroid carcinoma may show a miliary pattern of innumerable small nodules. In most cases, pulmonary spread of malignancy indicates a poor prognosis (**Fig. 5.28**).

Fig. 5.28a–f
a–d Nodular pulmonary metastases. (**a**) Ovarian carcinoma. (**b**) Parotid carcinoma. (**c,d**) Breast carcinoma.
e,f Lymphangitic carcinomatosis. Unilateral reticular and nodular interstitial thickening, mainly involving the right lower lobe.

6
Abdomen and Pelvis

◆ Approach

CT is the primary imaging study for evaluation of most patients with major trauma and acute abdominal pain. In multiorgan trauma, a chest radiograph, pelvis radiograph, and focused abdominal ultrasound are usually performed during initial clinical assessment to determine whether surgical exploration should precede further imaging. In the hemodynamically stable patient, CT is the next step, and several imaging strategies can be pursued depending on the mechanism of injury and clinical findings.

For trauma limited to the head, noncontrast head and cervical spine CT is performed, sometimes with the addition of cranial or neck CTA. Most patients with multiorgan trauma will require head, cervical spine, and abdominal CT. If there is clinical or radiographic evidence of thoracic injury, the chest should be imaged with the abdomen in a single acquisition. Extremity CT can be added for patients with complex orthopedic or vascular injuries.

Noncontrast CT of the head, face, and cervical spine are obtained first, usually in a single helical acquisition. If the chest is to be studied, images are obtained in the arterial phase of contrast enhancement, followed by a pause sufficiently long to image the abdomen and pelvis in the late arterial or early portal venous phase. Oral contrast is not routinely administered in the trauma setting, although oral and/or rectal contrast can be given to evaluate suspected penetrating injuries to the bowel. Delayed (excretory phase) images are valuable for detection of vascular extravasation and renal collecting system injuries.

For nontraumatic abdominal emergencies, ultrasound is used to investigate biliary colic, pelvic pain in women, scrotal pathology in men, suspected appendicitis or intussusception in children, and lower-extremity deep venous thrombosis. For most other acute conditions, CT is performed. Abdominal CT is obtained with intravenous contrast in the portal venous phase and oral contrast administered 45 to 90 minutes prior to the study. Imaging in the arterial phase can be performed to evaluate mesenteric ischemia, aortic dissection, or aneurysm, and can also be used to improve visualization of the pancreas in patients with upper abdominal pain.

Oral contrast is important for bowel visualization but may be omitted if clinical concern is limited to hepatic or pancreatic pathology, in which case water can be substituted immediately before scanning. Scans for hyperemergent conditions such as ruptured aneurysm, aortic dissection, or high-grade bowel obstruction with suspected ischemia should not be delayed for administration of oral contrast. Although it is controversial, some centers forgo the use of oral contrast material for abdominal CT in all emergency patients.

Patients who have had a prior life-threatening adverse reaction to any contrast agent, medication, or allergen should not receive intravenous contrast unless the clinical benefit of imaging with contrast outweighs the risks. Patients with prior anaphylactoid reactions can be premedicated with steroids and antihistamines, which reduce the risk of minor reactions and are presumed to reduce the risk of severe ones. Alternative imaging, such as MRI or ultrasound, should be considered in this group.

Patients with estimated glomerular filtration rate of 30–60 or serum creatinine 1.5–2.0 are at increased risk of contrast-induced renal injury and should receive no more than 75 mL intravenous contrast and 500–1,000 mL oral or intravenous hydration before and after the examination.

Patients with estimated glomerular filtration rate of < 30 or serum creatinine > 2.0 should not receive intravenous contrast unless an alternative study is not possible and the benefits and risks have been reviewed with the referring clinician. The decision to use intravenous contrast should be documented in the patient's chart.

Intravenous contrast is not necessary for investigation of uncomplicated renal colic and evaluation of most osseous abnormalities.

Anatomic Checklists

Radiograph

- Heart and lung bases
- Gas pattern (stomach, small bowel, colon)
- Soft tissues (liver, spleen, kidneys, psoas margins)
- Calcifications (gallstones, renal calculi, calcified masses)
- Bones

Computed Tomography

- Heart
- Lung bases
- Diaphragm
- Liver
- Gallbladder
- Biliary system
- Kidneys
- Adrenal glands
- Pancreas
- Spleen
- Esophagus
- Stomach
- Duodenum
- Small bowel
- Colon
- Appendix

- Mesenteric and retroperitoneal lymph nodes
- Blood vessels
- Spine, pelvis, and musculature
- Bladder
- Uterus and ovaries in women
- Prostate and seminal vesicles in men

Ultrasound

- Liver (including portal and hepatic veins)
- Gallbladder
- Common bile duct
- Kidneys
- Pancreas
- Spleen
- Abdominal aorta
- Bladder

◆ Imaging and Anatomy

Computed Tomography Protocols

Trauma

- Indications: Abdominal trauma.
- Technique: 300–700 mA, 120 kV
- Phase 1: arterial: bolus track to aorta 150 HU (symphysis to pubis)
- Phase 2: venous: 90 seconds (symphysis to pubis)
- Phase 3: delayed: 7 min (symphysis to pubis)—optional
- Oral contrast: none
- IV contrast: 1.5 mL/kg at 4 mL/sec, followed by 20 mL saline
- Images: 4-mm axial with coronal and sagittal reformation
- Approximate radiation dose: 700 mGy

Upper Abdominal Disease

- Indications: Epigastric pain, pancreatic mass, jaundice, cholecystitis.
- Technique: 300–700 mA, 120 kV
- Phase 1: arterial: 40 seconds (upper abdomen only)
- Phase 2: venous: 90 seconds (symphysis to pubis)

- Oral contrast: water (1 liter)
- IV contrast: 1.5 mL/kg at 4 mL/sec
- Images: 4-mm axial with coronal and sagittal reformation
- Approximate radiation dose: 700 mGy

Lower Abdominal Disease

- Indications: Appendicitis, diverticulitis, pelvic pain, acute abdomen.
- Technique: 300–700 mA, 120 kV
- Phase 1: venous: 90 seconds (symphysis to pubis)
- Oral contrast: Dilute diatrizoate meglumine (Gastrografin; 1 liter); water may be substituted for suspected pancreatitis
- IV contrast: 1.5 mL/kg at 3 mL/sec
- Images: 4-mm axial with coronal and sagittal reformation
- Approximate radiation dose: 700 mGy

Mesenteric Ischemia

- Indications: Suspected mesenteric ischemia.
- Technique: 300–700 mA, 120 kV
- Phase 1: arterial: bolus track to aorta 150 HU (symphysis to pubis)
- Phase 2: venous: 90 seconds (symphysis to pubis)
- Oral contrast: water (0.5 liters)
- IV contrast: 1.5 mL/kg at 4 mL/sec, followed by 20 mL saline
- Images: 4-mm axial with coronal and sagittal reformation
- Approximate radiation dose: 700 mGy

Abdominal Aortic Aneurysm or Dissection

- Indications: Suspected abdominal aortic aneurysm or dissection.
- Technique: 300–700 mA, 120 kV
- Phase 1: noncontrast (symphysis to pubis)
- Phase 2: arterial: bolus track to aorta 150 HU (symphysis to pubis)
- Oral contrast: water (0.5 liters)
- IV contrast: 1.5 mL/kg at 4 mL/sec, followed by 20 mL saline

- Images: 4-mm axial with coronal and sagittal reformation
- Approximate radiation dose: 700 mGy (1,600 mGy when combined with chest CT)

Renal Stone

- Indications: Renal colic.
- Technique: 300–700 mA, 120 kV
- Phase 1: noncontrast, prone position (symphysis to pubis)
- Oral contrast: None
- IV contrast: 1.5 mL/kg at 3 mL/sec
- Images: 4-mm axial with coronal and sagittal reformation
- Approximate radiation dose: 700 mGy

Ultrasound Protocols

FAST (Focused Assessment for Trauma)

- Indications: Blunt and penetrating abdominal trauma.
- Probe: Abdominal curvilinear (1–8 MHz)
- Views:
  - Subxiphoid (pericardium)
  - Right upper quadrant (Morrison pouch)
  - Left upper quadrant (perisplenic, left perirenal)
  - Suprapubic (perivesical)

Right Upper Quadrant

- Indications: Cholelithiasis, jaundice, upper abdominal pain.
- Probe: Abdominal curvilinear (1–8 MHz)
- Views:
  - Gallbladder (longitudinal and transverse)
  - Common bile duct/hepatic artery
  - Main portal vein (color and spectral Doppler)
  - Right kidney (longitudinal and transverse)
  - Pancreas (midline transverse)
  - Sonographic Murphy sign (presence or absence)
  - If gallstones are present, image in supine and decubitus positions for mobility

- Measurements:
  - Gallbladder diameter: maximum AP and lateral (normal < 4 cm)
  - Gall bladder wall thickness (normal < 3 mm)
  - Common bile duct (normal < 7 mm)

Renal

- Indications: Hydronephrosis, suspected renal mass, renal calculus.
- Probe: Abdominal curvilinear (1–8 MHz)
- Views:
  - Kidneys (sagittal and transverse, color Doppler of renal hilum)
  - Bladder (show urinary jets at ureteropelvic junction)
  - Prostate (males)
- Measurements:
  - Renal long axis, AP, transverse
  - Diameter of any cyst or mass

Scrotal

- Indications: Pain, mass, hernia.
- Probe: Linear probe (12 MHz or higher)
- Views:
  - Three transverse views of both testes on one image (upper, lower, mid)
  - Three sagittal views of each testicle
  - Epididymis (sagittal and transverse)
  - Color and arterial flow Doppler both testes (sagittal and transverse)
  - Inguinal region ± Valsalva for hernia
- Measurements:
  - Dimensions of each testis

Female Pelvic

- Indications: Pain, mass, hernia.
- Probes: Abdominal curvilinear (1–8 MHz), transvaginal
- Views:
  - Uterus (sagittal and transverse, transabdominal and transvaginal)
  - Endometrium
  - Ovaries with color and arterial flow Doppler
  - Any adnexal masses

- Measurements:
  - Uterus (sagittal and transverse)
  - Endometrium
  - Ovaries
  - Any mass or cyst > 1 cm

Obstetric First Trimester

- Indications: Pain, bleeding.
- Probes: Abdominal curvilinear (1–8 MHz), transvaginal
- Views:
  - Uterus (sagittal and transverse)
  - Gestational sac/yolk sac/embryo
  - Placenta (position)
  - Ovaries with color and arterial flow Doppler
  - Adnexa
- Measurements:
  - Record date of last menstrual period
  - Uterus (sagittal and transverse)
  - Cervical length
  - Ovaries
  - Any ovarian cysts > 1 cm
  - Gestational sac
  - Yolk sac
  - Embryo crown–rump length
  - Fetal heart rate by M-mode (avoid color Doppler)
  - If no heart rate and fetal pole is > 5 mm, check with color Doppler

Lower Extremity Venous Doppler

- Indications: Suspected deep venous thrombosis.
- Probes: Linear probe (5–12 MHz)
- Views:
  - Sagittal with Doppler and augmentation
  - Transverse with compression
  - Common femoral vein
  - Superficial femoral vein (proximal, mid, distal)
  - Popliteal vein
  - Posterior tibial and anterior tibial veins (color Doppler)

Anatomy

Hepatic Segmental and Subsegmental Anatomy

The liver is morphologically divided into a right lobe, left lobe, and caudate lobe. The right and left lobes can be divided into subsegments based on vascular supply and biliary drainage that permit partial hepatic resection for tumor (**Fig. 6.1**).

◆ Clinical Presentations and Differential Diagnosis

Clinical Presentations and Appropriate Initial Studies

Trauma

CT abdomen and pelvis with intravenous contrast.

- Diaphragmatic rupture
- Splenic, renal, or hepatic laceration

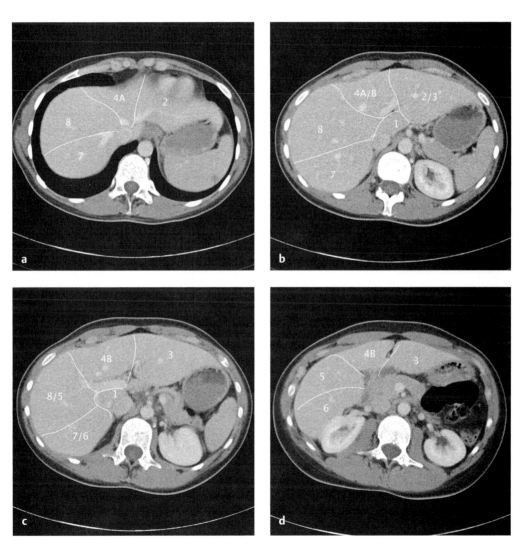

Fig. 6.1a–f
a–d Hepatic anatomy in the axial plane. The right and left lobes are separated by the middle hepatic vein. The left lobe is further subdivided into subsegments 2, 3, 4a, and 4b. The right lobe is subdivided into subsegments 5, 6, 7, and 8. The caudate lobe is segment 1. (**a**) Level of hepatic veins. (**b**) Level of left portal vein. (**c**) Level of right portal vein. (**d**) Inferior liver. (*Continued on page 274*)

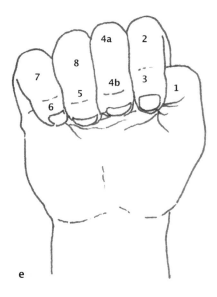

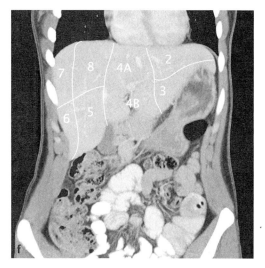

Fig. 6.1a–f (*Continued*)
e,f Hepatic anatomy in the coronal plane. Subsegmental anatomy can be remembered using the hand as a model. The thumb corresponds to segment 1. Subsegments 2–8 form a clockwise loop around the digits, with 4a and b located on the middle finger.

- Bowel contusion/perforation
- Hemoperitoneum
- Retroperitoneal hematoma
- Renal or hepatic arterial pseudoaneurysm
- Renal artery dissection
- Pelvic fracture/hematoma
- Intra- or extraperitoneal bladder rupture
- Spinal fracture

Upper Abdominal Pain

CT abdomen and pelvis with intravenous contrast (oral contrast material is usually not necessary, although water immediately prior to the examination improves gastric and duodenal distension). Ultrasound for biliary colic.

- Cholelithiasis/cholecystitis
- Gastritis
- Gastric or duodenal ulcer
- Pancreatitis
- Biliary obstruction
- Hepatic abscess
- Thoracic pathology
- Subphrenic abscess

Lower Abdominal Pain

CT abdomen and pelvis with intravenous and oral contrast.

- Appendicitis
- Diverticulitis
- Small-bowel obstruction
- Large-bowel obstruction
- Inflammatory bowel disease (ulcerative colitis, Crohn disease)
- Infectious enteritis/colitis
- Epiploic appendagitis/omental infarct
- Urolithiasis
- Colon carcinoma
- Abscess
- Pelvic inflammatory disease
- Ruptured or torsed ovarian cyst

Differential Diagnosis: CT

Pneumoperitoneum

- Recent surgery
- Peritoneal dialysis
- Perforated gastric ulcer
- Perforated duodenal ulcer
- Perforated diverticulitis

Gasless Abdomen on Plain Radiograph

- Proximal obstruction
- Ascites
- Vomiting
- Normal variation

Stomach Mass

- Malignant neoplasm (adenocarcinoma, lymphoma, gastrointestinal stromal tumor, metastasis)
- Leiomyoma
- Lipoma
- Bezoar (intraluminal)
- Hyperplastic, adenomatous, or hamartomatous polyp

Diffuse Gastric Wall Thickening

- Gastritis
- Pancreatitis
- Crohn disease
- Lymphoma

Diffuse Duodenal Wall Thickening or Mass

- Duodenitis
- Adenocarcinoma
- Lymphoma
- Metastasis
- Crohn disease
- Duodenal diverticulum
- Hematoma

Enhancing Small-Bowel Wall

- Shock bowel (avid mucosal enhancement)
- Inflammatory bowel disease
- Malignant neoplasm (adenocarcinoma, lymphoma, gastrointestinal stromal tumor, metastasis)
- Radiation enteritis

Concentric Enhancement (Halo or Target Signs): Almost Always Nonmalignant

- Inflammatory bowel disease
- Infectious enteritis
- Ischemic enteritis
- Vasculitis
- Angioedema
- Radiation

Focal Small-Bowel Wall Thickening

- Neoplasm (adenocarcinoma, lymphoma, gastrointestinal stromal tumor, metastasis)
- Perforation
- Crohn disease
- Diverticulitis

Segmental Small-Bowel Wall Thickening

- Crohn disease
- Enteritis
- Ischemia
- Lymphoma
- Hemorrhage

Diffuse Small-Bowel Wall Thickening

- Enteritis
- Ischemia
- Hypoalbuminemia
- Vasculitis

Terminal Ileal Wall Thickening/Inflammation

- Inflammatory bowel disease
- Tuberculosis
- Bacterial infection
- Lymphoma

Diffuse Colitis

- Pseudomembranous colitis
- Ulcerative colitis
- Other infectious colitis

Right-Sided Colitis

- Crohn disease
- Neutropenic enterocolitis
- Tuberculosis
- *Salmonella*
- *Yersinia*

Left-Sided Colitis

- Ulcerative colitis (contiguous, distal)
- Ischemic colitis (splenic flexure, sigmoid, tends to spare rectum)
- Diverticulitis

Cecal Mass

- Appendicitis
- Cecal carcinoma
- Appendiceal mucocele

Intestinal Pneumatosis

- Ischemia
- Obstruction
- Toxic megacolon
- Idiopathic (usually limited to colon)
- Postendoscopy
- Corticosteroids
- Chemotherapy

"Misty" Mesentery

- Pancreatitis
- Cholecystitis
- Diverticulitis
- Congestive heart failure
- Peritoneal carcinomatosis
- Lymphoma
- Sclerosing mesenteritis

Biliary Dilatation

- Age-related
- Postsurgical
- Cholangiocarcinoma
- Ampullary carcinoma
- Gallbladder carcinoma
- Pancreatic carcinoma
- Hepatic metastases
- Porta hepatis adenopathy
- Common duct stone
- Stricture
- Mirizzi syndrome (stone in cystic duct)
- Bile duct cyst

Gallbladder Wall Thickening (> 3 mm)

- Cholecystitis
- Hepatitis
- Hypoalbuminemia
- Cirrhosis
- Congestive heart failure
- Renal failure

Biliary System Gas

- Sphincterotomy
- Gallstone passage
- Age-related
- Postoperative
- Biliary enteric fistula
- Emphysematous cholecystitis (if air involves gallbladder wall)

Portal Venous Gas

- Bowel infarction
- Diverticulitis

Hepatomegaly

- Hepatoma
- Metastases
- Lymphoma
- Right-sided heart failure
- Hepatitis

Hepatic Lesion: Low Attenuation on Nonenhanced CT

- Hepatocellular carcinoma
- Adenoma
- Hemangioma
- Focal nodular hyperplasia
- Metastases
- Cyst
- Abscess

Hepatic Lesion: Arterial Phase Enhancing

- Hepatoma
- Hemangioma
- Focal nodular hyperplasia
- Adenoma
- Metastasis

Hepatic Lesion: Portal Venous Phase Enhancing

- Hepatoma
- Venous collaterals

Hepatic Lesion: Delayed (Equilibrium) Phase Enhancing

- Hemangioma
- Cholangiocarcinoma
- Treated metastases

Low-Attenuation Liver on Noncontrast CT

- Fatty infiltration
- Diffuse hepatoma or metastases
- Budd-Chiari syndrome
- Amyloid

Splenomegaly

- Portal hypertension
- Hemolytic anemias
- Leukemia/lymphoma
- Myelofibrosis
- Malaria
- Storage diseases
- Sarcoidosis
- Amyloidosis
- Mononucleosis and other infections

Splenic Lesion

- Lymphoma
- Metastases
- Hamartoma
- Hemangioma
- Sarcoid
- Developmental or posttraumatic cyst
- Abscess

Cystic Pancreatic Mass

- Pseudocyst
- Intraductal papillary mucinous neoplasm
- Cystadenoma
- Simple cyst
- Metastasis
- Abscess

Solid Pancreatic Mass

- Adenocarcinoma
- Focal pancreatitis
- Metastasis
- Islet cell tumor
- Solid and papillary epithelial tumors

Solid Renal Mass

- Renal cell carcinoma
- Oncocytoma
- Angiomyolipoma
- Metastasis
- Abscess
- Infarct

Cystic Renal Mass

- Simple cyst
- Complex cyst
- Renal cell carcinoma (mixed solid/cystic)
- Abscess

Pelvic Mass

- Ovarian cyst (simple, hemorrhagic, corpus luteum)
- Ovarian neoplasm
- Tubo-ovarian abscess
- Uterine neoplasm
- Rectal or sigmoid carcinoma
- Prostate carcinoma
- Bladder carcinoma

Differential Diagnosis: Ultrasound

Enlarged Ovary

- Ovarian torsion
- Ovarian neoplasm
- Tubo-ovarian abscess
- Hemorrhagic cyst

Hyperechoic Hepatic Mass

- Hemangioma
- Focal fatty infiltration
- Metastasis
- Hepatocellular carcinoma
- Focal nodular hyperplasia
- Hepatic adenoma

Hypoechoic Hepatic Mass

- Hepatocellular carcinoma
- Abscess
- Focal fatty sparing

"Starry Sky" Liver

- Acute hepatitis
- Hepatocellular carcinoma
- Diffuse metastatic disease
- Hepatic congestion
- Biliary or portal venous gas

Portal Vein Thrombosis

- Cirrhosis
- Hepatocellular carcinoma
- Diffuse metastatic disease
- Hypercoagulable state
- Periportal infection

Common Bile Duct Dilatation

- Choledocholithiasis
- Chronic pancreatitis
- Obstructing pancreatic or biliary malignancy
- Cholangitis

Gallbladder Wall Thickening

- Acute cholecystitis
- Wall edema (hydration, congestive heart failure)
- Hepatitis
- HIV
- Gallbladder carcinoma
- Adenomyomatosis

Hyperechoic Renal Mass

- Angiomyolipoma
- Renal cell carcinoma
- Complex cyst

Hypoechoic Renal Mass

- Simple cyst
- Lymphoma
- Renal abscess
- Renal cell carcinoma

Extratesticular Fluid Collection

- Hydrocele
- Varicocele
- Hematocele
- Pyocele

Adnexal Mass

- Ectopic pregnancy (+ beta-hCG)
- Corpus luteum cyst
- Hemorrhagic cyst
- Tubo-ovarian abscess
- Endometrioma
- Ovarian neoplasm

Enlarged Painless Testicle

- Testicular neoplasm
- Lymphoma/leukemia
- Intratesticular cyst

Enlarged Painful Testicle

- Orchitis/epididymitis
- Torsion
- Trauma (hematoma/fracture)

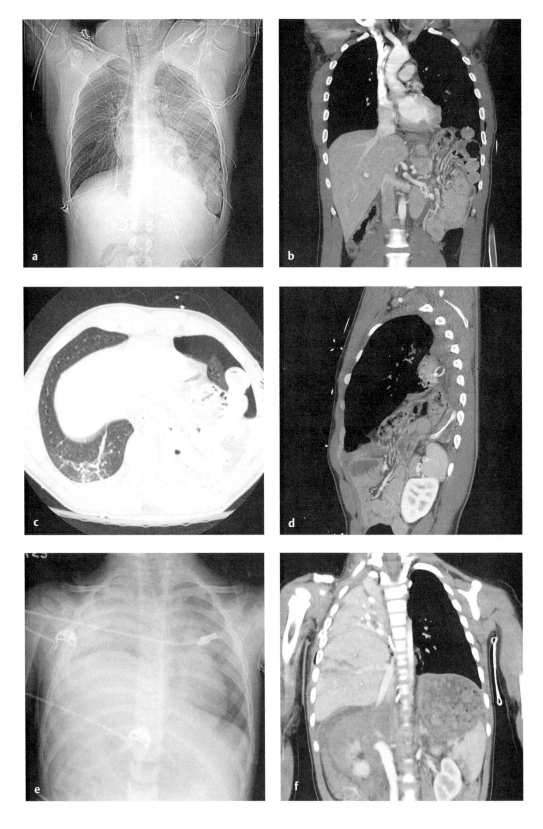

◆ Diaphragm Rupture

Blunt impact to the abdomen can cause an abrupt elevation of intra-abdominal pressure and result in diaphragmatic rupture. Abdominal viscera can herniate through the defect, with acute or delayed bowel obstruction. Penetrating trauma to the back or upper abdomen can also result in diaphragm laceration. In both cases, the diagnosis can be missed or delayed, especially in patients who are placed on assisted ventilation immediately after resuscitation. Because positive intrathoracic pressure serves to prevent visceral herniation through any small diaphragmatic defect, the integrity of the diaphragm should be directly assessed, particularly in the ventilated patient. Remote diaphragmatic injury is a consideration in any patient with acute bowel obstruction and a past history of significant torso trauma.

Sagittal and coronal CT reformations best evaluate the diaphragm. Direct imaging signs of rupture or laceration include diaphragmatic discontinuity, waistlike constriction of herniated viscus (collar sign), and the dependent viscera sign, in which abdominal viscera appear to contact the posterior thoracic wall. Indirect findings include diaphragmatic thickening, injury on both sides of the diaphragm, or hemothorax without obvious thoracic injury, all of which indicate potential rupture. Penetrating injuries are less likely than blunt injuries to result in organ herniation, as the diaphragmatic defect is smaller (1 cm for penetrating injury compared with 5–6 cm in blunt trauma) (**Fig. 6.2**).

Fig. 6.2a–f
a–d Traumatic left-sided diaphragm rupture. (**a**) CT scout shows left thoracostomy tube, small pneumothorax, and lobulated mass in the left lower thorax. The nasogastric tube is looped and superimposed on the cardiac shadow. (**b–d**) Multiplanar CT shows herniated small-bowel loops in left posterior hemithorax. The stomach, which contains a looped NG tube, is apposed against the posterior thoracic wall.
e,f Hepatic herniation through ruptured diaphragm. Markedly elevated apparent right hemidiaphragm (plain radiograph). Discontinuous right hemidiaphragm with displacement of the liver into the right hemithorax, hepatic laceration, and compressive atelectasis of right lung.

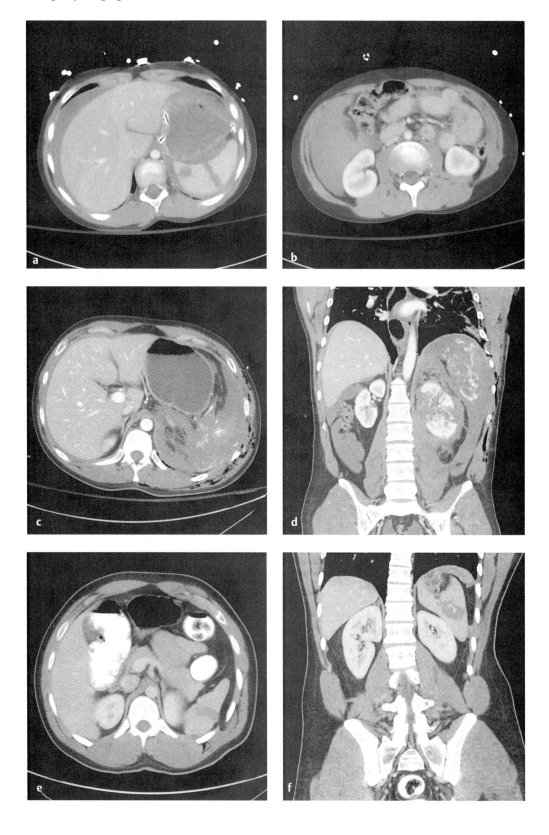

◆ Splenic Injury

Splenic hematoma, laceration, devascular- ization, or frank rupture are potential con- sequences of blunt or penetrating injuries to the left torso. In patients with mono- nucleosis, the spleen is often enlarged and predisposed to rupture in minor abdomi- nal trauma. Patients may present follow- ing trauma with diffuse abdominal pain or left upper quadrant tenderness. Associated left shoulder pain is referred to as the Kehr sign. Leukocytosis and hyperamylasemia may also be seen. Hemodynamic stability, rather than grade of injury, directs initial management and surgical decision making.

During initial evaluation and resuscita- tion, FAST (Focused Assessment with So- nography in Trauma) quickly identifies any intraperitoneal hemorrhage or obvious visceral injury. Contrast-enhanced CT scan is the most accurate test for evaluating the spleen and should be obtained in the he- modynamically stable patient.

On CT, lacerations appear as nonen- hancing linear or jagged lesions, often at the splenic periphery. They are associated with pericapsular or subcapsular hemato- mas, a crescent-shaped soft tissue–attenu- ation fluid collection. This finding permits differentiation from splenic clefts, a nor- mal variant. Splenic hematomas appear as low-attenuation intrasplenic masses. Acute contrast extravasation, particularly if increased on 5-minute delayed images, indicates active hemorrhage. Splenic ar- tery pseudoaneurysms are contained vas- cular injuries that appear as small round or oval lesions with attenuation identical to that of other arteries on postcontrast studies. Extravasation and pseudoaneu- rysm are indications for emergent visceral arteriography.

Most classification systems grade splen- ic injury based on the size and location of subcapsular or parenchymal hematoma, length and depth of any laceration, and the presence or absence of active bleeding. In- juries that involve the vascular hilum may require embolization or splenectomy to control hemorrhage. Absent life-threaten- ing hemorrhage, trauma surgeons increas- ingly prefer nonoperative management for splenic salvage. The American Association for the Surgery of Trauma (AAST) grading for splenic injury can be seen in **Table 6.1**.

Depending on hemodynamic stability, most grade I–III injuries, as well as some of higher grade, can be managed nonopera- tively. Grade IV and V injuries may require either arteriography/embolization or sple- nectomy (**Fig. 6.3**).

Table 6.1   AAST (American Association for the Surgery of Trauma) Grading for Splenic Injury

I	Subcapsular hematoma involving < 10% of surface area, or laceration < 1 cm depth
II	Subcapsular hematoma involving 10–50% of surface area, intraparenchymal hematoma < 5 cm in diameter, or laceration 1–3 cm in depth not involving trabecular vessels
III	Subcapsular hematoma involving > 50% of surface area, intraparenchymal hematoma > 5 cm, any expanding hematoma, laceration > 3 cm depth or involving trabecular vessels, or ruptured subcap- sular or parenchymal hematoma
IV	Laceration involving segmental or hilar vessels with > 25% devascularization
V	Shattered spleen or hilar vascular injury with devascularization

Fig. 6.3a–f
a,b Blunt trauma, AAST grade III splenic injury. 5-cm laceration extending to splenic hilum with extensive hemoperitoneum.
c,d Blunt trauma, grade V injury. Shattered spleen with associated grade V renal injury and extensive hemoperitoneum.
e,f Stab wound to flank, grade III injury. Laceration with no subcapsular hematoma or hemoperitoneum.

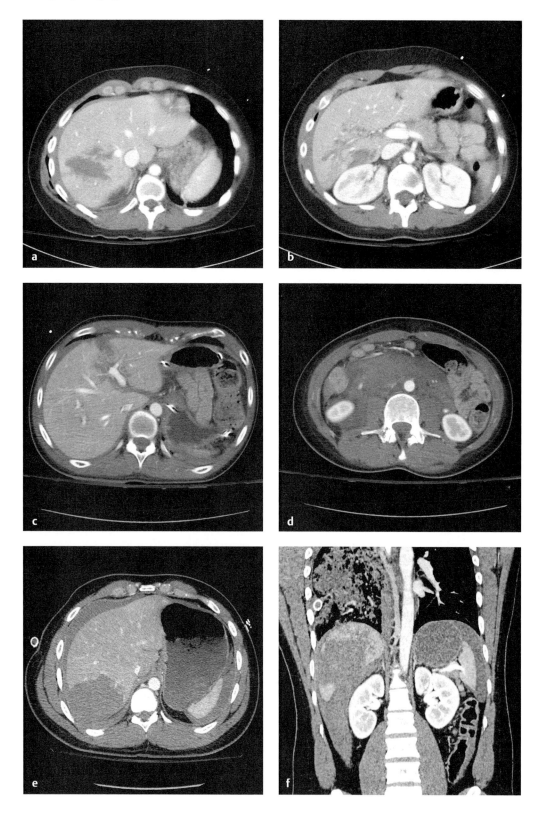

◆ Hepatic Injury

The liver is the second most frequently injured organ in the abdomen, and hepatic injury is the most common cause of death in abdominal trauma. Blunt injuries include subcapsular or intraparenchymal hematoma, contusion, capsular disruption, laceration, and biliary disruption. Penetrating injuries from stab or gunshot wounds are usually managed nonoperatively or by angioembolization.

Contrast-enhanced CT localizes and characterizes parenchymal injury and detects other associated visceral injuries. As in the case of splenic injury, angiography and embolization are indicated for active extravasation or hepatic artery pseudoaneurysm. Similarly, the decision to operate or observe is dictated by the patient's hemodynamic stability, the presence of active extravasation, or a decreasing hematocrit. Nonoperative management is generally preferred. High-grade injuries (IV–VI) should, if managed nonoperatively, be reimaged in 7 to 10 days, or sooner if there is a change in the patient's clinical status. AAST grading for hepatic injury can be seen in **Table 6.2** (**Fig. 6.4**).

Table 6.2   AAST Grading for Hepatic Injury

I	Subcapsular hematoma < 10% surface area or capsular tear < 1 cm depth
II	Subcapsular hematoma 10–50% surface area, intraparenchymal hematoma < 10 cm diameter, or capsular tear, 1–3 cm depth and < 10 cm length
III	Subcapsular hematoma >50% surface area, active bleeding, intraparenchymal hematoma > 10 cm diameter, or capsular tear > 3 cm depth
IV	Intraparenchymal hematoma with active bleeding, parenchymal disruption involving either 25–75% hepatic lobes or 1–3 Couinaud segments within one lobe
V	Parenchymal disruption involving > 75% of one hepatic lobe or > 3 Couinaud segments within one lobe, inferior vena cava laceration, or hepatic vein laceration
VI	Hepatic avulsion

Fig. 6.4a–f
a,b   Grade II–III hepatic laceration, right lobe. ~ 8 cm laceration involving hepatic segments 5–8 (right hepatic lobe). Minimal perihepatic hematoma without active hemorrhage.
c,d   Grade III hepatic laceration, left lobe. Laceration involving the junction of the right and left hepatic lobes. Large associated mesenteric hematoma and hyperenhancing (shock) bowel.
e,f   Hepatic parenchymal hematoma. Peripheral hematoma involving hepatic segments 5–8 (right hepatic lobe). Large amount of perihepatic and perisplenic intraperitoneal hemorrhage.

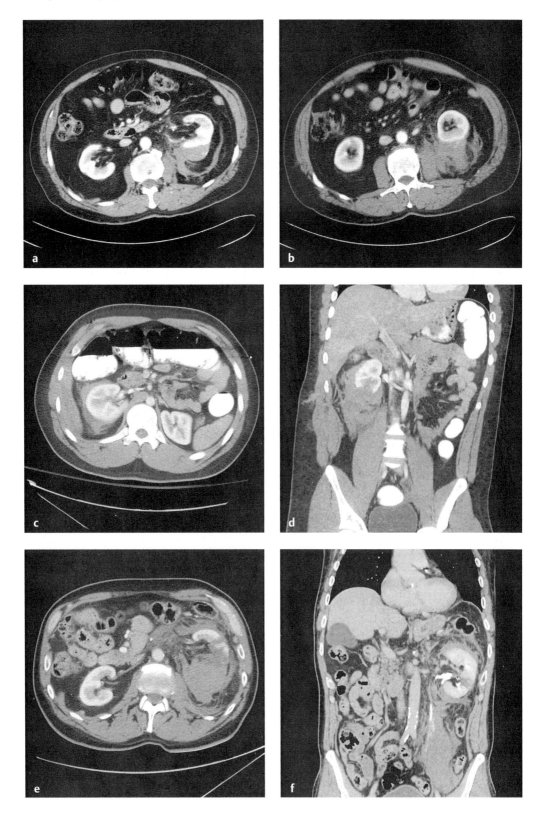

◆ Renal Injury

Most renal injuries are due to blunt trauma, and concomitant visceral or skeletal injuries are often present. CT identifies subcapsular and parenchymal hematomas (contusion), renal lacerations, arterial extravasation, pseudoaneurysms, and collecting system injury. If a renal abnormality is found on initial workstation review, delayed images through the kidneys and collecting system should be obtained to detect arterial or urine extravasation.

Renal contusions are poorly defined, round, or ovoid low-attenuation areas and should be distinguished from renal infarcts, which are sharply delineated, usually peripheral, and wedge-shaped. Subcapsular hematomas are elliptical hemorrhages interposed between the renal capsule and the kidney parenchyma.

Major injuries comprise approximately 10% of renal injuries and include lacerations that extend from the cortex to the collecting system, multiple renal lacerations (known as shattered kidney), segmental infarcts, and vascular injury to the renal pedicle (often with active hemorrhage).

Sudden deceleration can disrupt the ureteropelvic or ureterovesical junctions. Surgical mishap, ureteroscopy, gunshot, and penetrating trauma are other causes. Disruption of the collecting system is confirmed by detecting contrast medial to the kidney or along the course of the ureter, and injuries are classified as complete (avulsion) or incomplete (laceration). Consequences of delayed diagnosis include urinoma, abscess, and stricture. AAST grading for renal injury is seen in **Table 6.3**.

All grade I and II injuries and 90% of grade III and IV injuries are managed conservatively. Grade V injuries usually require nephrectomy (**Fig. 6.5**).

Table 6.3 AAST Grading for Renal Injury

I	Hematuria with normal kidney, renal contusion or nonexpanding subcapsular hematoma
II	Nonexpanding perirenal hematoma, confined to the retroperitoneum. Laceration < 1 cm in depth, no urinary extravasation
III	Laceration > 1 cm parenchymal depth, without collecting system rupture or urinary extravasation
IV	Laceration through renal cortex, medulla, and collecting system; renal artery or vein injury with contained hemorrhage
V	Completely shattered kidney; renal hilum avulsion with devascularized kidney

Fig. 6.5a–f
a,b Subcapsular hematoma (grade II). Left subcapsular and inferior posterior perirenal hematoma confined to the retroperitoneum. No parenchymal laceration.
c,d Stab wound to flank with renal laceration (grade III). 2-cm inferior renal laceration with retroperitoneal hematoma.
e,f Collecting system disruption (grade IV–V). Initial axial shows large parenchymal hematoma. Delayed coronal image shows contrast and urine extravasation inferomedial to the kidney.

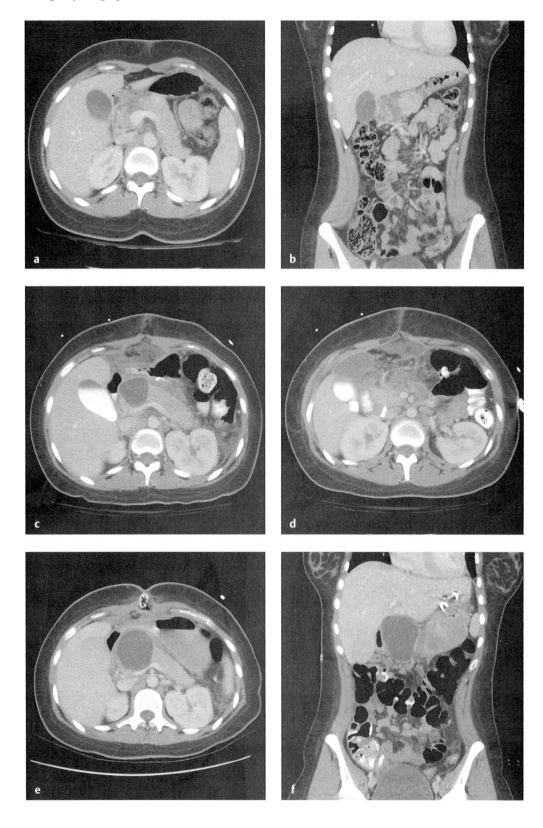

◆ Pancreatic Trauma

Traumatic pancreatic injuries are rare, but missed or delayed diagnosis can result in significant morbidity and mortality. In blunt trauma with rapid deceleration, the midbody of the pancreas can be compressed against the spine and contused or transected. Unrestrained drivers and bicyclists who hit handlebars are both at particular risk for this injury. Patients may have few symptoms at presentation, and initial CT scans can even be normal. However, even in apparently minor injuries, symptoms can develop after several days as digestive pancreatic enzymes are released into retroperitoneal tissues.

Ultrasonography is of limited utility in the acute setting for evaluation of pancreatic injuries, but if performed, it may show hypoechoic defects within the parenchyma. CT is much more sensitive for detection of pancreatic injuries and reveals focal or diffuse edema, low-attenuation lesions, peripancreatic fluid, fat stranding, retroperitoneal hematoma, or combinations of these findings.

One should specifically examine the main pancreatic duct to assess for transection, as such injuries often require endoscopic retrograde cholangiopancreatography (ERCP) with stent placement. In other cases of pancreatic injury, surgical intervention may be required.

Complications of pancreatic trauma include pancreatitis, fistula, retroperitoneal abscess, pseudoaneurysm, or pseudocyst formation (**Fig. 6.6**).

Fig. 6.6a–f
a,b Isolated pancreatic injury following a bicycle accident, initial examination. Well-defined low-attenuation lesion at junction of head and body of pancreas. Minimal associated peripancreatic edema. The pancreatic duct is not visible. Liver, kidneys, and spleen are normal.
c,d Intra-abdominal fluid collections 2 weeks after injury. Intrapancreatic collection at the site of pancreas fracture and multiple intraperitoneal fluid collections, several of which required surgical/interventional drainage.
e,f Pseudocyst formation 8 weeks after injury. The intrapancreatic collection remains well defined, consistent with pseudocyst formation. Abscess drainage catheters are located between the stomach and left hepatic lobe and deep to the umbilicus.

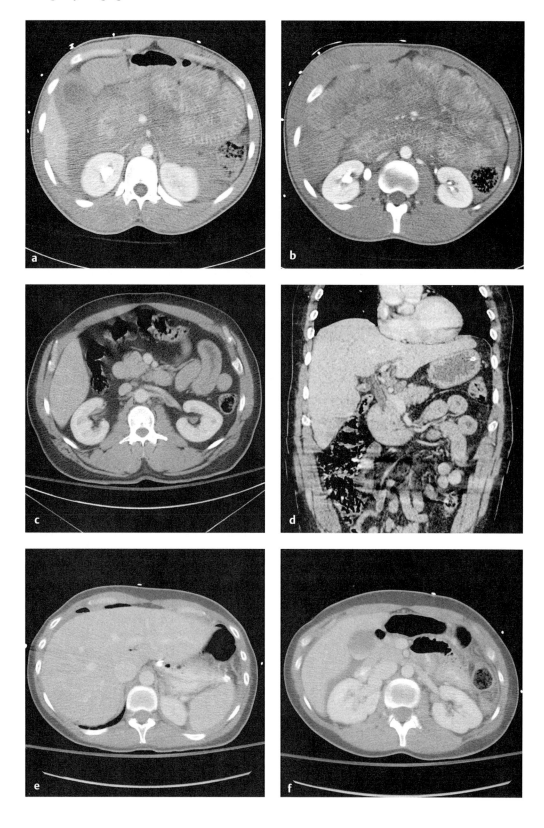

◆ Shock Bowel and Small-Bowel Injury

The term *shock bowel* describes the intestinal CT findings seen in those trauma patients who are initially hypotensive and hypovolemic. Shock bowel is characterized by diffuse small-bowel wall thickening; fluid-filled, dilated small-bowel loops; and pronounced mucosal enhancement. The large bowel, in contrast, usually appears normal. Other visceral manifestations of hypotension include a flattened inferior vena cava (IVC), small-caliber aorta, and intense renal enhancement, the latter due to hypoperfusion. These generally resolve completely with effective fluid management.

Small-bowel injuries are often clinically subtle. Distracting injuries, intoxication, and depressed consciousness limit the sensitivity of physical examination. Free fluid may be missed on initial FAST examination, and peritoneal signs may be delayed. Witnessed or suspected abdominal impact and abdominal wall bruising should raise suspicion for bowel contusion or other gastrointestinal injury.

CT has decreased the historic need for exploratory laparotomies after blunt abdominal trauma and should be obtained in any stable patient. Focal small-bowel thickening indicates a probable contusion, and a discrete intramural or mesenteric hematoma may also be seen. Underdistended bowel can have a similar appearance.

The consequences of small-bowel laceration are blood loss and peritoneal contamination. Spillage of the intestinal contents into the abdomen ultimately produces a suppurative peritonitis that may take up to 8 hours to manifest clinically, or longer if the patient is unconscious or sedated. Concomitant mesenteric and visceral injuries are often present.

Pneumoperitoneum, oral contrast extravasation, bowel wall discontinuity, or mesenteric vascular extravasation indicate urgent operative exploration. In contrast to most solid organ injuries (e.g., spleen or liver), which are often observed, bowel perforation must be managed surgically.

Small amounts of free fluid, bowel wall thickening, mesenteric stranding, and bowel mucosal enhancement are suggestive findings, and surgery should be considered if two or more of these are present. In penetrating trauma, such as stab wounds, small amounts of extraluminal gas are nonspecific and can be due to air from the wound tract (**Fig. 6.7**).

Fig. 6.7a–f
a,b Shock bowel (two patients). The small bowel wall is diffusely edematous with dramatic mucosal enhancement, most pronounced in the proximal small bowel. In both cases, the inferior vena cava is flattened and the kidneys enhance intensely into the excretory phase. Intraperitoneal and intramesenteric fluid are present.
c,d Small-bowel injury. Thickened proximal small-bowel loops with the appearance of "Cheerios" in transverse section.
e,f Small-bowel laceration. Free intraperitoneal air and fluid interposed between the duodenum and gallbladder.

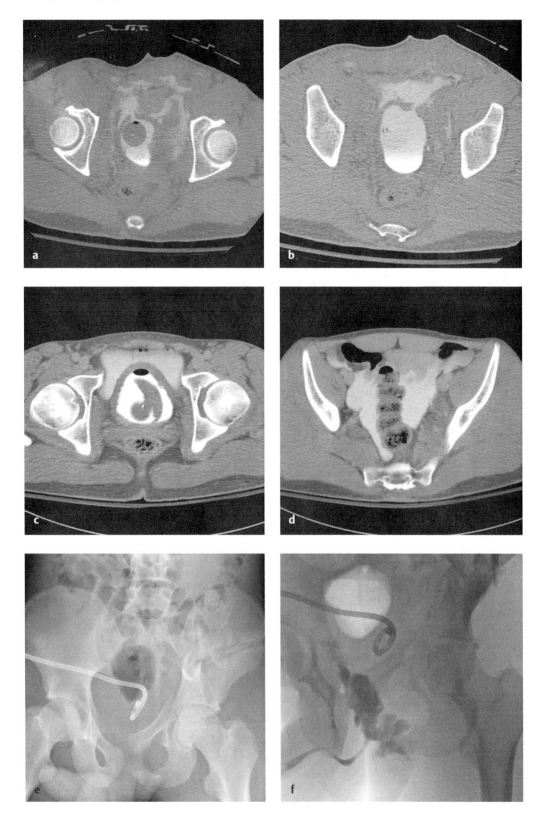

◆ Bladder and Urethral Injury

Bladder injury in abdominal trauma is indicated by suprapubic pain, inability to void, gross hematuria, or microscopic hematuria greater than 25 red blood cells (RBC)/high-power field. Most injuries result from blunt external impact, frequently in conjunction with pelvic fractures.

Bladder rupture is classified as extraperitoneal, intraperitoneal, or combined intra- and extraperitoneal. Most are extraperitoneal and result from shearing forces that deform the pelvic ring or direct puncture by pelvic bone fragments. If the bladder laceration is below the peritoneal reflection, urine extravasation is limited to the extraperitoneal space. Intraperitoneal extravasation results from disruption of the bladder dome, above the peritoneal reflection, and is often due to a direct blow to the lower abdomen in patients with a distended bladder. Intraperitoneal rupture tends to occur in intoxicated patients and belted passengers in motor vehicle accidents.

Bladder contusions and mural bladder hematomas are relatively benign and are diagnoses of exclusion. The bladder may appear normal or teardrop-shaped on cystography; management is conservative with observation for resolution of hematuria.

Standard abdominal CT scanning for trauma readily identifies perivesical fluid or pelvic fractures adjacent to the bladder, but it is insensitive for detection of small leaks.

A dedicated CT or plain film cystogram, in which contrast is directly instilled into the bladder via a Foley catheter, more accurately excludes small bladder ruptures. In severe polytrauma requiring immediate laparotomy, cystography is usually bypassed, and the bladder is directly evaluated intraoperatively.

Urethral injuries, while uncommon, contribute to significant long-term morbidity from complications including impotence, stricture formation, urinary retention, or incontinence. They most commonly involve the posterior urethra and are seen less frequently in women, primarily because of shorter urethral length. In blunt trauma, posterior urethral injury is almost always associated with pelvic fractures. Anterior urethral injuries (penile, bulbar urethra) are more frequently due to blunt trauma to the perineum (straddle injuries) and may present years later with complications from stricture formation.

The male patient with pelvic trauma who presents with gross hematuria, blood at the urethral meatus, edema or hematoma of the perineum or penis, or with a "high-riding" or boggy prostate after a pelvic fracture is likely to have a urethral injury. In these patients, a retrograde urethrogram should be performed prior to the insertion of a Foley catheter, which could enlarge a laceration or contaminate a previously sterile hematoma (**Fig. 6.8**).

Fig. 6.8a–f
a,b Extraperitoneal bladder rupture. Contrast fills the prevesical space via two anterior defects in the bladder wall.
c,d Intraperitoneal bladder rupture. Contrast is present in the bladder and surrounds the sigmoid colon in the peritoneal cavity. A large clot is evident in the bladder.
e,f Traumatic urethral disruption. (**e**) Open book–type pelvis fracture with left acetabular, iliac, and superior and inferior pubic ramus fractures and pubic symphysis diastasis. (**f**) Retrograde urethrogram showing extravasation of contrast material into extraperitoneal space without any filling of the urinary bladder.

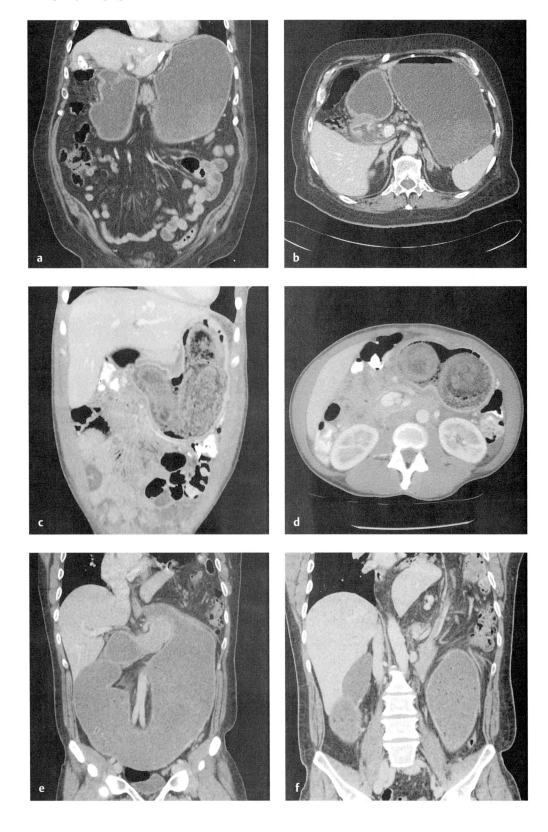

◆ Gastric Ulcer/Gastric Outlet Obstruction

Causes of mechanical gastric outlet obstruction include pyloric or distal gastric malignancy, peptic ulcer disease, gastric polyps, diaphragmatic hernia, caustic ingestion and scarring, pancreatic pseudocysts, and bezoars. Delayed gastric emptying (gastroparesis) can result in distention and is most often due to diabetes, Parkinson disease, or multiple sclerosis. In both extrinsic and intrinsic obstruction, patients present with intermittent symptoms of vomiting and nausea, which worsen until obstruction is complete. Initially, patients tolerate liquids better than solid food. Progressive obstruction may lead to dehydration, electrolyte abnormalities, and malnutrition. Congenital pyloric stenosis occurs in infants aged 2–6 weeks who develop projectile vomiting after feeding.

Plain abdominal radiographs, upper GI contrast studies with Gastrografin or barium, and CT with oral contrast show gastric dilatation and contrast within an enlarged stomach and can identify gastric neoplasm, ulceration, and adenopathy.

Bezoars are concretions of ingested vegetable matter (phytobezoar) or hair (trichobezoar) that accumulate in the stomach and can form an obstructing cast. Poor gastric motility, as well as ingestion of indigestible plant fiber, can predispose to phytobezoars. Trichobezoars are seen in patients with psychiatric disorders due to compulsive hair pulling and ingestion. Radiographs show an enlarged gastric outline with a mottled intragastric mass. On barium studies, the bezoar is visible as an intraluminal filling defect that is not attached to the bowel wall. Delayed imaging is helpful, as barium is often trapped within the mass for hours. CT shows an intragastric mass with mixed density due to entrapped air and food in the bezoar's interstices (**Fig. 6.9**).

Fig. 6.9a–f
a,b Gastric outlet obstruction due to antral ulcer. The stomach is distended due to pyloric edema associated with a small ulcer. The small bowel and large bowel are collapsed.
c,d Gastric outlet obstruction due to trichobezoar. The stomach is obstructed at the pylorus by a heterogeneous intraluminal gastric mass containing innumerable tiny air pockets due to compulsive hair ingestion.
e,f Gastric outlet obstruction due to diaphragmatic hernia. The duodenum and proximal small bowel have herniated through a diaphragmatic defect, resulting in massive gastric dilatation from obstruction just distal to the antrum.

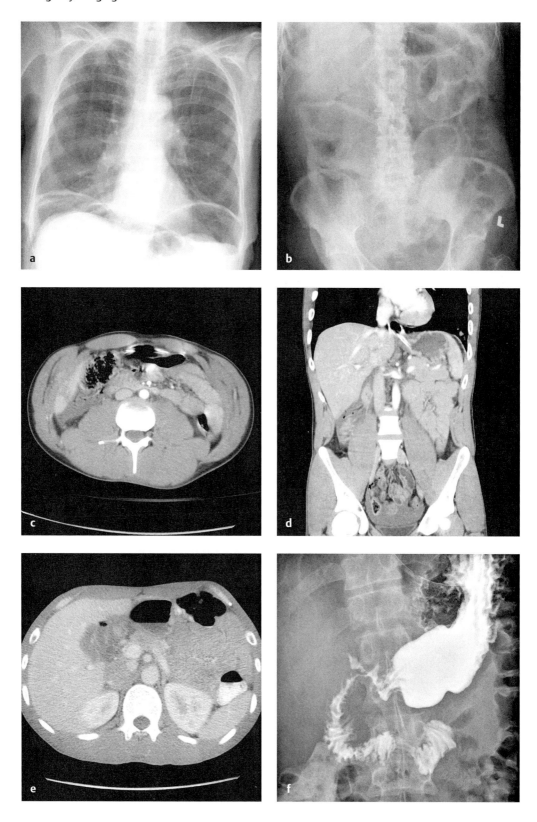

◆ Duodenal Perforation

Duodenal perforation is usually a consequence of peptic ulcer disease, but it can also result from blunt abdominal trauma and can complicate endoscopy or other instrumentation. In peptic ulcer disease, duodenal perforation is two to three times as common as gastric perforation. Intestinal contents can spill into the peritoneal cavity (free perforation) or can be contained by adjacent organs. Diffuse peritonitis can complicate free perforation.

Free intraperitoneal air is detectable on plain radiographs in about two-thirds of patients with bowel perforation. When visible, it appears as small lucent crescents below the diaphragm on upright radiograph or below the antidependent abdominal wall on decubitus or CT examinations.

On supine radiographs, larger quantities of air may outline the falciform ligament as well as the inner and outer surfaces of the bowel wall (Rigler sign). The most common causes of nontraumatic intraperitoneal air on plain radiographs are perforated duodenal ulcer, perforated diverticulitis, and less commonly, perforated colon carcinoma. Recent abdominal surgery is another etiology of free air, but that should be evident from the patient's history.

Abdominal CT sensitively identifies free air, intra-abdominal fluid collections, and any contrast extravasation, and it can often delineate the location and morphology of the perforated viscus. Upper gastrointestinal series can identify ulcers, luminal narrowing, or irregularity and extravasation (**Fig. 6.10**).

Fig. 6.10a–f
a,b Duodenal perforation with intra-peritoneal air. Extensive free subdiaphragmatic air on upright chest radiograph. Air outlines the inner and outer small-bowel wall on supine abdominal radiograph (Rigler sign).
c,d Duodenal rupture in blunt abdominal trauma. Small amount of fluid and several tiny bubbles of air adjacent to the second part of the duodenum.
e,f Perforated duodenum due to peptic ulcer disease. Small, contained fluid collection with a focus of air adjacent to the proximal duodenum. On upper gastrointestinal series, contrast extravasates from the narrowed first portion of the duodenum.

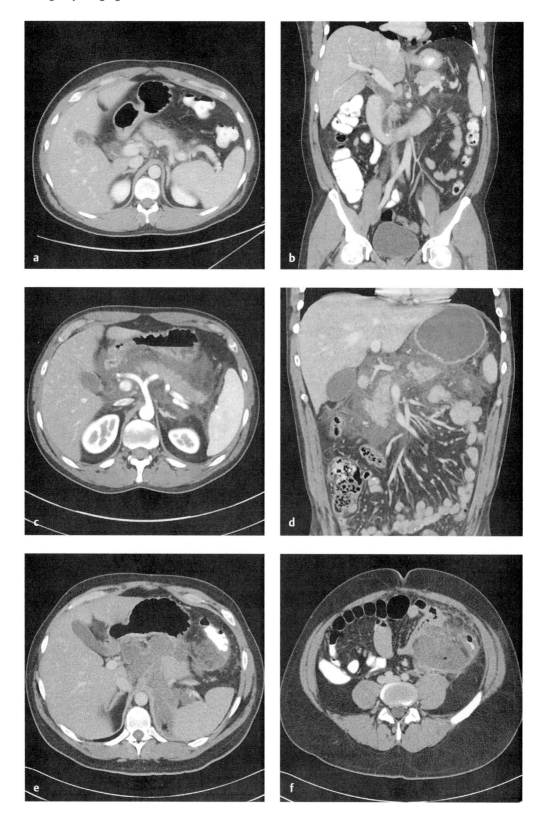

◆ Acute Pancreatitis

Acute pancreatic injury, inflammation, or ductal obstruction can lead to intrapancreatic enzyme activation, disruption of pancreatic ducts, and leakage of pancreatic secretions with autodigestion of adjacent tissues. The most common causes of acute pancreatitis are chronic alcohol consumption and acute pancreatic duct obstruction from biliary stone disease. Less common causes include hypertriglyceridemia, medications, and trauma.

The diagnosis is based on clinical and laboratory findings, severe upper abdominal pain in a patient at risk for pancreatitis, and elevated serum lipase. The role of CT in acute pancreatitis is to confirm the diagnosis, assess severity, and point to a cause (e.g., obstructing gallstone, pancreatic mass, cirrhosis). Imaging may be normal in mild or early disease, and its greatest value is in identifying subacute and late complications, such as necrosis, pseudocyst, and abscess formation.

Contrast-enhanced CT shows the edema and inflammation of acute pancreatitis as parenchymal enlargement, heterogenous attenuation, indistinct pancreatic margins, retroperitoneal fat stranding, and, if severe, peripancreatic fluid collections or frank pancreatic necrosis.

Ultrasound is less sensitive and specific for evaluating the pancreas than is CT, but it can be useful for detecting or following peripancreatic collections. When imaged by ultrasound, acute pancreatitis appears as an enlarged, hypoechoic pancreas, sometimes with an adjacent fluid collection.

CT grading (Balthazar) is seen in **Table 6.4**. Patients with grades A through C have a 0% mortality and 4% complication rate, whereas patients with grade D or E pancreatitis have a 14% mortality and a 54% complication rate (**Fig. 6.11**).

Table 6.4   CT Grading (Balthazar) for acute pancreatitis

A	Normal pancreas
B	Pancreatic enlargement
C	Pancreatic and or peripancreatic fat inflammation
D	Single peripancreatic fluid collection
E	Two or more peripancreatic fluid collections and/or retroperitoneal air

Fig. 6.11a–f
a,b   Gallstone pancreatitis. Mild peripancreatic edema anterior to the body of the pancreas. Distended common bile duct with tiny calcification at the ampulla of Vater (grade C).
c,d   Moderately severe acute pancreatitis. Peripancreatic edema with retroperitoneal fluid surrounding the head and body of pancreas (grade D).
e,f   Severe acute pancreatitis. Multiple large peripancreatic fluid collections, including a well-defined left lower quadrant collection containing bubbles of gas (grade E).

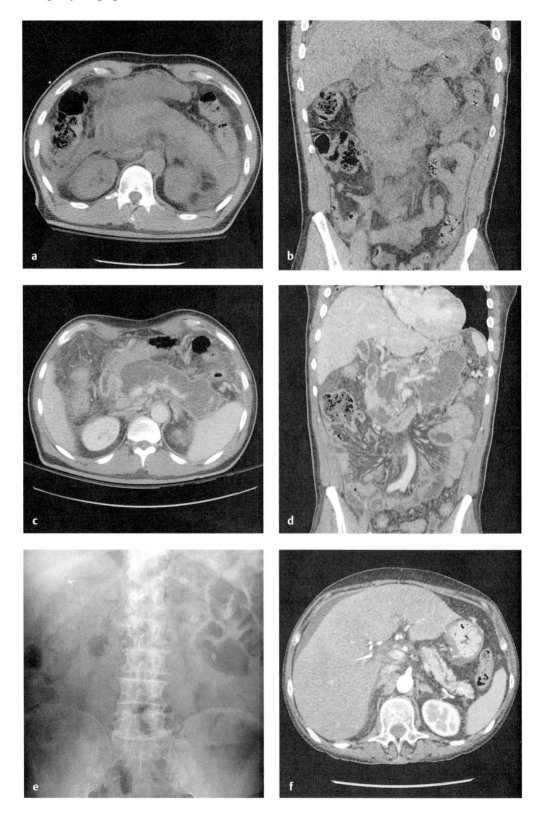

◆ Pancreatic Necrosis and Chronic Pancreatitis

Pancreatic necrosis is one of the severe complications of acute pancreatitis and is associated with increased morbidity and mortality. Inflammation severe enough to cause cell death and liquefactive necrosis typically develops 24 to 48 hours after symptom onset. Consequently, CT scans obtained in the first 12 hours may be falsely reassuring. Contrast-enhanced CT 3 days after symptom onset will more accurately detect necrosis than studies obtained at initial presentation will.

In severe pancreatitis, a pseudocyst forms when necrotic tissue is sequestered within a fibrous capsule over a period of 3 to 4 weeks. The contained necrotic tissue is prone to infection and abscess development. There are three potential outcomes for pancreatic necrosis: resolution, formation of noninfected pseudocyst, or abscess.

Portions of the pancreas that fail to enhance after the administration of intravenous contrast are considered necrotic. Intra- or peripancreatic gas bubbles may also be seen. Pancreatic necrosis may be accompanied by peripancreatic fat necrosis, which appears as a heterogenous fluid collection adjacent to the pancreas.

Chronic pancreatitis is the consequence of continuing, chronic pancreatic inflammation with eventual glandular fibrosis, atrophy, and dystrophic calcification. Patients report a long history of intermittent epigastric pain that radiates to the back or recurrent episodes of acute pancreatitis. With sufficient pancreatic damage, the gland's endocrine and exocrine functions fail, leading to malabsorption and diabetes. In contrast to the laboratory abnormalities seen in acute pancreatitis, lipase and amylase may be normal or only mildly elevated.

Abdominal or chest radiographs often show punctate or coarse upper abdominal calcifications distributed transversely across the epigastrium. These are primarily intraductal, located either within the main pancreatic duct or in the small pancreatic duct radicles. CT and ultrasound may show focal enlargement or atrophy of the gland, parenchymal calcifications, and pancreatic duct dilatation with ductal width greater than 5 mm at the head and 2 mm in the body and tail (**Fig. 6.12**).

Fig. 6.12a–f
a–d Acute pancreatitis with pancreatic necrosis. (**a,b**) The pancreas is diffusely enlarged with extensive surrounding edema. Fluid is present in both anterior pararenal spaces. (**c,d**) At 18 days after symptom onset, most of the pancreas has been replaced by low-attenuation necrotic tissue contained by a thin, well-defined capsule. Mesenteric inflammatory changes persist.
e Chronic pancreatitis. Abdominal radiograph with multiple small calcifications overlying the L1 and L2 vertebral bodies.
f Chronic pancreatitis. Atrophic pancreas with multiple punctate calcifications and mild pancreatic ductal dilatation. Small amount of perihepatic ascites.

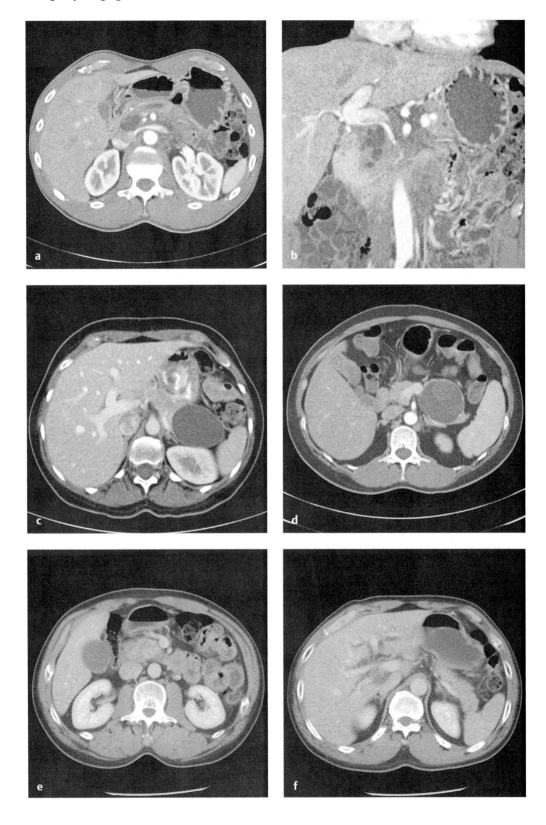

◆ Pancreatic Masses and Pancreatic Adenocarcinoma

Pancreatic cysts are usually asymptomatic and incidentally discovered. Most of these are benign or indolent and include serous cystadenomas, mucinous cystic neoplasms, intraductal papillary mucinous neoplasms (IPMN), and pseudocysts. Ductal adenocarcinomas represent about 2.5% of incidentally discovered pancreatic cysts, and mucinous neoplasms, which have a malignant potential, represent about 55%.

Simple cysts < 2 cm should be reimaged in one year and, if stable, are considered benign.

Simple cysts 2–3 cm (and those that have grown from < 2 cm) should be characterized by MRI. Uncharacterized masses should be followed yearly. Cysts consistent with branch-duct IPMNs should be followed every 6 months for 2 years and annually thereafter. Cysts consistent with serous cystadenomas should be followed every 2 years and resection considered if they grow to > 4 cm.

Cysts > 3 cm should be characterized by MRI; most should be considered for cyst aspiration and resection depending on risk and comorbidities. Serous cystadenomas should be considered for resection when they reach 4 cm.

Solid pancreatic masses include true neoplasms, most notably adenocarcinoma and neuroendocrine tumors, and nonneoplastic conditions that can mimic tumors, such as autoimmune pancreatitis, intrapancreatic spleen, or sarcoidosis. Solid tumors and cysts with solid components should generally be resected.

Pancreatic adenocarcinoma is the most common primary pancreatic malignancy and affects patients in the seventh and eighth decades who typically present with pain, jaundice, and weight loss. Unfortunately, most have unresectable disease at the time of diagnosis, due to hepatic and peritoneal metastases. Five-year survival is ~ 5%. Thin-section CT in both arterial and portal venous phases is the best technique for evaluating solid pancreatic tumors, and most will appear as low-attenuation lesions within the normally enhancing pancreas. Criteria for resectability include lack of distant metastases; clear fat planes around the hepatic, celiac, and superior mesenteric arteries; and tumor that does not abut the portal or superior mesenteric veins (**Fig. 6.13**).

Fig. 6.13a–f
a,b Intraductal papillary mucinous neoplasm. ~ 2.5-cm cystic mass in the pancreatic head with associated pancreatic duct dilatation.
c Serous cystadenoma. Simple 5-cm cyst in the pancreatic tail.
d Mucinous cystadenoma. Complex cyst in the pancreatic tail with internal septations and intermediate-attenuation component.
e,f Pancreatic carcinoma. Solid, enhancing mass in head of pancreas with associated intra- and extrahepatic biliary dilatation.

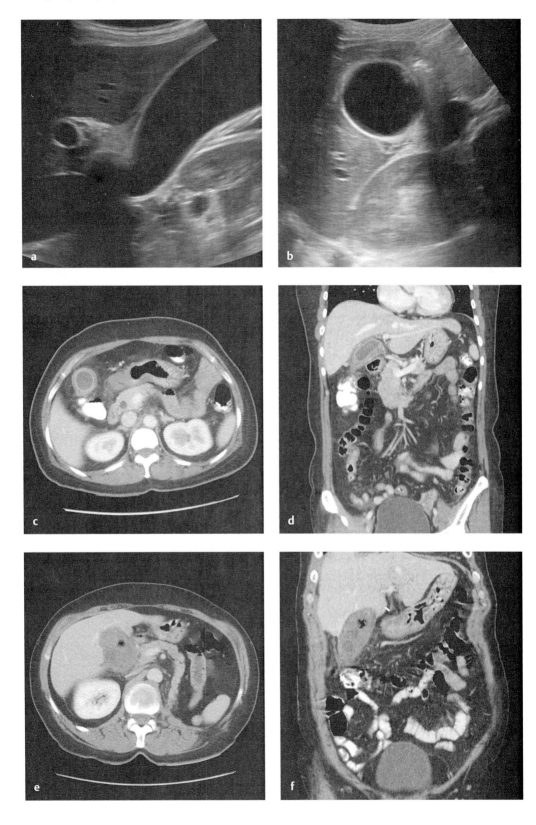

◆ Acute Cholecystitis

Cystic duct obstruction by a calculus or by sludge in the gallbladder neck is the usual etiology for acute cholecystitis. Patients present with right upper quadrant pain that radiates to the back, nausea, and anorexia. Early laboratory findings may be normal, but leukocytosis and mild transaminase elevation eventually occur and reflect biliary obstruction and inflammation.

Ultrasound is the primary imaging approach to detection of gallstones and gallbladder inflammation. Gallstones, pericholecystic fluid, luminal distention, gallbladder wall thickening, and pain on compression of the gallbladder under visualization (the sonographic Murphy sign) make up the constellation of supportive findings. The normal gallbladder should be less than 4 cm in diameter, and its wall should be less than 3 mm thick. The best evidence of acute cholecystitis is detection of gallstones in conjunction with a sonographic Murphy sign. Gallbladder wall thickening and pericholecystic fluid are less definitive findings and can be seen in other conditions such as hepatitis, pancreatitis, or colitis.

Cholecystitis is often diagnosed on CT obtained for abdominal pain that is less typical of acute cholecystitis or in patients whose ultrasound is nondiagnostic due to obesity or other technical factors. It is less sensitive then ultrasound for detecting gallstones, which may be isodense to bile in some cases. In patients with equivocal ultrasound or CT findings, hepatobiliary iminodiacetic acid (HIDA) scan can be obtained and is considered diagnostic of acute cholecystitis if the gallbladder does not fill 4 hours after radionuclide administration (**Fig. 6.14**).

Fig. 6.14a–f
a,b Acute cholecystitis. The gallbladder is markedly distended with minimal wall thickening but without pericholecystic fluid. A shadowing mass (gallstone) is located in the gallbladder neck.
c,d Acute cholecystitis. The gallbladder wall is thickened, with associated pericholecystic inflammatory stranding and pericholecystic fluid. The common bile duct is mildly distended.
e,f Acute cholecystitis and cholelithiasis. The gallbladder is distended with sludge and near isodense gallstones, one of which contains gas. Mild pericholecystic inflammatory fat stranding.

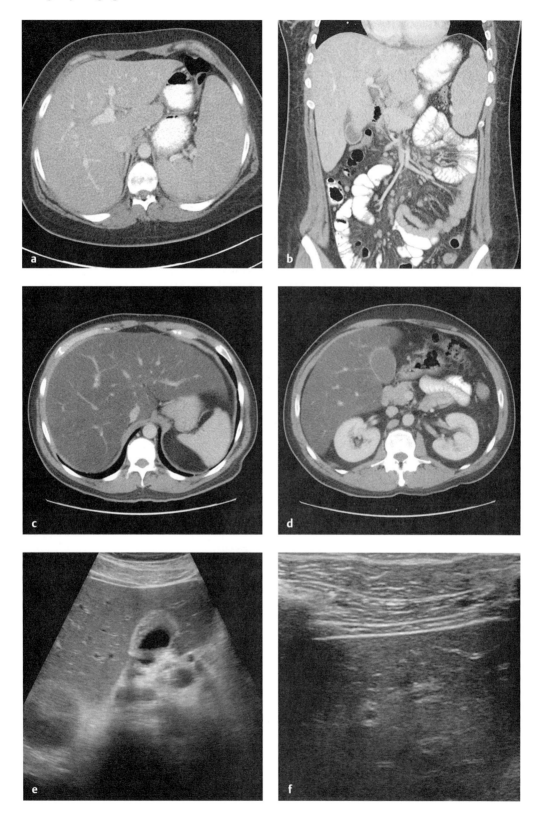

◆ Hepatitis

Generalized inflammation of the liver is most often due to alcohol, medications, viral infection, and autoimmune disease. Signs and symptoms of hepatitis range from mild abdominal discomfort to fulminant hepatic failure. Many patients experience anorexia, nausea, vomiting, and variable degrees of jaundice.

Alanine aminotransferase (ALT), aspartate transaminase (AST), and alkaline phosphatase can be helpful in grouping patients into those with primarily hepatocellular disease and those with biliary obstruction/cholestatic disease. In hepatocellular disease, AST or ALT levels are typically elevated to a greater extent than alkaline phosphatase levels, whereas in patients with cholestatic disease, alkaline phosphatase is elevated to a greater extent than AST and ALT. In acute alcoholic hepatitis, ALT and AST are modestly elevated with an AST/ALT ratio > 2:1. Extremely high levels of AST and ALT are seen in hepatic necrosis, as in acetaminophen poisoning.

While imaging is not necessary to establish clinical diagnosis of hepatitis, CT or ultrasound is often obtained for evaluation of upper abdominal pain, and recognition of liver parenchymal abnormalities can suggest the diagnosis as other considerations, such as cholecystitis or hepatic abscess, are excluded. CT findings are nonspecific and include hepatomegaly, ascites, and periportal edema. The latter reflects fluid accumulation or lymphatic dilation surrounding the portal triads and is seen in many conditions besides hepatitis.

Two distinct parenchymal ultrasound patterns have been described. With a "starry sky" appearance, hepatocellular edema leads to a general decrease in liver echogenicity highlighting the echogenic portal venules. Another pattern, called the bright liver, refers to increased parenchymal echogenicity and attenuation of the diffusely inflamed liver parenchyma. These patterns can also be seen in acute alcoholic hepatitis, cirrhosis, chronic hepatitis, and diffuse fatty infiltration of the liver. Viral hepatitis is frequently associated with gallbladder wall thickening and periportal lymphadenopathy (**Fig. 6.15**).

Fig. 6.15a–f
a,b   Hepatitis. Nonspecific CT findings of hepatomegaly with portal adenopathy, mild periportal edema, and pericholecystic fluid.
c,d   Severe fulminant hepatitis. Marked hepatomegaly and diffusely decreased attenuation. Mild reactive gallbladder wall thickening.
e,f   Hepatitis. Ultrasound showing conspicuous echogenic portal venules and mild associated gallbladder wall thickening.

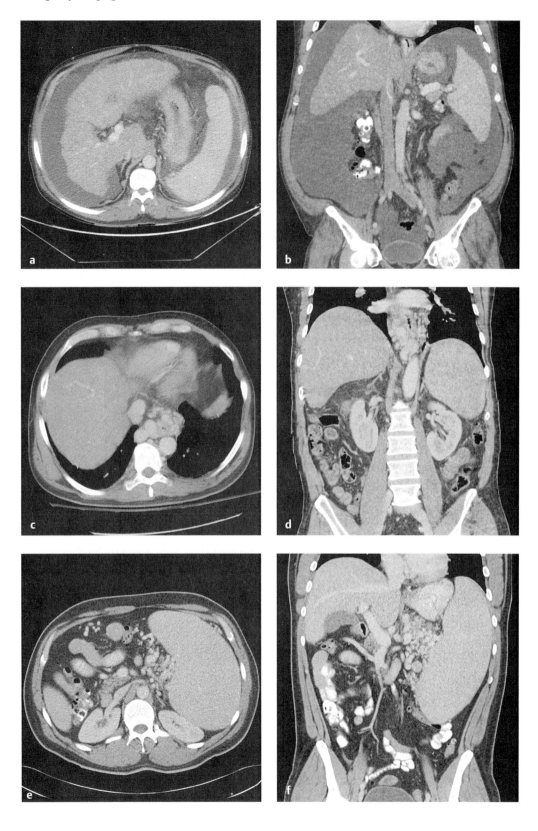

◆ Cirrhosis and Portal Venous Hypertension

Cirrhosis is a late consequence of chronic or recurrent hepatocyte injury and is characterized by partial regeneration and fibrosis of the liver. Longstanding alcohol use, hepatitis, biliary disease, hemochromatosis, Wilson disease, and alpha-1-antitrypsin deficiency are some of the more common causes.

Gross morphological changes can be recognized on a variety of imaging techniques. Left hepatic and caudate lobe hypertrophy may be seen on CT, MRI, and ultrasound. The caudate lobe is frequently enlarged, defined by a ratio of the caudate lobe width to right hepatic lobe width > 0.65. On ultrasound, diffuse or focal fatty infiltration leads to a coarse parenchymal appearance. The liver surface and parenchyma may also appear nodular, particularly in more advanced cases. CT findings include a small liver with lobulated or crenulated surface, variable fatty change, and isodense or hyperdense regenerative nodules.

Portal venous hypertension is due to impaired portal venous flow through the liver and is defined by portal venous pressures that exceed 12 mm Hg; it is classified as presinusoidal, sinusoidal, or postsinusoidal, depending on the point of venous obstruction. Persistently elevated portal venous pressure leads to enlargement of normally minuscule venous collaterals that shunt blood from the portal to the systemic venous circulation, bypassing the liver.

Presinusoidal portal hypertension is due to portal vein thrombosis, schistosomiasis, or any extrinsic compression of the portal vein proximal to its intrahepatic capillary network. Isolated splenic vein thrombus can result in splenomegaly and varices isolated to the gastrosplenic collateral bed. Hepatic parenchymal fibrosis results in sinusoidal portal venous hypertension. Cirrhosis is the most common etiology, but others include hepatitis, liver metastases, and hepatocellular carcinoma. Postsinusoidal portal hypertension may result from Budd-Chiari syndrome, hepatic venoocclusive disease, or cardiac failure.

CT and MRI can establish the etiology of portal venous hypertension and can define the collateral vessels associated with portosystemic shunting. The most common portosystemic shunt is the coronary–gastroesophageal route, which gives rise to lower esophageal and gastric varices. Other manifestations of portal venous hypertension include umbilical vein recanalization, hemorrhoids and abdominal wall varices, splenomegaly, ascites, and mottled hepatic parenchymal enhancement with contrast administration. Esophageal varices are particularly prone to life-threatening upper gastrointestinal hemorrhage.

Ultrasound frequently shows a dilated portal vein (> 13 mm), but this is a nonspecific finding. Biphasic or reversed flow in the portal vein as well as recanalization of the paraumbilical vein are pathognomonic for portal venous hypertension but are seen in advanced disease (**Fig. 6.16**).

Fig. 6.16a–f
a,b Cirrhosis with ascites. The liver is small with an irregular, nodular surface. Extensive intraperitoneal fluid. Marked splenomegaly.
c,d Cirrhosis with portal hypertension, splenomegaly, and esophageal varices. The liver is normal in size. The spleen is enlarged. Numerous tubular, serpiginous, dilated veins surround the distal esophagus and gastroesophageal junction.
e,f Isolated left-sided portal venous hypertension due to splenic vein thrombosis. Marked splenomegaly with large gastrosplenic varices. The liver and portal vein are normal.

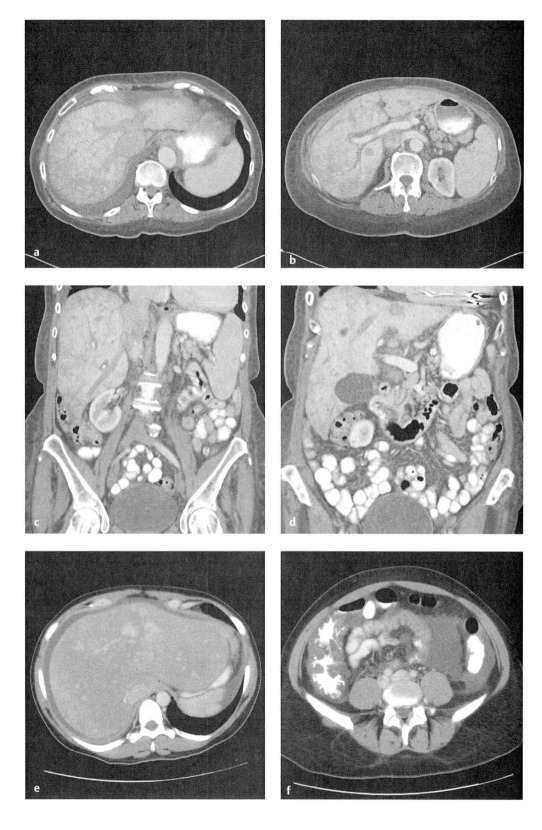

◆ Postsinusoidal Portal Venous Hypertension

Passive hepatic congestion is a complication of right heart failure, which can be seen in pericardial effusion, constrictive pericarditis, cardiomyopathy, and tricuspid or pulmonic valvular disease. Decompensated right ventricular or biventricular function causes transmission of elevated central venous pressure to the liver via the IVC and hepatic veins. The accumulation and stasis of deoxygenated blood within the liver sinusoids leads to parenchymal atrophy, necrosis, and ultimately fibrosis, referred to as cardiac cirrhosis.

On contrast-enhanced CT scans, the liver appears inhomogeneous, with a mottled, reticulated pattern that reflects delayed enhancement of small and medium-sized hepatic veins, often associated with retrograde opacification and enhancement of the IVC and hepatic veins. Other nonspecific findings include hepatomegaly, ascites, pleural effusion, IVC distention, and splenomegaly. CT and MRI can often identify or confirm the cardiac etiology.

Budd-Chiari syndrome is an uncommon malady in which hepatic vein occlusion compromises hepatic venous outflow. In acute cases, thrombosis of the IVC or main hepatic vein leads to rapidly developing ascites. Predisposing conditions include hypercoagulability, blood dyscrasias, malignancy, and oral contraceptive use. Patients present with abdominal pain, hepatosplenomegaly, massive ascites, and clinical and laboratory signs of liver failure. Budd-Chiari syndrome can also develop insidiously, from intrahepatic venous thrombosis related to chronic inflammation or tumor invasion.

Ultrasound evaluation with color flow Doppler will show absent or inappropriately directed flow in the hepatic veins and heterogenous liver echotexture, often with associated gallbladder wall thickening, splenomegaly, and caudate lobe hypertrophy.

CT and MRI both can identify absent hepatic vein enhancement and heterogeneous, patchy enhancement of the liver parenchyma. This characteristic mottled appearance is often referred to as "nutmeg" liver and generally spares the caudate lobe because of its separate, direct drainage to the IVC.

Management is directed at reversing the specific etiology, and options include long-term anticoagulation, hepatic vein angioplasty and stenting, or placement of a transjugular intrahepatic portosystemic shunt (TIPS) (**Fig. 6.17**).

Fig. 6.17a–f
a–d Passive hepatic congestion in cardiac failure. The heart is massively enlarged, as is the intrahepatic inferior vena cava. The liver is mildly enlarged with mottled parenchyma. Moderate periportal edema; small right pleural effusion.
e,f Budd-Chiari syndrome. The liver is enlarged with inapparent hepatic veins. Ascites and colonic wall thickening (portal colopathy) reflect portal venous hypertension.

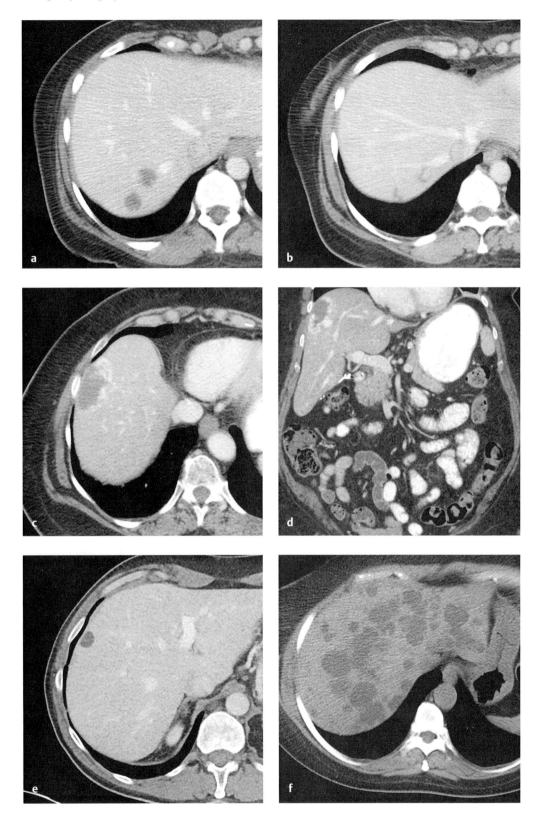

◆ Incidental Liver Masses

Hepatic cysts, hemangiomas, and hamartomas are frequently encountered on abdominal CT and may be difficult to distinguish from more concerning lesions, such as metastatic disease or primary hepatobiliary malignancy. Strategies for further evaluation in ambiguous cases depend on the lesion's appearance and the patient's general risk of malignancy and overall clinical condition. Clinically, patients can be divided into low-, normal-, and high-risk categories.

Low-risk patients are < 40 years without hepatic disease or other malignancy risk factor. *Normal-risk patients* are > 40 years without hepatic disease or other malignancy risk factor. *High-risk patients* have a known primary malignancy that has a propensity to metastasize to the liver or an underlying hepatic disease that predisposes to hepatic malignancy such as cirrhosis, hepatitis, chronic active hepatitis, hemochromatosis, sclerosing cholangitis, primary biliary sclerosis, or hemosiderosis (**Fig. 6.18**).

Benign Imaging Features

- Typical hemangioma: discontinuous nodular peripheral enhancement with delayed enlargement of enhancing foci
- Sharply marginated
- Low attenuation (< 20 HU)
- No enhancement: cyst, hemangioma, hamartoma

Suspicious Imaging Features

- Poorly defined margins
- Enhancement (> 20 HU)
- Heterogeneity
- Enlargement over time

Approach to the Incidental Hepatic Lesion Based on Size, Appearance, and Risk Factors

- < 0.5 cm:
  - Follow in high-risk patients only
- 0.5–1.5 cm:
  - Follow low-attenuation lesions with suspicious imaging features
  - Follow flash filling lesions in high-risk patients only
- > 1.5 cm:
  - Low attenuation with benign features: no follow-up necessary
  - Low attenuation with suspicious features: follow-up or biopsy
  - Flash filling with benign features: no follow-up necessary
  - Flash filling with no benign features: follow-up or biopsy

Fig. 6.18a–f
a–d Hemangioma. (**a,b**) Two small, well-defined lesions that measure 50 HU and show nodular enhancement at their upper margins. (**c,d**) Large segment 8 mass with peripheral nodular enhancement.
e,f Simple hepatic cysts. (**e**) 1-cm subcapsular cyst measuring 15 HU with sharply defined margins and no enhancement. (**f**) Innumerable simple hepatic cysts in a patient with polycystic kidney disease.

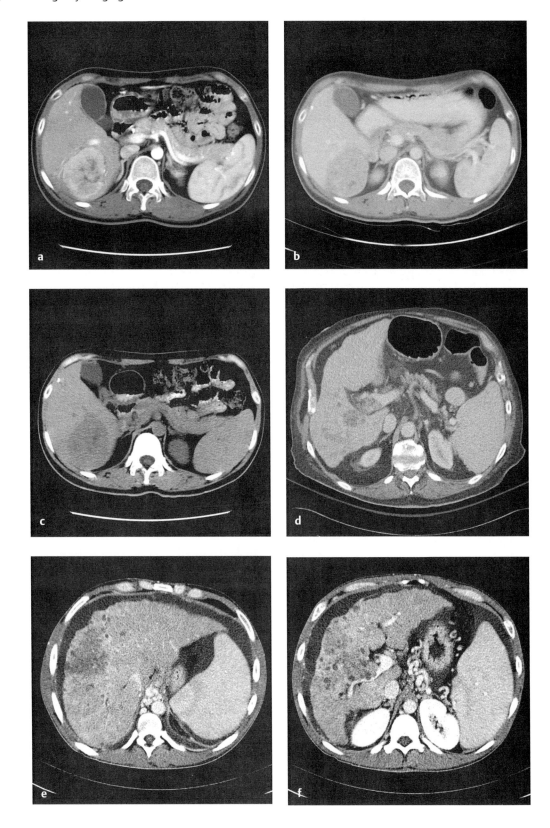

◆ Hepatocellular Carcinoma

Hepatocellular carcinoma (HCC) is a primary malignancy of the liver seen in patients with underlying chronic liver disease, mainly hepatitis C or cirrhosis. HCC may appear as either a solitary mass or diffuse hepatic infiltration, which on imaging studies can sometimes be difficult to differentiate from surrounding cirrhotic liver or regenerating liver nodules.

Accurate diagnosis and surgical planning usually requires multimodality cross-sectional imaging. While ultrasound is commonly used for screening, its sensitivity and specificity are limited, particularly as interpretation is made more difficult by underlying cirrhosis. Nor does ultrasound provide sufficient anatomic detail for surgical planning or ablation. When detected on ultrasound, tumors are generally round or oval with sharp, smooth boundaries and variable echogenicity relative to the remainder of the liver parenchyma. Doppler ultrasound may show neovascularization compared with neighboring regenerative nodules, as well as vascular occlusion or invasion.

Contrast-enhanced CT with images obtained in arterial, portal venous, and late washout phases is optimal for characterization of HCC. The tumor appears as a mass with dense arterial-phase enhancement and rapid washout in the portal venous phase, becoming indistinct or hypodense compared to the rest of the liver. In contrast, regenerative nodules generally appear isodense or hypodense relative to surrounding parenchyma on all phases. HCC may be associated with a halo of focal fatty sparing in the setting of an otherwise fatty liver. Other specific findings of HCC include visualization of a tumor capsule, hepatic and portal vein invasion, and portal vein tumor thrombus (**Fig. 6.19**).

Fig. 6.19a–f
a–c Hepatocellular carcinoma. Well-defined heterogeneously enhancing mass in segments 5 and 6 with typical enhancement characteristics of hepatocellular carcinoma. The mass is hyperdense on arterial phase and slightly hypodense on portal venous phase and late washout phase imaging.
d Hepatocellular carcinoma with portal venous invasion. Low-attenuation mass involving segments 5 and 6 with invasion of the right and main portal veins. Nodular hepatic contour.
e,f Hepatocellular carcinoma in cirrhosis. Poorly defined low-attenuation mass mainly involving segment 8. Small, nodular liver with splenomegaly and gastroesophageal varices.

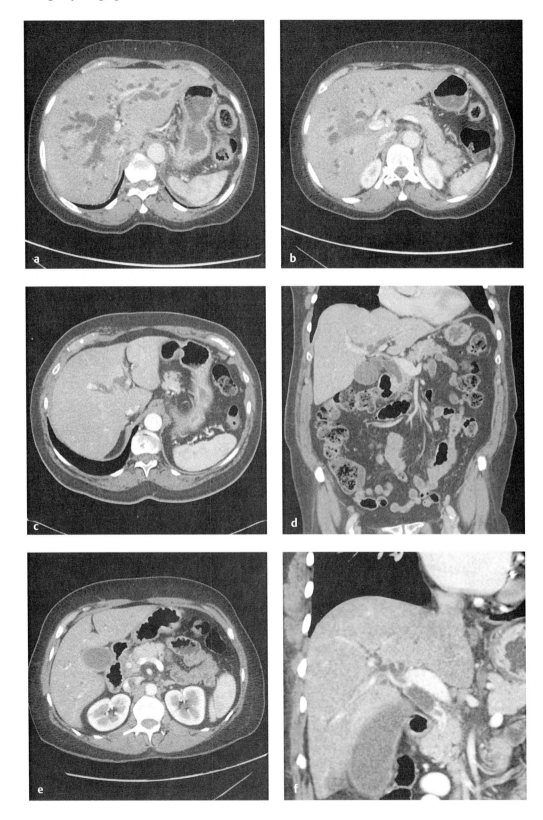

◆ Cholangiocarcinoma

Cholangiocarcinoma is a rare, malignant tumor that arises from the intrahepatic, extrahepatic (perihilar), or distal extrahepatic segments of the biliary tree. Perihilar tumors are most common and are located at the bifurcation of the left and right hepatic ducts. The highest prevalence of this cancer occurs in the sixth and seventh decades of life, and its incidence is increased in patients with long-standing biliary inflammation, whether the result of parasitic infection (*Clonorchis* or *Opisthorchis*), primary sclerosing cholangitis, or recurrent pyogenic cholangitis.

Signs and symptoms include painless jaundice, clay-colored stools, hyperbilirubinuria, pruritus, weight loss, and abdominal pain.

Right upper quadrant ultrasound usually shows biliary duct dilatation and may identify the level of obstruction but rarely identifies a discrete mass. CT, using a dedicated pancreatic protocol with thin-section arterial-phase postcontrast imaging, or MRI cholangiography can characterize the size and location of any mass or stricture. Ampullary or pancreatic carcinoma can result in symptoms identical to those of cholangiocarcinoma, and this is also best evaluated using these methods.

Endoscopic retrograde cholangiopancreatography (ERCP) is generally performed for both diagnostic biopsy and therapeutic biliary stenting. Cholangiocarcinoma has a poor prognosis, as many patients present with unresectable or metastatic disease (**Fig. 6.20**).

Fig. 6.20a–f
a,b Cholangiocarcinoma involving the hepatic duct bifurcation (Klatskin tumor). Marked right and left intrahepatic biliary ductal dilatation. Low-attenuation infiltrative mass adjacent to main portal vein.
c–f Cholangiocarcinoma with obstruction at distal common bile duct (CBD). (**c,d**) Mild intrahepatic ductal dilatation with distal CBD wall thickening and obstruction at the ampulla of Vater. (**e,f**) Similar patient with more clearly defined CBD wall enhancement.

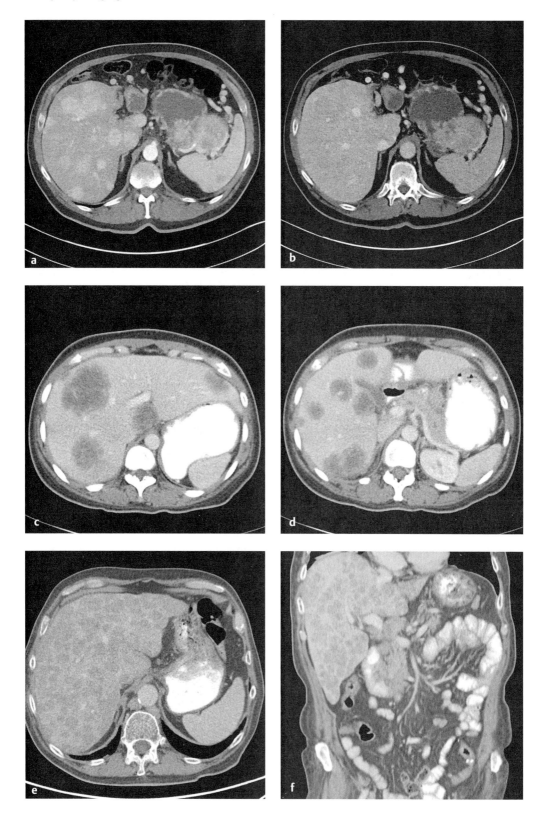

◆ Hepatic Metastases

Because of its rich, dual blood supply, the liver is a frequent site of metastases, and metastatic disease is considerably more common than primary hepatic malignancy. Most hepatic metastases originate from tumors of the gastrointestinal tract and spread to the liver via the portal circulation, but other primary sites include the breast, ovaries, lung, and pancreas.

Postcontrast CT with images obtained in arterial and portal venous phases is the optimal examination for detecting hepatic metastases. An important obstacle in CT imaging for liver metastases is the high prevalence of benign liver lesions that resemble metastatic disease, most notably atypical hemangiomas and focal nodular hyperplasia (FNH). Most liver metastases are hypovascular and will appear as low-attenuation lesions against a background of normal hepatic enhancement.

Ultrasound is also a reasonable screening modality for suspected liver metastases, which can be seen as focal or diffuse parenchymal changes in the liver. While less specific than CT, multiple hepatic nodules of differing sizes and echogenicity suggest metastatic disease.

MRI is typically reserved for diagnostically challenging cases or when iodinated contrast material is contraindicated. Most liver tumors, both benign and malignant, appear hypointense on T1-weighted images and hyperintense on T2-weighted images. Metastatic melanoma, however, is an exception, as melanin exhibits a high signal intensity on T1 compared with that of the adjacent hepatic parenchyma (**Fig. 6.21**).

Fig. 6.21a–f
a,b Hepatic metastases (pancreatic carcinoma). Multiple hyperdense intrahepatic masses on arterial-phase imaging that become hypodense to liver parenchyma on portal venous-phase images. Large distal pancreatic mass interposed between the stomach and spleen.
c,d Hepatic metastases (colon carcinoma). Multiple, poorly marginated, round low-attenuation masses within all hepatic lobes and segments.
e,f Hepatic metastases (prostate carcinoma). Innumerable small, round low-attenuation masses throughout the liver. Multiple enlarged periportal lymph nodes.

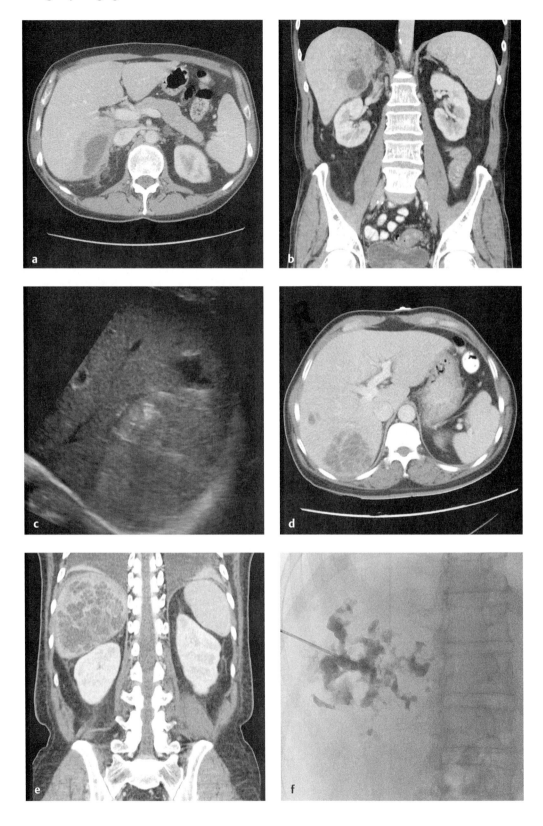

◆ Hepatic Abscess

Hepatic abscess is a potential consequence of bacterial seeding of the liver either via arterial, venous, or biliary routes or by direct inoculation. As such, it can result from transient bacteremia and no source may be identified, or it can be due to portal vein thrombophlebitis, biliary obstruction, traumatic injury, or peritonitis. Hepatic abscess can complicate abdominal surgery or biliary endoscopic intervention. Approximately 80% of hepatic abscesses in developed countries are pyogenic; the remainder are fungal, amebic (*Entamoeba histolytica*), or parasitic (*Echinococcus granulosus*). The right lobe of the liver is more commonly involved than the left.

Advanced age, diabetes, HIV disease, and immunosuppression predispose to bacterial or fungal abscesses. Patients most frequently present with fever and abdominal pain, which may be associated with right upper quadrant pain, nausea, vomit-

ing, and weight loss. Laboratory findings include elevated white blood cells, serum bilirubin, liver enzymes, and anemia.

The diagnosis is made by ultrasound or CT by detecting one or more intrahepatic fluid collections. Ultrasound will show a complex cystic mass, which may contain septa, debris, and/or gas. CT most frequently shows a peripherally enhancing cystic mass, often with surrounding edema. Pyogenic abscesses are often multiple and may contain gas; fungal or amebic abscesses are more likely solitary. Echinococcal cysts may show peripheral calcification. The primary imaging differential considerations are simple liver cysts, necrotic metastases, and hepatocellular carcinoma.

Prior to the advent of effective surgical management, pyogenic hepatic abscess was almost always fatal. Current treatment involves a combination of interventional drainage and antibiotic therapy (**Fig. 6.22**).

Fig. 6.22a–f
a,b Hepatic abscess. Low-attenuation mass in hepatic segment 5/6 with surrounding low-attenuation change and small daughter abscesses.
c–f Hepatic abscess in another patient. Ultrasound shows heterogeneous mass in hepatic segment 7. Corresponding CT shows complex, multiseptate, low-attenuation mass. Fluoroscopy shows contrast filling the interstices of the abscess cavity during placement of catheter for drainage.

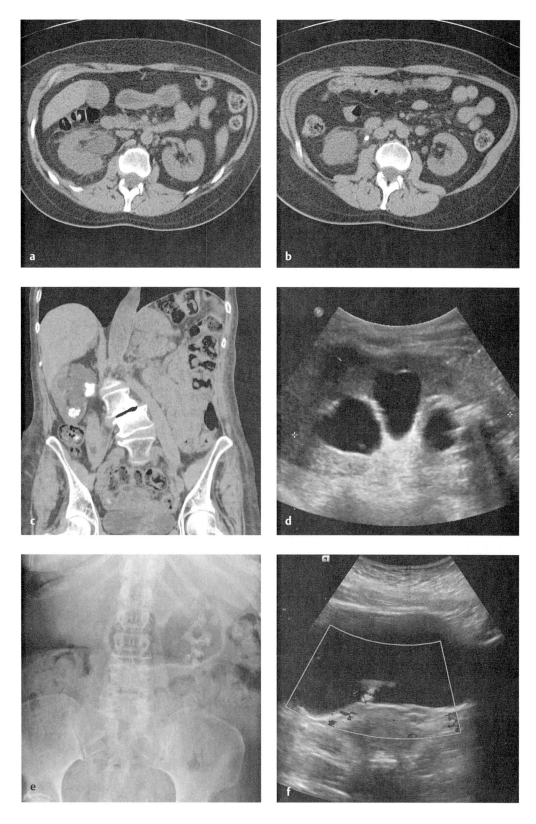

◆ Nephrolithiasis

Renal colic is characterized by acute, severe, and intermittent flank pain that may radiate to the groin and is often associated with nausea or vomiting. Costovertebral tenderness is variably present, and many, but not all, patients will show microscopic hematuria. The aim of emergent imaging is to detect and characterize calculi, which may be located anywhere along the course of the urinary tract, to evaluate for hydronephrosis or other complications of ureteral obstruction, and to diagnose or exclude other conditions that could mimic stone disease.

Fewer than half of renal calculi are visible on plain radiographs, but almost all are visible on CT. The few calculi that are invisible even on CT include those associated with Indinavir antiretroviral therapy and mucous aggregates (matrix stones). Calculi may be intrarenal, intraureteral, or intravesicular. While most are radio-opaque on CT, they vary considerably in density. Calcium oxalate and calcium phosphate stones are typically 400 to 600 HU. In contrast, cystine and urate stones have CT attenuation in the range of 100 to 400 HU.

Stones most commonly lodge at the ureterovesicular junction (UVJ), and 80% of stones less than 4 mm in diameter will spontaneously pass into the bladder. Prone imaging can be performed to distinguish between a true obstructing UVJ stone and an intravesical stone, as stones that have passed into the bladder lie along its dependent, anterior wall in the prone patient. Larger calculi may require ureteral stent placement or percutaneous nephrostomy if analgesia and hydration are not sufficient to permit passage.

Staghorn calculi are large calcifications that form a cast of the renal collecting system. Most are composed of struvite (magnesium aluminum phosphate). Staghorn calculi form in alkaline urine and are seen in patients with chronic or recurrent infection with urease-producing bacteria such as *Proteus*, *Klebsiella*, and *Pseudomonas*.

CT findings in cases of obstructing ureteral calculi include hydroureter, hydronephrosis, perinephric stranding, and focal ureteral thickening surrounding the stone. This finding, the "soft tissue rim sign," can be helpful in distinguishing a ureteric calculus from a phlebolith in patients with little retroperitoneal fat. Phleboliths tend to have imperceptible walls and may demonstrate a soft tissue "tail" representing a scarred or thrombosed vein extending from the calcified phlebolith.

Because it does not utilize ionizing radiation, ultrasound is preferred in children or pregnant women. Stones may be difficult to detect, but hydronephrosis is easily identified. With color flow Doppler evaluation of the UVJ, absence of the normal peristaltic jet of urine into the bladder indirectly confirms ureteral obstruction (**Fig. 6.23**).

Fig. 6.23a–f
a,b Obstructing ureteral and nonobstructing renal calculi. A 7-mm calculus is located in the right proximal ureter. Mild pelvocaliectasis and perinephric stranding.
c,d Ureteropelvic junction calculus with hydronephrosis. A bulky (staghorn) calculus is located at the ureteropelvic junction. A second, popcorn-shaped calculus is located at the lower renal pole. Ultrasound shows hydronephrosis as well as the lower pole shadowing stone.
e Staghorn calculus on plain radiograph. The left renal collecting system is completely filled with a calcified cast resembling the antlers of a stag.
f Ureteral jet at the left ureterovesical junction. This finding, when present, excludes an obstructing calculus.

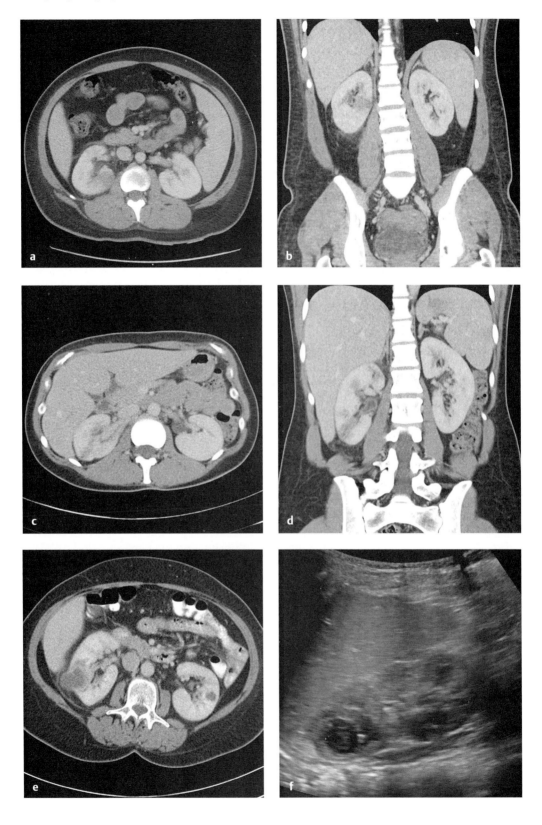

◆ Pyelonephritis and Renal Abscess

Pyelonephritis, renal parenchymal infection characterized by pyuria, fever, and costovertebral angle tenderness, is generally diagnosed and treated on clinical findings alone. CT imaging is not indicated in acute pyelonephritis but may be obtained if a patient does not improve after 72 hours of appropriate antibiotic treatment. In this situation, CT can detect or exclude complications such as an infected renal calculus or obstruction, renal abscess, or emphysematous pyelonephritis. Pyelonephritis is often identified on CT obtained for evaluation of abdominal pain when the diagnosis is not clinically evident.

CT with intravenous contrast will usually show an enlarged kidney with poor vascular perfusion. A "striated" nephrogram with well-defined areas of hypoenhancement results from focal inflammation that reduces vascular perfusion in portions of the infected kidney. Ultrasound will similarly show areas of heterogeneous perfusion characterized by areas of differing renal parenchymal echotexture and poor definition of the normal corticomedullary interface. The collecting system urothelium, which is normally imperceptibly thin on CT, may appear thickened and can enhance after contrast administration.

Renal abscesses can complicate ascending pyelonephritis and, when present, are usually located in the corticomedullary parenchyma. If an abscess is due to hematogenous spread from a distant infection, it is more frequently located at the renal cortex. Medical management is reasonable if the patient is hemodynamically stable and the abscess is smaller than 3 cm. Larger abscesses and abscess associated with sepsis with hypotension usually require percutaneous drainage. Predisposing factors include advanced age, diabetes mellitus, and obstructing renal calculus (**Fig. 6.24**).

Fig. 6.24a–f
a,b Pyelonephritis. Right-sided round, poorly defined low-attenuation parenchymal change. Mild perinephric stranding.
c,d Pyelonephritis and pyelitis. Poorly marginated, radially oriented areas of low attenuation within the right kidney parenchyma. Mild enhancement of the central renal collecting system urothelium. No hydronephrosis.
e Renal abscess. Well-defined low-attenuation mass centered in the right renal cortex with enhancing walls. A lesion in the right kidney is indeterminate and likely a simple cyst.
f Renal abscess in 15-month-old infant. Low-attenuation cystic masses with internal echoes in the corticomedullary portions of the upper pole and mid portion of the right kidney.

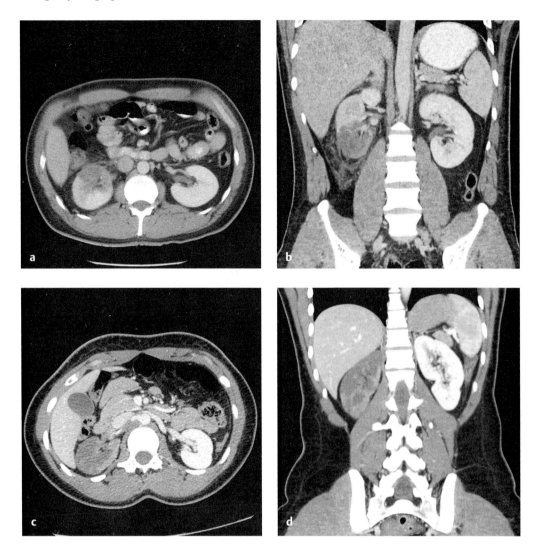

◆ Renal Infarct

Most renal infarcts are due to thromboemboli from valvular heart disease. They can also result from aortic dissection, traumatic renal artery dissection, vasculitis, and malignant hypertension. Renal infarcts may be asymptomatic or can present with acute flank or back pain, hematuria, and proteinuria.

Each renal segment is supplied by its own branch of the renal artery. The most common location for a segmental infarct is the upper pole of the kidney, but any part of the kidney can be involved. The base of the infarct is typically at the periphery, with the apex at the hilum.

On abdominal CT, a renal infarct is most easily identified on arterial or nephrographic postcontrast phases as a well-defined, wedge-shaped parenchymal lesion that involves both the cortex and medulla. If the main renal artery is occluded, the entire kidney may fail to enhance. CT obtained several hours after an acute renal artery occlusion will often show a thin rim of enhancing renal cortex, indicating collateral capsular perfusion (cortical rim sign).

Ultrasound is occasionally used in the emergency department if the diagnosis is uncertain. Acute infarction is identified by finding absent perfusion on color Doppler examination and may be either complete or focal depending on the location of occlusion. Doppler interrogation of the renal artery or vein can sometimes confirm thrombosis (**Fig. 6.25**).

Fig. 6.25a–d
a,b Renal infarct. A sharply defined area of low-attenuation involves the lower pole of the right kidney with moderate adjacent retroperitoneal fat stranding. The left kidney is normal.
c,d Traumatic right renal artery dissection and infarct. The right renal artery is occluded 1 cm from its origin. The kidney shows minimal peripheral enhancement related to capsular vessels and multiple areas of parenchymal infarction. The left kidney enhances normally.

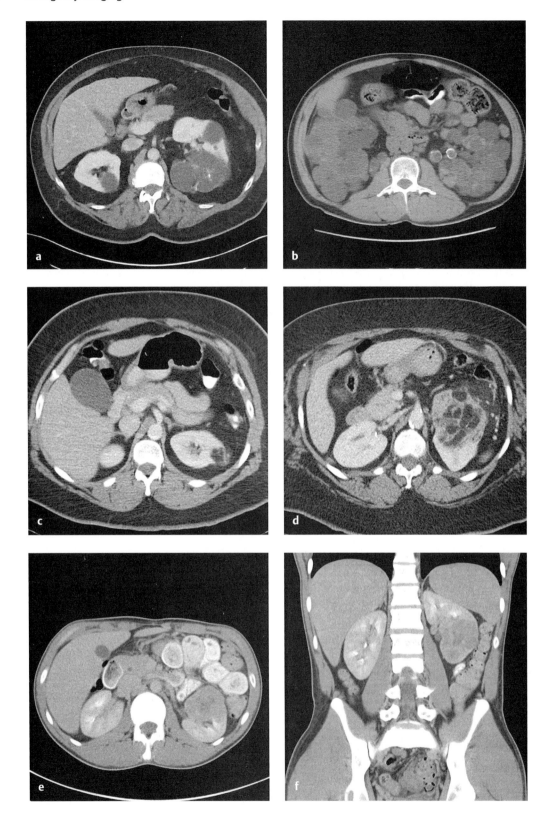

◆ Renal Masses and Renal Cell Carcinoma

Renal lesions of some sort are present in 50% of patients over age 50. While most malignant renal masses are incidentally discovered, most incidentally discovered lesions are benign. A renal mass that contains bulk fat is a benign angiomyolipoma. Solid renal masses that do not contain visible fat < 1 cm should be followed. In most cases, solid renal masses larger than 1 cm should be resected.

The malignant potential of an incidentally discovered renal cyst is based on their morphology. The Bosniak classification system allows management according to the following categories, shown in **Table 6.5**.

Category I and II lesions are benign and require no follow-up. Category IIF lesions are followed, with consideration of surgery if there is a change in morphology. Category III and IV masses are resected except in patients with limited life expectancy or significant comorbidities (**Table 6.6**).

For the general population, masses > 1 cm should be biopsied or resected, and masses < 1 cm should be followed until > 1 cm, then resected. Observation should be considered in all groups for patients with limited life expectancy or significant comorbidities.

Renal cell carcinoma (RCC), the most common malignant renal neoplasm in adults, is derived from the tubular epithelium of the kidney. While RCC can present clinically with macroscopic hematuria, flank pain, and a palpable flank mass, in most cases the diagnosis is made incidentally during CT or ultrasound assessment for nonspecific abdominal complaints. CT will show a solid renal mass, sometimes with necrosis, calcification, or hemorrhage. Renal vein invasion and upper abdominal adenopathy may be seen (**Fig. 6.26**).

Table 6.5 Bosniak classification system of renal cyst categories

I	Simple cyst with thin wall; no septa, calcification, or solid component; no enhancement; density = water
II	Few thin septa ± fine calcifications, or hyperdense cyst < 3 cm
IIF	Well-marginated with several thin septa ± calcification, no enhancing soft tissue, or hyperdense cyst > 3 cm
III	Cystic mass with thick, enhancing, irregular septa
IV	All elements of category III and enhancing soft-tissue components independent of but adjacent to septa

Table 6.6 Solid renal masses

> 3 cm	Renal cell carcinoma
> 1 cm	Renal cell carcinoma versus minimal fat angiomyolipoma
< 1 cm	Renal cell carcinoma, oncocytoma, angiomyolipoma

Fig. 6.26a–f
a Simple and complex renal cysts. Simple right renal cyst (category I). Complex left renal cyst with thin septations and calcification (category II).
b Polycystic kidney disease. Innumerable renal cysts, some of which are hyperdense; others contain peripheral calcifications. Pancreatic and hepatic cysts are also commonly seen in this condition.
c,d Small and large renal angiomyolipomas. (**c**) Small, peripheral, exophytic renal mass containing fat. (**d**) Large heterogenous fat-containing renal mass.
e,f Renal cell carcinoma. ~ 5 cm diameter solid left lower pole mass. No perinephric extension.

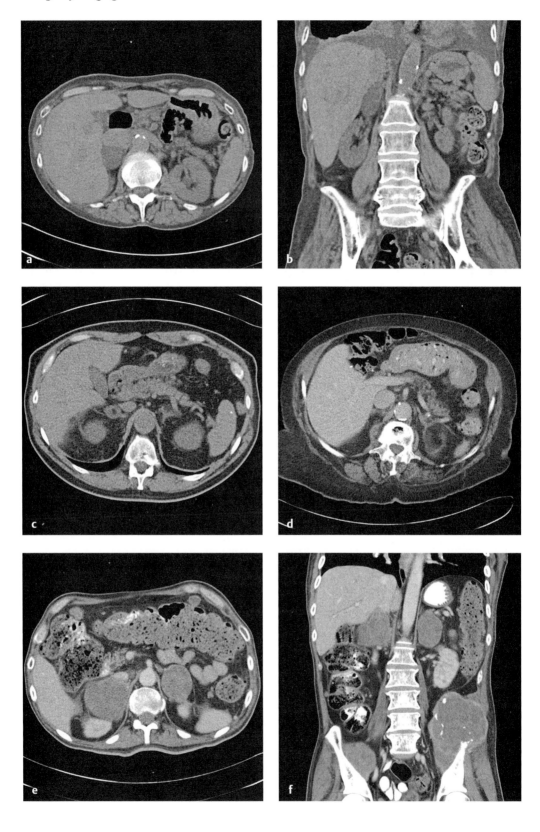

◆ Adrenal Nodules and Masses

Adrenal nodules are frequent incidental findings on abdominal CT. In patients with a known extra-adrenal malignancy, approximately 30–40% of adrenal masses will be metastatic. In patients without an underlying malignancy, a nodule or mass can be characterized by size and appearance as likely benign, indeterminate-risk, or highly suspicious for malignancy. Generally, larger masses and those with nodules that display persistent enhancement on delayed-contrast CT scans are more likely malignant.

Any mass larger than 5 cm that does not have visible fat on CT is likely malignant. Clearly identifiable fat within an adrenal mass is diagnostic of myelolipoma, and these require no further workup. Small, in-determinate nodules in patients without a history of malignancy can be followed up in 6 months to assess for stability.

On nonenhanced CT, the average attenuation of an adrenal adenoma is – 2 HU, while that of a metastasis is ~ 30 HU. On postcontrast CT, nodules with attenuation < 30 HU are almost always benign. For adrenal masses with attenuation > 10 HU on nonenhanced CT, or an initial attenuation > 30 HU on postcontrast CT, dynamic contrast washout can be determined. The patient is scanned immediately and 15 minutes after contrast administration; washout = (Initial HU – delayed HU)/(Initial HU). Greater than 50% washout indicates a benign adenoma (**Fig. 6.27**).

Fig. 6.27a–f
a,b Adrenal adenoma. 3-cm smooth, round, homogeneous right adrenal mass that measures 14 HU in attenuation on nonenhanced CT. Because this mass measures > 10 HU, dynamic CT with delayed imaging could be performed to determine percent washout and better characterize the mass as a benign adenoma.
c,d Adrenal myelolipomas. (**c**) Right adrenal mass containing bulk focal fat. The low-attenuation center of the enlarged right adrenal gland measures – 50 HU. (**d**) Large left adrenal mass composed primarily of fat.
e,f Adrenal metastasis from melanoma. 6-cm right and 5-cm left adrenal masses measuring 30 HU on postcontrast CT. Bilateral iliac wing metastases with large soft tissue components.

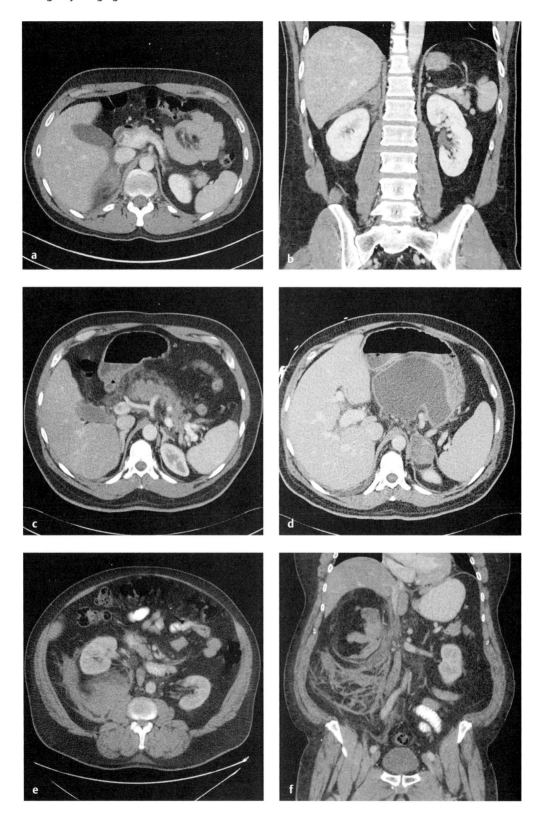

◆ Adrenal Hemorrhage

Adrenal hemorrhage can be a consequence of trauma, physiologic stresses, hypocoagulable states, and infection (meningococcemia). Unilateral adrenal hemorrhage is often asymptomatic and usually discovered as a focus of dystrophic calcification long after it has occurred. Acute bilateral hemorrhage is potentially catastrophic, as it can trigger an adrenal crisis leading to coma or death if not detected and treated.

CT identifies adrenal hemorrhage but cannot reliably differentiate a simple bleed from hemorrhagic tumor within the gland. Acute adrenal hemorrhage appears as a hyperdense (50 to 75 HU), round or oval intra-adrenal mass with perihemorrhagic fat stranding on noncontrast CT. If the apparent mass is larger than 5 cm or enhances with contrast, further evaluation is indicated to exclude hemorrhagic adrenal carcinoma or metastasis (**Fig. 6.28**).

Fig. 6.28a–f
a,b Acute adrenal hemorrhage. Ill-defined right adrenal enlargement with periadrenal stranding.
c,d Adrenal hemorrhage complicating pancreatitis. (**c**) Initial CT shows peripancreatic inflammation and normal left adrenal gland. (**d**) Follow-up examination shows a large pancreatic pseudocyst along lesser gastric curvature and a new left adrenal mass corresponding to interval hemorrhage.
e,f Hemorrhagic adrenal myelolipoma. Fat-containing right adrenal mass with large adjacent periadrenal and retroperitoneal hematoma.

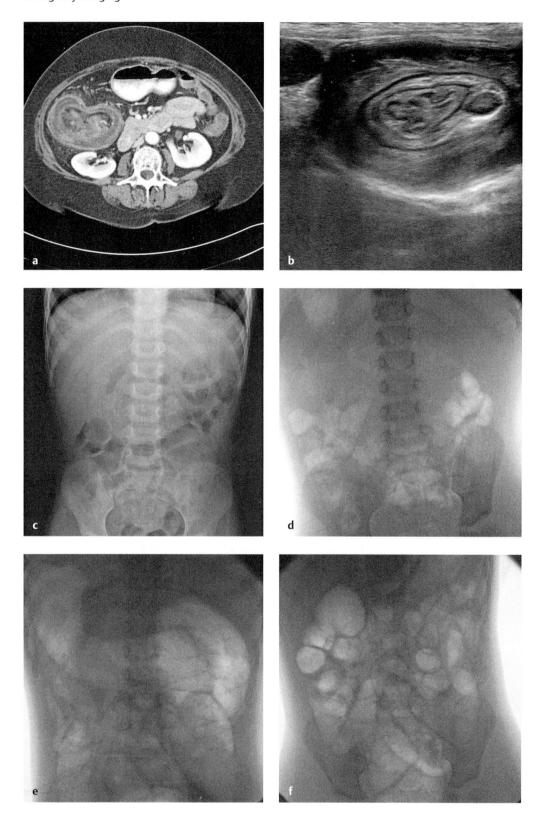

◆ Intussusception

In intussusception, peristalsis causes one segment of bowel (the intussusceptum) to invaginate into the lumen of the more distal bowel (the intussuscipiens). It is an uncommon cause of colonic and distal small-bowel obstruction in adults but is seen frequently in young children. In adults, it is usually caused by a mucosal or submucosal mass that acts as a lead point for the telescoping bowel. Such masses include lipomas, adenomatous polyps, leiomyoma, lymphoma, or metastases. Patients present with acute, severe, colicky abdominal pain, nausea, and vomiting. Transient intussusception is an asymptomatic, benign condition that usually involves the proximal small bowel and can be seen incidentally on CT examinations. A pathologic "lead point" is not identified, bowel obstruction does not occur, and the condition resolves spontaneously.

Adult intussusception appears on CT as a mass, contiguous with the bowel, with concentric, hyperdense, enhancing rings of tissue in transverse section. These correspond to the mucosa of the intussuscipiens and the superimposed edges of the folded serosa. Mesenteric fat and vessels may be pulled in with the telescoping proximal bowel, appearing as an eccentric mass alongside the intussuscipiens. High-grade obstruction, if present, and definitive diagnosis of any leading mass usually require laparotomy.

Pediatric intussusception most commonly involves the ileocolic junction, with most children presenting at between 3 months and 2 years of age. Often, no leading mass is identified, and in these cases, intussusception is usually due to lymphatic hypertrophy related to viral enteric infection. Rarely a Meckel diverticulum or polyp can create a pathologic lead point. Since the "classic" triad of abdominal pain, currant-jelly stools, and a palpable abdominal mass is present in fewer than 50% of children with intussusception, the diagnosis should be considered in any infant or toddler with sudden onset of severe and intermittent abdominal pain.

Abdominal plain films may show an elongated mass in the right upper quadrant with an air-filled cecum and collapsed distal colon. Ultrasound findings include the "target sign," in which concentric hypoechoic rings surround a hyperechoic core on transverse images, or the "crescent in donut sign," in which mesentery has been pulled into the intussuscipiens, forming an echogenic crescent on one side of the intussuscepted bowel. The longitudinal equivalent of the latter is referred to as the "pseudokidney" of intussusception; fat-containing mesentery appears similar to the normal renal hilum, and the adjacent edematous bowel to the normal renal parenchyma. A combination of plain radiograph and ultrasound is usually adequate to make the diagnosis, followed by fluoroscopically guided air enema, which is both diagnostic and therapeutic. Plain radiographs can exclude the diagnosis by revealing a completely normal air- or stool-filled colon (**Fig. 6.29**).

Fig. 6.29a–f
a Adult colo-colic intussusception due to cecal carcinoma. Large right upper quadrant mass containing rings of both mesenteric fat and soft tissue corresponding to both colon and intussuscepting tumor.
b–f Pediatric intussusception. (**b**) Ultrasound showing the "target sign." (**c**) Abnormal plain radiographic bowel gas pattern with gas limited to the small bowel and paucity of gas in the right upper quadrant. (**d–f**) Progressive insufflation of air per rectum with filling of the colon and reflux of air into the small bowel after the intussusception is reduced.

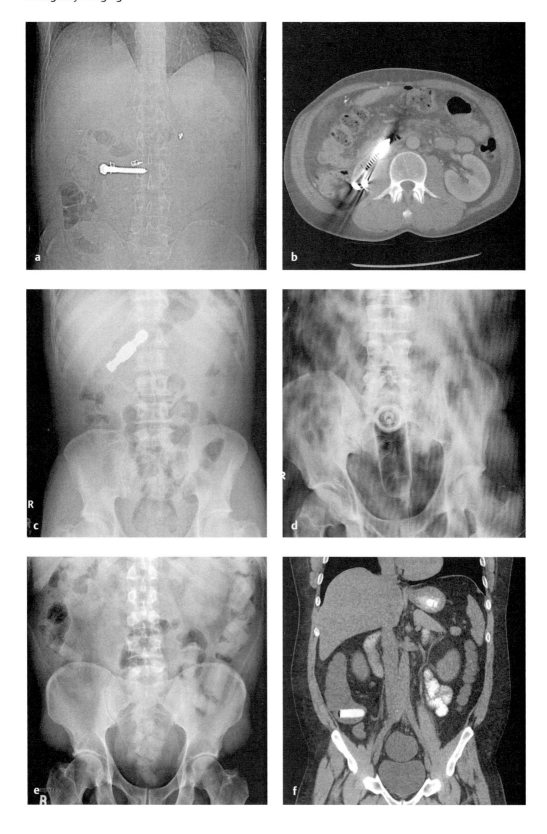

◆ Abdominal Foreign Bodies and Body Packing

Foreign objects that have been either ingested or inserted per rectum are often encountered in emergency practice, and most are easily localizable on plain radiographs. CT is occasionally necessary for identification of non-radiodense objects. Commonly swallowed objects include coins, batteries, pens, paper clips, toothbrushes, razor blades (often wrapped in tape), and illegal drugs secured within balloons or condoms for the purpose of smuggling.

Most small ingested objects will pass uneventfully through the gastrointestinal tract. Elongated or sharp objects can cause perforation and should be removed by endoscopy if they are located in the stomach or esophagus. "Button" batteries that have lodged in the esophagus can cause tissue necrosis in a relatively short period of time and should also be removed promptly. Those that have passed into the stomach can usually be observed as they transit through the GI tract.

Objects inserted in the rectum are frequently "plastic novelties" but can comprise a diverse group that includes vegetables, aerosol cans, jars, cooking spoons, and lightbulbs, among many others. Removal of some objects can be challenging, and CT is occasionally useful for precise localization.

The primary concern is perforation and studies should be carefully evaluated for signs of free intraperitoneal air, especially in patients with abdominal pain.

Rarely, instruments or sponges are retained after surgery, especially in obese individuals and following emergent operations. If unrecognized, these may cause late adhesions, obstruction, abscess, or perforation.

Body packing is the concealment of illegal drugs within the abdomen. Drugs are typically carefully packed, wrapped into a sheathlike glove finger, plastic bag, condom, or balloon for transport across national borders. Smugglers usually employ constipating agents to prolong transit time. Laxatives or other promotility medications may be used upon arrival to help pass the packets.

On abdominal radiograph, ingested packets may be visible as oval or round radio-opaque foreign bodies surrounded by a gas halo. Noncontrast CT is the imaging modality of choice and provides critical information on the number, location, size, and shape of packets. Most patients are managed conservatively with laxatives and observation for passage of packets. Symptomatic or unstable patients may require laparotomy (**Fig. 6.30**).

Fig. 6.30a–f
a–c Ingested foreign bodies. (**a,b**) A large screw as well as several small metallic foreign bodies are located in the duodenum. (**c**) Ingested crack cocaine pipe in distal stomach or proximal duodenum.
d Inserted foreign body per rectum. An aerosol canister is located in the rectosigmoid.
e,f Body packing. (**e**) Abdominal radiograph shows numerous tubular packets of heroin surrounded by gas within the colon. (**f**) After passage of most of the packets, CT reveals that one is left in the cecum.

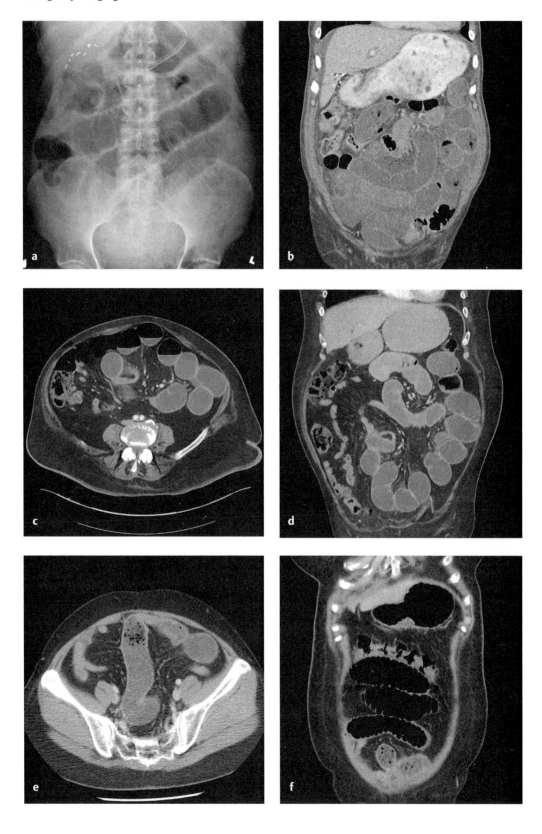

◆ Small-Bowel Obstruction I

Small-bowel obstruction (SBO) is a common cause of acute abdominal pain and a frequent indication for abdominal imaging. The most common causes are adhesions from prior surgery, malignancy, acute inflammatory bowel disease, and internal or external hernias. Rarely, SBO follows perforation of the gallbladder with passage of a gallstone into adherent small bowel (gallstone ileus) or intussusception.

Intermittent abdominal pain, nausea, vomiting, and distention are presenting symptoms, with severity and progression dependent upon whether the obstruction is partial or complete, obstructed at a single point (simple) or "closed loop," in which a segment of small bowel is torsed about itself, creating an isolated loop of bowel obstructed at both ends. If not diagnosed and properly treated, SBO can lead to dehydration, metabolic abnormalities, and bowel ischemia from vascular compromise. In contrast to colonic obstruction, constipation and the absence of flatus are usually late features.

Plain abdominal radiographs show distended loops of small bowel provided they are at least partially filled with air. If the distended bowel is completely fluid-filled, the appearance will be that of a gasless abdomen. Thickened edematous plicae circularis may be seen, and with severe distention these may become completely effaced. Small-bowel loops are generally located centrally in the abdomen and should be less than 3 cm in diameter. On upright radiographs, three or more air-fluid levels suggests obstruction. A "string of pearls" appearance sometimes results from nearly completely fluid-filled bowel with small bubbles of air trapped against the plicae.

CT confirms disproportionate small-bowel distention and can usually locate a transition point between the proximally distended and distally collapsed bowel. The "small-bowel feces" sign refers to a bubbly appearance of air and fluid that resembles colonic contents and is often located in small bowel immediately proximal to the point of obstruction. Provided enough time has been permitted for oral contrast to reach the colon by the time the patient is scanned, contrast beyond the ileocecal valve excludes complete small-bowel obstruction.

Bowel wall thickening, segmental lack of mucosal contrast enhancement, frank ascites, or interloop fluid are all signs of ischemia. These are more commonly seen in closed-loop obstruction. Serum lactate is usually elevated in bowel ischemia and is a useful confirmatory test (**Fig. 6.31**).

Fig. 6.31a–f
a,b Small-bowel obstruction with ischemic bowel. Supine radiograph shows markedly dilated air-filled small bowel without colonic gas. On coronal CT, oral contrast fills only the stomach, the small bowel is filled with fluid, and a distal segment of bowel in the right lower quadrant has a thick edematous wall, consistent with ischemia.
c,d Transition point in small-bowel obstruction. The proximal small bowel is moderately dilated and filled with fluid on axial and coronal images. A transition point between dilated proximal and collapsed distal small bowel is located in the mid-abdomen anterior to the spine.
e,f Small-bowel feces sign. High grade obstruction due to an adhesion along the anterior abdominal wall showing the typical bubbly appearance of fecalized small-bowel contents immediately proximal to the obstruction.

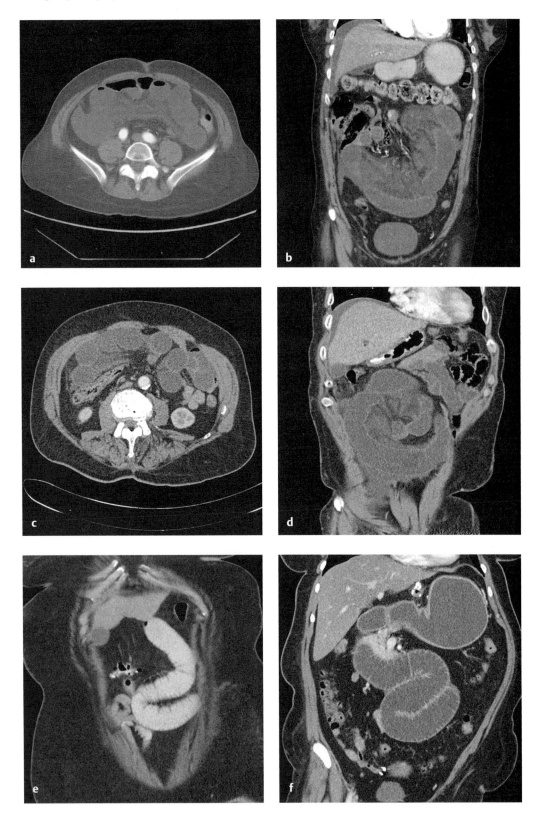

◆ Small-Bowel Obstruction II

Closed-loop obstruction results when a single point of obstruction isolates a loop of bowel from the remainder of the intestine. This usually occurs when a portion of bowel torses, passes through a mesenteric herniation, or is obstructed at two points by a single adhesion. In closed-loop obstruction there is a high risk of bowel ischemia and perforation.

CT identifies c- or u-shaped small-bowel loops in a radial orientation or twisting of mesenteric vessels about the point of obstruction. Wall thickening, hypoenhancement, and ascites all indicate bowel ischemia.

Roux-en-Y gastrojejunostomy is commonly performed for obesity and involves the division of the proximal jejunum distal to the ligament of Treatise and the creation of two anastomoses. The more proximal anastomosis is located between a pouch created from the gastric cardia and the distal jejunal segment (gastrojejunonostomy).

The second is between the excluded stomach/duodenal/jejunal segment and the small bowel (enteroenteric anastomosis). The reconnected bowel forms a y in which one limb bypasses the stomach and duodenum, limiting food absorption (the "Roux" or efferent limb) and the other carries intestinal secretions, pancreatic enzymes, and bile into the more distal small bowel (the biliopancreatic or afferent limb). Either of these two limbs can become obstructed at the enteroenteric anastomosis, and patients may present with a complete or partial obstruction at any time from immediately after surgery to decades after the operation.

Abdominal CT directly visualizes both segments and can distinguish between Roux limb, biliopancreatic limb, and distal obstruction. Radiography is nonspecific and will show distended loops of small bowel but usually cannot show the type of obstruction (**Fig. 6.32**).

Fig. 6.32a–f
a–d Closed-loop obstruction in two patients. Multiple loops of distended, mildly thick walled, hypoenhancing bowel radiate from a point in the mid mesentery in a u-shaped conformation. Moderate interloop and perihepatic fluid.
e,f Obstruction in gastric bypass. (**e**) Roux (efferent) limb obstruction with contrast-filled distended jejunum leading from the upper abdomen distally. (**f**) Pancreaticobiliary (afferent) limb obstruction. The excluded portion of the stomach, duodenum, and proximal jejunum are distended with fluid that does not contain oral contrast. The Roux limb and distal small bowel are collapsed.

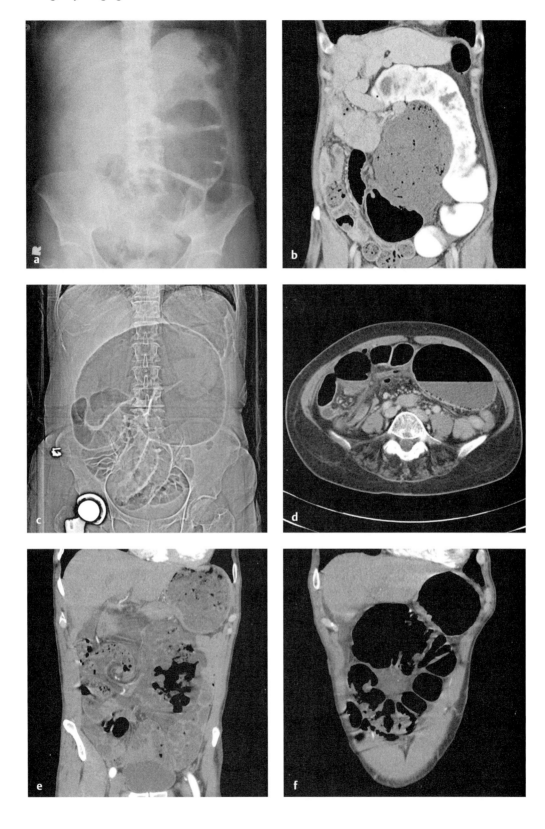

◆ Cecal Volvulus

If the cecal attachment to the posterior abdominal wall is deficient, the cecum and ascending colon can twist around its mesentery, effectively forming a closed-loop obstruction, or the cecum can simply fold upon itself (cecal bascule). In the latter situation, the cecum is obstructed distally by the fold and proximally by a competent ileocecal valve. Patients present with acute pain, constipation, and inability to pass flatus, often with a distended and tympanitic abdomen.

When the cecum simply twists along its long axis, the focally distended bowel is located in the right lower quadrant. If the mesentery supporting the cecum and distal small bowel twists as well, the distended loop tends to be located in the left upper quadrant. With upward folding of the cecum (bascule), the distended loop is usually in the mid, lower abdomen.

Adhesions, masses, or scarring can all act as a point of fixation and an axis for rotation. Predisposition to volvulus is probably due to developmental failure of cecal fixation to the posterior abdominal wall.

Plain radiographs show a gas-filled, distended loop of bowel that can resemble a coffee bean as it extends from the right lower quadrant to the left upper quadrant. CT will show beaking, or tapering of afferent and efferent loops, as well as the "whirl" sign common to all forms of colonic volvulus. The whirl is formed by the engorged mesenteric fat and vasculature radiating outward from the nidus of twisted bowel.

In contrast to sigmoid volvulus, which can be reduced by colonoscopy, cecal volvulus is managed surgically (**Fig. 6.33**).

Fig. 6.33a–f
a,b Cecal volvulus. Distended, air and fluid filled cecum located in the left abdomen. CT after rectal contrast administration confirms obstruction at the hepatic flexure.
c,d CT localizer shows massively distended cecal loop in left upper quadrant with moderately distended, air-filled small bowel loops in the right lower quadrant. This pattern conforms to twisting of mesentery supplying both large and distal small bowel.
e,f Mesenteric twisting in cecal volvulus. Large loop of distended ascending colon with the cecum located in the upper abdomen. Right upper quadrant swirl of vessels, mesentery, and small bowel.

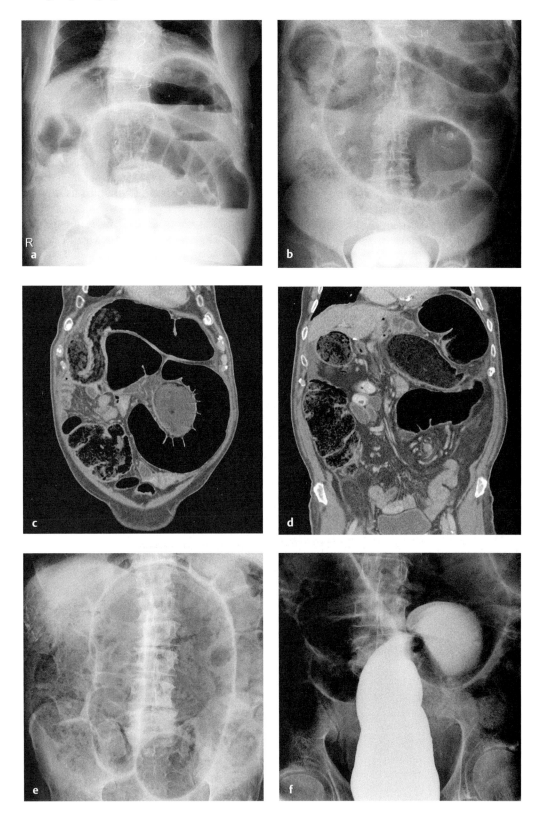

◆ Sigmoid Volvulus

Sigmoid volvulus is the most common form of gastrointestinal volvulus and occurs when the sigmoid colon twists on its mesentery, the sigmoid mesocolon. Patients present with acute colicky abdominal pain and distention. Constipation, inability to pass flatus, and borborygmus are other signs that may accompany sigmoid volvulus, but such findings are common and often not sufficiently reliable for clinical diagnosis.

Plain radiographs may show the "beak" sign at tapering of the afferent and efferent loops leading to the dilated segment of sigmoid colon. An inverted u-shaped "coffee bean sign" is often seen as the distended closed loop of air-filled bowel extends from the left lower quadrant toward the mid-abdomen. CT imaging will show beaking at the point of obstruction as well as distended sigmoid colon proximal to the volvulus. The "whirl" sign, formed by the engorged mesenteric fat and vasculature leading into the twisted bowel segment, may be seen in sigmoid volvulus as in midgut and cecal volvulus.

Sigmoid volvulus can usually be reduced by careful passage of an endoscope or rectal tube (**Fig. 6.34** and **Fig. 6.35**).

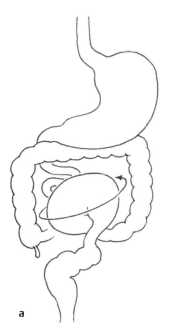
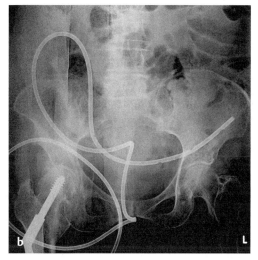

Fig. 6.35a,b
a,b Anatomy of sigmoid volvulus. (**a**) Torsion of redundant or mobile sigmoid results in closed-loop obstruction. This can usually be reduced by passage of a rectal tube or endoscope. (**b**) Rectal tube looping within and extending beyond a sigmoid volvulus.

Fig. 6.34a–f
a–f Sigmoid volvulus. (**a–d**) Air-filled, distended loop of sigmoid colon in the left lower quadrant. CT shows distended sigmoid with haustra and swirling mesenteric vessels. (**e,f**) Another patient shows a similar "coffee bean" sign of markedly distended loop. Barium enema shows point of torsion in left lower quadrant.

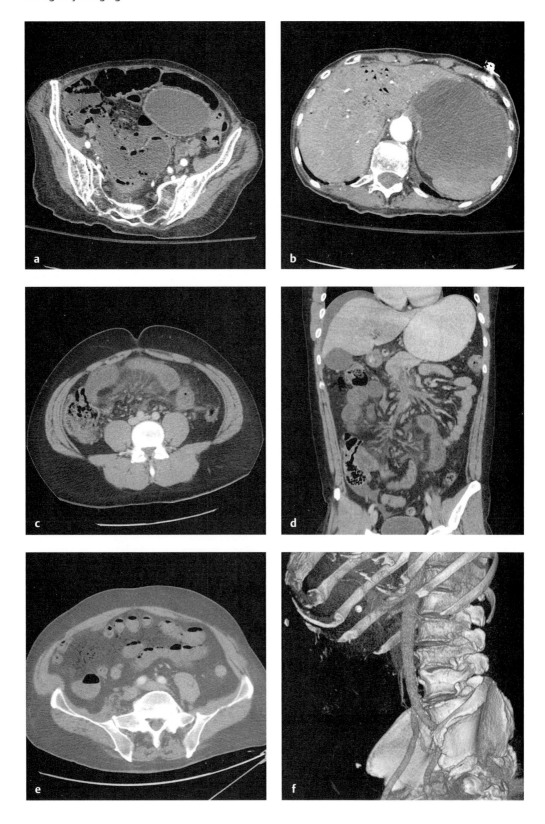

◆ Acute Bowel Ischemia and Necrosis

Acute bowel ischemia results from sudden compromise of the arterial supply or venous drainage to the large or small bowel. Injury may be segmental or diffuse and range in severity from superficial mucosal ischemia to full-thickness bowel wall necrosis. Etiologies include mechanical bowel obstruction, atherosclerosis, thromboembolic disease, vasculitis, aortic aneurysm, and low-flow states such as hypovolemic shock and cardiac failure. Acute periumbilical pain in an elderly patient, with little or no tenderness or rebound pain is a common presentation.

Ischemia due to small-bowel obstruction appears on radiographs and CT as segmental small bowel dilatation with wall thickening, hypoenhancement, and ascites. In contrast, ischemia due to arterial or venous occlusion usually shows a normal, or nonspecifically abnormal gas pattern on radiographs. Air in the intrahepatic portal venous system, the portal and mesenteric veins, and the bowel wall (pneumatosis intestinalis) may be seen in severe ischemia. Air in the portal venous system appears as fine linear and branching lucencies at the periphery of the liver, in contrast to pneumobilia, which is centrally located and is commonly seen in patients who have had prior ERCP or biliary stenting.

Contrast-enhanced CT with arterial-phase imaging best evaluates the patency of mesenteric vessels and the extent of bowel ischemia and can identify alternative causes of abdominal pain. Bowel wall thickening (> 5 mm) with decreased enhancement is a specific finding of bowel ischemia. Supportive findings include mesenteric or portal arterial and venous thrombosis, intramural gas, mesenteric fat stranding, portal venous gas, mucosal edema, and dilation of the bowel proximal to the region of ischemia (**Fig. 6.36**).

Fig. 6.36a–f
a,b Ischemic bowel due to superior mesenteric artery thrombus. Pneumatosis intestinalis, air within the peripheral branches of the portal venous system and bowel wall hypoenhancement.
c,d Superior mesenteric vein thrombus. Thickened small-bowel wall with mesenteric edema and vascular engorgement. The superior mesenteric and portal veins do not opacify.
e,f Superior mesenteric artery thrombus. Pneumatosis intestinalis and air within the small bowel wall and mesenteric veins. 3D CT reformation shows abrupt cutoff of the proximal superior mesenteric artery ~ 4 cm from its origin.

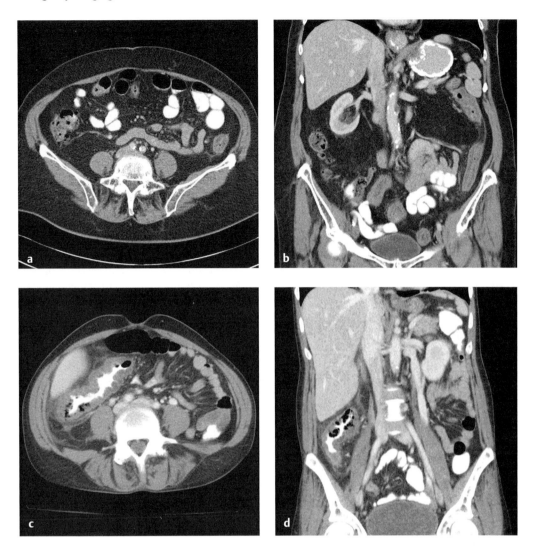

◆ Ischemic Colitis

Ischemic colitis results from inadequate colonic perfusion, usually subacute or chronic. Causes include arterial insufficiency, mesenteric venous thrombosis, arterial embolism, hypotension, vasospasm, or vasculitis. The consequence of poor perfusion is inflammation and injury, most commonly involving the border zone between the superior and inferior mesenteric artery circulations: the descending colon and splenic flexure.

The severity and consequences of the disease are highly variable. Ischemic colitis or intestinal ischemia is typically a disease of the elderly with most patients 60 years or older. In younger patients, the disease is usually a consequence of vasculitis or hypercoagulable states. Patients present with generalized or left-sided abdominal pain and bloody diarrhea. If the colitis has progressed to necrosis and perforation, peritoneal signs may be present.

Plain abdominal radiographs are either normal or nonspecifically abnormal, often demonstrating an ileus pattern with dilated, fluid-filled loops of bowel and thumbprinting due to mucosal edema. Contrast-enhanced CT identifies the segment of bowel affected, and images obtained in arterial phase can detect thromboemboli to the proximal mesenteric arteries. Positive findings include segmental colitis, particularly in the setting of visceral or lower aortic atherosclerotic disease, left colon location, and arterial or venous thrombosis. In severe ischemia, pneumatosis coli and portal venous gas may be seen.

Prognosis is variable, depending on the etiology, severity, and presence of any complication. Arterial or venous thrombosis can be treated with anticoagulation or thrombolysis, either systemically or locally, and percutaneous interventions may be employed in cases of embolic occlusion. Emergent surgical intervention is indicated for peritonitis, perforation, and obstructing stricture (**Fig. 6.37**).

Fig. 6.37a–d
a,b Chronic ischemic colitis. Left-sided segmental bowel wall thickening without pericolonic inflammatory changes.
c,d Acute right-sided ischemic colitis. Marked focal ascending colon wall thickening with areas of pneumatosis and pericolonic inflammation.

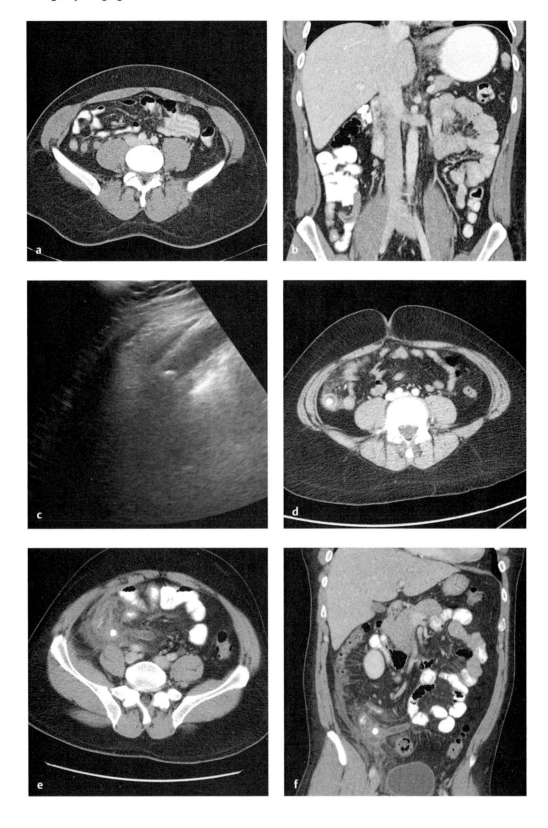

◆ Acute and Perforated Appendicitis

Acute appendicitis is the most common reason for emergency abdominal surgery. Appendiceal luminal occlusion by an appendicolith (fecalith) or by lymphoid hyperplasia causes an increase in intraluminal and intramural pressures that compromise local venous and lymphatic drainage. Bacterial invasion of the appendiceal wall follows. Anorexia and periumbilical pain localize over a period of hours to the right lower quadrant, with associated leukocytosis, fever, and signs of peritoneal irritation.

CT is the most appropriate imaging modality for evaluation of acute appendicitis in adults. The diagnosis is made by finding an enlarged, fluid-filled appendix, often with wall enhancement and surrounding fat stranding. The normal appendiceal wall thickness is less than 2 mm, and the normal diameter is 6 mm or less. An appendicolith may or may not be present and can be incidentally seen in patients scanned for other reasons. In the setting of right lower quadrant pain, detecting an appendicolith is usually diagnostic of acute appendicitis.

Ultrasonography is the preferred initial study for children and pregnant women in order both to avoid ionizing radiation and to exclude potentially confounding gynecologic pathology. A noncompressible, blind-ending tubular structure that arises from the cecum and has a diameter greater than 6 mm is diagnostic. An obstructing appendicolith, periappendiceal fluid, and echogenic pericecal fat support the diagnosis. Locating the appendix can sometimes be challenging, and failure to identify an abnormal appendix does not exclude appendicitis in the patient with typical symptoms. The sensitivity and specificity of ultrasound is reduced in obese patients and varies depending on the operator's expertise. MRI without gadolinium is an alternative to CT and may be used in pregnant patients to avoid exposure to ionizing radiation.

Perforated appendicitis complicates acute appendicitis in up to a third of cases and, if it occurs, is associated with significant morbidity due to wound infection, urinary retention, ileus, small-bowel obstruction, and abscess.

In both ruptured and unruptured appendicitis, the abnormal appendix is distended and thick-walled with periappendiceal inflammatory changes. Findings indicating perforation include a gap in the appendiceal wall, adjacent free fluid or extraluminal air, an appendicolith outside of the bowel lumen, large phlegmon, or a frank pericecal abscess. While contrast-enhanced CT detects acute appendicitis with high sensitivity and specificity, very early or subtle perforation may not always be distinguishable from unruptured appendicitis.

Distinguishing perforated from nonperforated appendicitis is important because it often precludes immediate surgery in favor of antibiotic treatment and, if an abscess has formed, percutaneous drainage. If urgent appendectomy is contemplated, evidence of perforation usually indicates an open rather than a laparoscopic approach (**Fig. 6.38**).

Fig. 6.38a–f
a,b Acute appendicitis. The appendix is thick-walled with overall diameter 1.5 cm and minimal periappendiceal inflammatory changes. The lumen does not fill with oral contrast.
c,d Ultrasound of acute appendicitis. Dilated, noncompressible blind-ending tubular structure with shadowing echogenic calcification at the apex. Corresponding CT shows a dilated, thick-walled appendix containing an appendicolith with surrounding inflammatory changes.
e,f Perforated appendicitis. Periappendiceal phlegmon. The appendix is dilated, with enhancing but incomplete wall and periappendiceal inflammatory changes. A 1.5-cm appendicolith is located adjacent to the cecum in an area of inflammatory change. While there is a small amount of free fluid, there is no well-defined abscess.

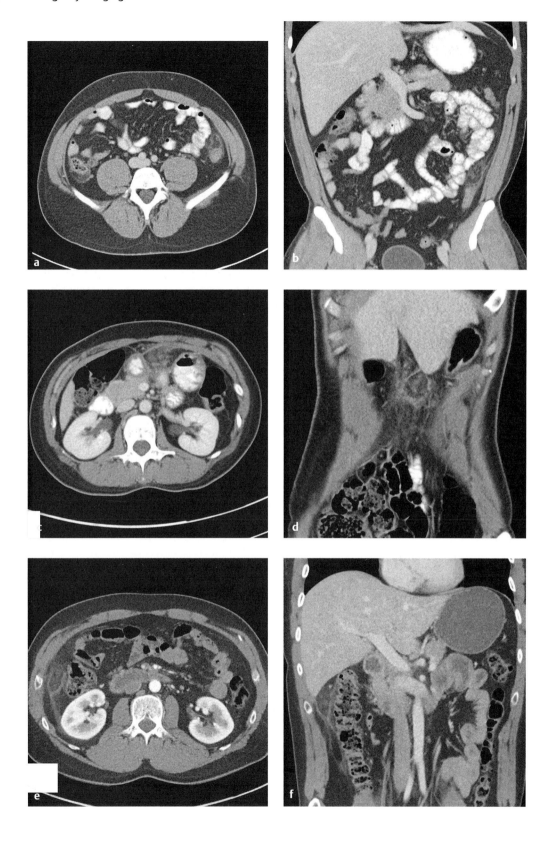

◆ Epiploic Appendagitis and Omental Infarct

Epiploic appendagitis refers to infarction and inflammation of small, fat-filled, peritoneal outpouchings found along the serosal surface of the colon, known as the epiploic appendages. These are not normally visible on CT imaging, but if they are torsed, venous obstruction and thrombosis of the vascular stalk leads to edema and inflammation. Epiploic appendagitis presents clinically with abdominal pain similar to that of appendicitis or diverticulitis: acute pain localized to the right or left flank. In contrast to appendicitis or diverticulitis, nausea, fever, and leukocytosis are uncommon. Epiploic appendagitis typically occurs in middle-aged patients, especially women and obese individuals.

CT findings are diagnostic and consist of a hyperdense halo of inflammatory stranding surrounding a 0.5- to 5-cm oval nidus of normal fat, closely related to the serosal surface of the colon. A central thrombosed vessel may or may not be visible. Appendagitis can occur anywhere along the colon, but most often involves the rectosigmoid junction.

Symptoms resolve spontaneously within 2 weeks, and treatment, when necessary for pain, is with nonsteroidal anti-inflammatory drugs (NSAIDs). CT findings may take up to 6 months to return to normal.

Omental infarction is due to vascular compromise of a portion of the omentum from adhesion, torsion, or an anomalous blood supply. It can occur spontaneously, following intra-abdominal surgery, and in patients with omentum-containing inguinal hernias. Symptoms include sharp, constant right-sided abdominal pain, often with low-grade fever and leukocytosis.

CT is diagnostic and reveals a focal, heterogeneous area of increased attenuation within the fatty omentum, usually ventral to the transverse colon or anteromedial to the ascending colon, that extends over an area greater than 5 cm in diameter. Fat stranding, parietal peritoneal thickening, and mild bowel wall thickening may also be seen. While imaging findings are similar to those of epiploic appendagitis, omental infarction typically involves a larger area, has a different distribution, and less commonly demonstrates a well-defined enhancing ring.

While omental infarct can mimic the symptoms of acute appendicitis or diverticulitis, it is, like epiploic appendagitis, a benign, self-limited condition, and its management is similarly limited to pain control. Only with severe or prolonged symptoms might operative management be considered (**Fig. 6.39**).

Fig. 6.39a–f
a,b Epiploic appendagitis. A well-defined oval, ~ 2-cm area of fat with surrounding inflammatory changes abuts the anterior wall of the descending colon.
c,d Omental infarction, ascending colon. Focal inflammatory changes involve an oblong portion of right subhepatic fat along the antimesenteric border of the ascending colon; thickening of the adjacent transversalis fascia.
e,f Omental infarction, transverse colon. Focal inflammatory changes involve the transverse colonic omentum in the midline subjacent to the rectus abdominis.

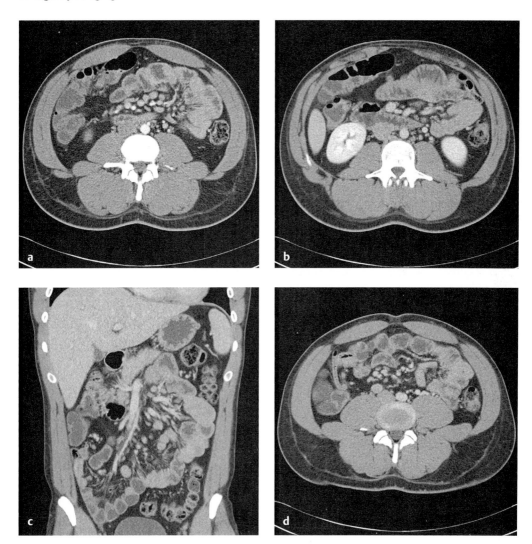

◆ Mesenteric Adenitis

Mesenteric adenitis is commonly seen in children and young adults and can clinically mimic acute appendicitis, with acute right lower quadrant pain, fever, and leukocytosis. Reactive, painful adenopathy involves the central and right lower quadrant mesentery, often as a consequence of viral enteritis. Mildly thickened loops of jejunum are a common associated finding.

CT shows conspicuous mesenteric lymph nodes, the largest of which typically measure between 5 and 15 mm. While mesenteric lymphadenopathy can be seen in many conditions, including malignancy, AIDS, amyloidosis, sarcoidosis, and myco-bacterial infections, most of these conditions affect older adults and are usually one manifestation of an otherwise systemic disease. In an otherwise healthy child or young adult with acute abdominal pain, the most likely diagnoses are appendicitis or inflammatory bowel disease. These should be excluded before making the presumptive diagnosis of mesenteric adenitis. Uncomplicated appendicitis is not usually associated with prominent adenopathy.

Mesenteric adenitis is treated conservatively. Pain and inflammation typically abate over the course of a few weeks, and most patients do not require hospitalization (**Fig. 6.40**).

Fig. 6.40a–d
a–d Mesenteric adenitis. (**a–c**) Multiple enlarged intramesenteric lymph nodes. Thickened jejunum. (**d**) Normal air-containing appendix.

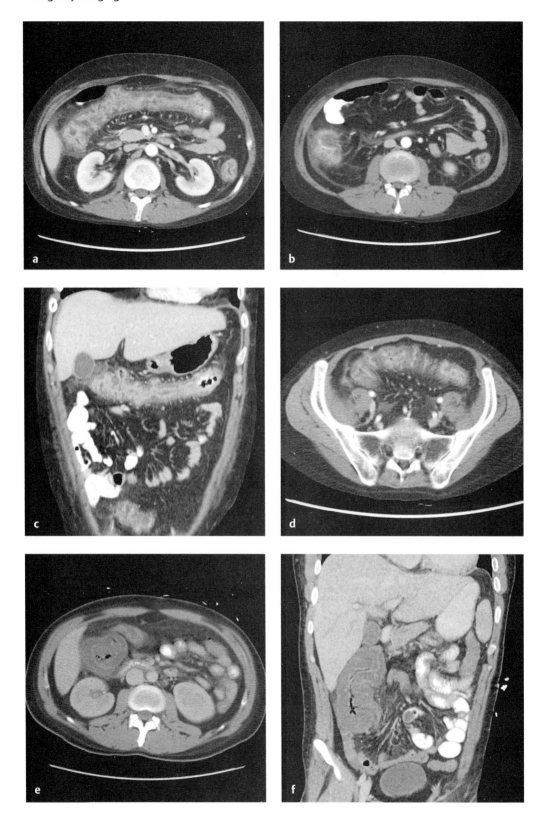

◆ Pseudomembranous and Neutropenic Colitis

Pseudomembranous colitis is an infectious colitis that results from proliferation of *Clostridium difficile,* often as a consequence of recent antibiotic therapy or chemotherapy that displaces the patient's normal gut bacteria. Clinical features are diffuse, crampy abdominal pain, diarrhea, fever, and leukocytosis. It is usually seen in hospitalized patients and can have a high morbidity and mortality, as untreated or refractory pseudomembranous colitis can progress to toxic megacolon, perforation, and peritonitis.

Radiographs are nonspecific, but bowel dilatation with mural and haustral thickening may be seen. Pseudomembranous colitis characteristically shows severe bowel wall thickening involving most or all of the colon. Edematous haustral folds divide the colonic lumen into narrow contrast-filled spaces with the appearance of accordion bellows. Rectal involvement with pericolic stranding is common. Diagnosis is by identification of *C. difficile* antigen and toxin.

Oral vancomycin or intravenous metronidazole are primary treatments. Fecal bacteriotherapy (stool transplant) has been employed with success. In severe cases, colectomy may be necessary.

Neutropenic colitis, or cecitis, is a circumferential cecal or right-sided colitis seen in patients undergoing chemotherapy or immunosuppressive treatment. It is associated with bowel distention that can progress to necrosis and perforation. Apart from its predilection for the proximal colon, neutropenic colitis appears much like any other colitis, with segmental bowel-wall thickening and variable adjacent inflammatory fat stranding and fluid.

Clinically, neutropenic colitis can mimic acute appendicitis with right lower quadrant pain and fever. In contrast to most patients with acute appendicitis, patients with neutropenic colitis have very low WBC counts (less than 1,000 cells/mm^3 with total neutrophil count less than 500 per milliliter) and often have diarrhea. Oral and pharyngeal mucositis may manifest before the onset of colonic symptoms.

Management is supportive and consists of bowel rest, intravenous hydration, and broad-spectrum antibiotic therapy. Close clinical monitoring for signs of abscess, necrosis, or perforation is necessary to avoid delay in surgery should it become necessary. CT can serve as both a baseline examination and follow-up study in the event of clinical deterioration (**Fig. 6.41**).

Fig. 6.41a–f
a–d Pseudomembranous colitis. (**a–c**) The entire colonic wall is edematous with enlarged pericolonic lymphatic vessels and inflammatory changes in the adjacent fat. (**d**) The "accordion" sign, formed by thickened haustra in the sigmoid colon.
e,f Neutropenic colitis. Marked mucosal and submucosal colonic thickening, limited to the cecum. Normal small bowel.

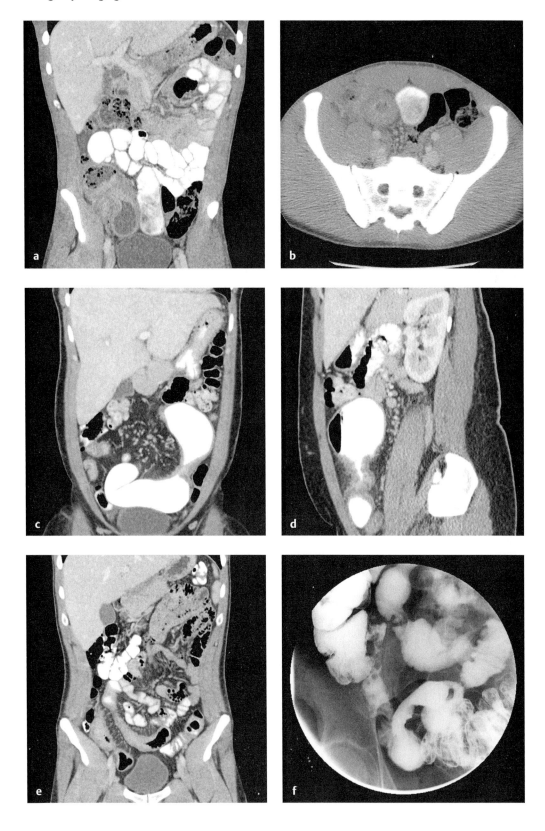

◆ Crohn Disease

Crohn disease is an inflammatory bowel disease with granulomatous, transmural inflammation affecting noncontinuous segments (skip lesions) in any part of the gastrointestinal tract. The disease preferentially involves the ileocolic junction. Crohn disease tends to present more insidiously than ulcerative colitis; patients often report vague symptoms for years prior to diagnosis.

Barium studies with small-bowel follow-through may show deep transmural ulcerations, which may be either longitudinal or circumferential, in the bowel wall. The sparing of intervening normal mucosa results in a cobblestone appearance. Intramural edema produces thickened folds (thumbprinting).

CT is commonly performed in the emergency department for patients with acute abdominal pain, and a first diagnosis of Crohn disease is often made in this setting. If colitis is suspected, both intravenous and intraluminal oral contrast should be given in order to best detect bowel wall thickening and enhancement as well as to identify any associated abscess or fistula.

Patients with established disease may show fibrofatty proliferation along the mesenteric small bowel border and enlarged vasa recta, giving the appearance of a comb (the "comb" sign). Subserosal fat can be seen in areas of remote quiescent disease.

Complications of severe or longstanding disease include fibrotic stricture with bowel obstruction and potential perforation, abdominal abscesses, toxic colitis, fistulae (enteroenteric, enterovesicular, or enterocutaneous), and bleeding. Perianal disease is common and associated with local abscess, fistula, and sinus tract formation and is a frequent reason for emergency department visits.

Patients with Crohn disease tend to receive many abdominal CT examinations over time. While CT is optimal for diagnosis and primary evaluation, MRI can be used as an alternative to reduce the cumulative radiation dose in patients with known disease (**Fig. 6.42**).

Fig. 6.42a–f
a,b   Crohn disease involving terminal ileum. Marked focal terminal ileal transmural thickening with stricture at the ileocecal junction. The remainder of the small and large bowel is normal.
c,d   Crohn disease with sigmoid colon stricture. CT with rectal contrast shows segmental sigmoid wall thickening, mild pericolonic inflammatory changes, and several mesenteric lymph nodes.
e,f   Ileal and cecal Crohn disease. Severe distal ileal and cecal transmural thickening with "comb sign" on CT and "cobblestoning" on small-bowel contrast examination.

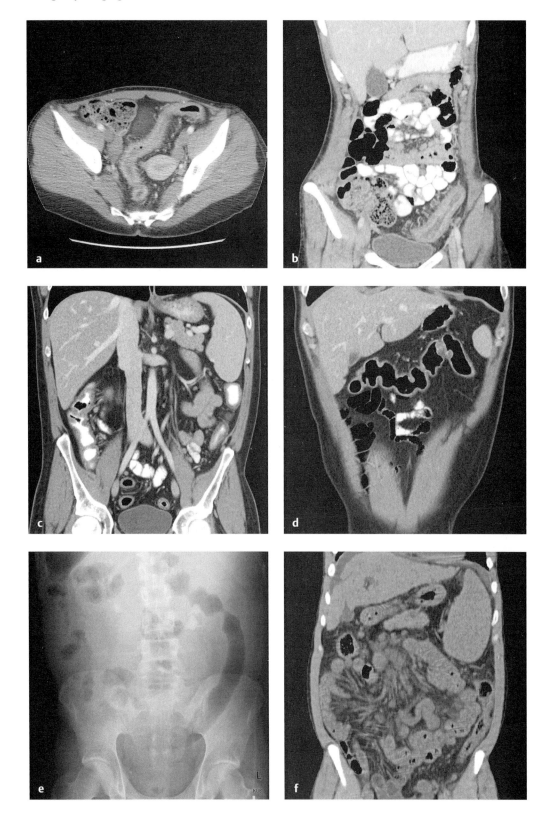

◆ Ulcerative Colitis

Ulcerative colitis, like Crohn disease, is an inflammatory bowel disorder with systemic manifestations. In contrast to Crohn colitis, inflammation in ulcerative colitis tends to involve the colonic mucosa and submucosa most severely, resulting in ulceration and the formation of shallow crypt abscesses. Ulcerative colitis typically involves the rectum with variable but usually contiguous extension to the more proximal colon, and patients present with abdominal pain, tenesmus, fecal urgency, and bloody diarrhea.

While the diagnosis is usually made by endoscopy and biopsy, radiographs, fluoroscopy and cross-sectional imaging can accurately evaluate the extent of colonic involvement. Radiographs may show mural thickening of the bowel wall with intramural edema, or thumbprinting, in more severe cases. If no contraindication exists, double-contrast barium enema can provide exquisite detail of the colonic mucosa and may show a granular appearance with scattered islands of normal mucosa remaining, sometimes referred to as pseudopolyps. In longstanding disease, the bowel may become featureless, resembling a lead pipe with luminal narrowing and bowel shortening.

While CT is less sensitive than endoscopy or barium enema for detecting the subtle mucosal abnormalities seen in mild or early disease, it is often obtained for evaluation of lower abdominal pain in the emergency department and therefore may be the first diagnostic study in a patient with new-onset ulcerative colitis. CT readily distinguishes inflammatory colon disease from appendicitis or diverticulitis. Findings include contiguous distal wall thickening, mild pericolonic inflammatory changes, and the "target sign" of concentric mural inflammation. It also identifies complications of ulcerative colitis: perforation, abscess, and stricture.

Ulcerative colitis is a risk factor for colorectal carcinoma, which is frequently sessile and may appear as a simple stricture on CT or barium enema. Patients with a history of ulcerative colitis are generally screened at intervals by colonoscopy. Primary sclerosing cholangitis (PSC), an autoimmune inflammatory disorder of the bile ducts, is strongly associated; approximately 5% of patients with ulcerative colitis develop PSC, and 70–80% of patients with primary sclerosing cholangitis have a history of ulcerative colitis. Arthritis is also strongly associated with ulcerative colitis, affecting up to a quarter of patients (**Fig. 6.43**).

Fig. 6.43a–f
a,b Active ulcerative colitis. Contiguous distal colon wall inflammation with loss of haustra and pericolonic fat-stranding/edema.
c,d Ulcerative colitis. Mildly thickened ascending and descending colon wall with loss of transverse colonic haustra.
e,f Longstanding ulcerative colitis. Featureless ("lead pipe") descending colon on radiograph and coronal CT. Multiple small reactive mesenteric lymph nodes (CT). No inflammatory thickening or pericolonic inflammation.

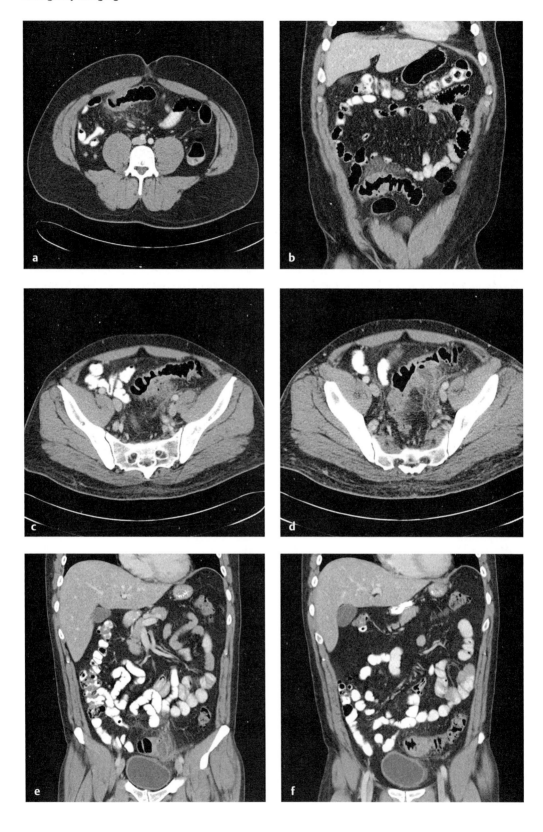

◆ Diverticulitis

Diverticulosis, small outpouchings of colonic mucosa that protrude through the muscularis, is a common condition due to elevated colonic pressure, usually in the sigmoid, and correlated with age and chronic constipation. Diverticulitis is the consequence of fecal impaction in diverticula with subsequent inflammatory response. While diverticulitis can involve any part of the gastrointestinal tract, it most commonly involves the sigmoid colon.

Patients present with colicky abdominal pain, often localized to the left lower quadrant and associated with fever, vomiting, dysuria, and tenderness. Sometimes a mass can be palpated, corresponding to an inflammatory phlegmon. Complications include perforation, bleeding, and abscess formation, and patients with neglected or severe diverticulitis can develop peritonitis.

CT for left lower quadrant pain should be performed with intravenous and oral contrast material if possible. Findings of diverticulitis include segmental bowel wall thickening and inflammation, similar to that seen in colitis, but with visible diverticula. Adjacent fat stranding is often out of proportion to the extent of local bowel wall thickening and enhancement. Extraluminal air should be carefully sought, as it indicates microperforation and more severe disease. Excluding recent abdominal surgery, perforated diverticulitis and perforated gastric or duodenal ulcer are the two most common etiologies of free intraperitoneal air detected on imaging examinations.

Treatment for localized disease consists of conservative management with intravenous antibiotics, bowel rest, and fluid therapy. Percutaneous drainage may be necessary for diverticular abscesses. Surgery is reserved for patients who fail to improve with medical management or who have severe disease, usually with perforation or peritonitis (**Fig. 6.44**).

Fig. 6.44a–f
a,b Uncomplicated sigmoid diverticulitis. The bowel wall and haustra are thickened adjacent to a small, air-filled diverticulum. Marked pericolonic inflammatory fat stranding.
c–f Sigmoid diverticulitis with microperforation and diverticular abscess. A 2-cm, low-attenuation fluid collection with enhancing rim is along the mesenteric border of the sigmoid colon. Secondary inflammation of the adjacent bladder wall. Several dots of extraluminal air within the pericolonic phlegmon.

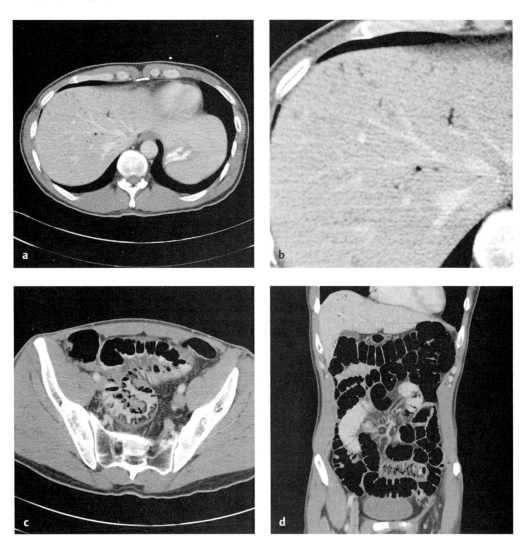

◆ Benign Pneumatosis Coli

Air within the large bowel wall, pneumatosis coli, can be a manifestation of life-threatening ischemia or a benign, incidental finding. The pathogenesis is not well understood, and possibilities include dissection of gas into the bowel wall due to increased intraluminal pressure and gas produced in the bowel wall as a byproduct of bacterial metabolism.

While pneumatosis coli is sometimes seen on plain radiographs, CT is the most sensitive test for its identification. On both radiographs and CT, pneumatosis coli appears as air-attenuation linear or bubble-like gas foci in the bowel wall. It can be an incidental and benign finding in healthy adults and in patients who have recently received systemic chemotherapy. When associated with bowel wall thickening, absent or intense mucosal enhancement, dilated bowel, ascites, and mesenteric or portal venous gas, pneumatosis is more likely due to bowel ischemia. In the pediatric population, pneumatosis coli is frequently seen in premature infants and considered an indication of early necrotizing enterocolitis (**Fig. 6.45**).

Fig. 6.45a–d
a–d   Benign pneumatosis in a patient who had received chemotherapy 1 week prior to imaging. (**a,b**) Air within the hepatic branches of the portal vein. (**c,d**) Submucosal air in the wall of the sigmoid colon.

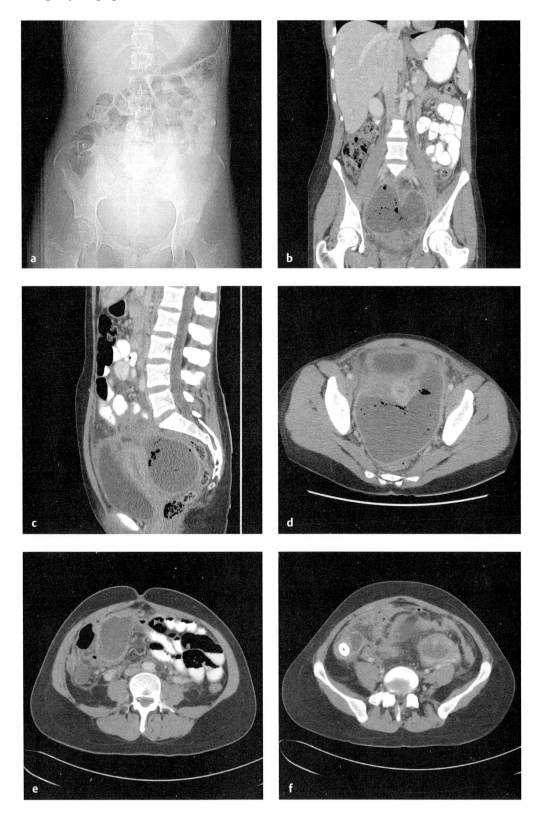

◆ Abdominal Abscess

Intra-abdominal abscess is a fairly common postoperative complication, often related to penetrating trauma, bowel perforation (peptic ulcer, appendicitis, diverticulitis, or colon carcinoma), gangrenous cholecystitis, or bowel infarction. Pancreatitis, inflammatory bowel disease, and pelvic inflammatory disease are other frequent causes.

Symptoms are often vague and include abdominal pain, fever, general malaise, and weight loss. A suspected abscess is best evaluated by CT with oral and intravenous contrast and with attention to the intraperitoneal compartments: the pelvis, the right and left pericolic gutters, the infradiaphrag- matic space, the lesser sac, and the potential spaces between loops of small intestine.

While ultrasound can detect complicated fluid collections, particularly in the pelvis, contrast-enhanced CT is generally better for locating and characterizing abdominal abscesses. These appear as low-attenuation extraintestinal abdominal fluid collections, often (but not always) with an enhancing rim. Gas bubbles may be seen within the lumen of the abscess. CT can guide percutaneous drainage or operative strategy, evaluate the patient's response to interventional and antibiotic therapy, and detect recurrent or undrained collections (**Fig. 6.46**).

Fig. 6.46a–f
a–d Abdominopelvic abscess. Gas-filled bowel is displaced craniad by a pelvic soft tissue mass on CT scout image. CT shows a large, peripherally enhancing, pelvic fluid collection containing multiple small suspended gas bubbles interposed between the uterus and rectum.
e,f Perforated appendicitis complicated by abscesses. Large right lower quadrant appendicolith. Multiple surrounding lower abdominal fluid collections with thick, enhancing walls.

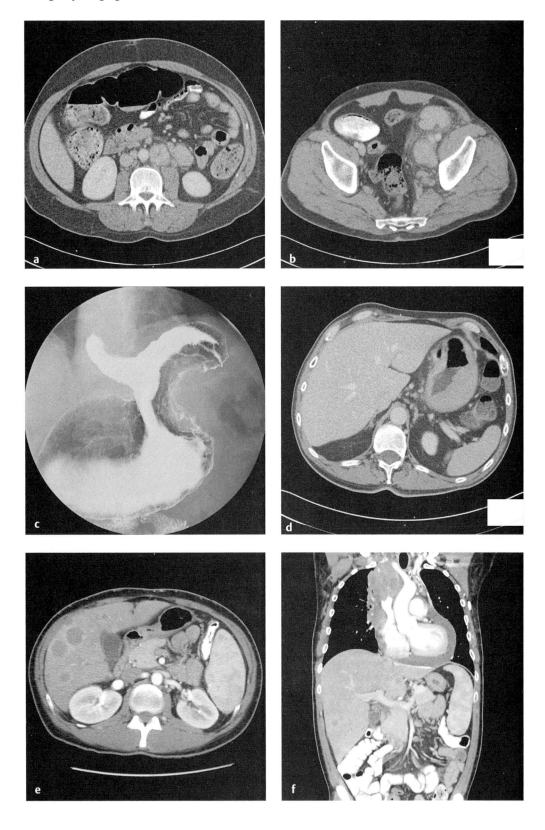

◆ Abdominal Lymphoma

Lymphomas are a heterogenous group of malignancies that arise in different nodal and extranodal sites. Most lymphomas are either Hodgkin lymphoma (HL) or non-Hodgkin lymphoma (NHL). Immuno-deficiency-associated lymphoproliferative disorders represent a third group but are much less common. Most patients with NHL and a smaller percentage of HL patients will have abdominal involvement, most commonly para-aortic adenopathy. Other manifestations include single or multiple abdominal masses, diffuse adenopathy, or diffuse tissue infiltration.

Ultrasound, CT, and MR can be used for detection, staging, and follow-up of lymphoma. In general, abdominal lymphomas produce symptoms by compression or displacement of adjacent structures rather than by direct invasion. On CT, lymphomas are often denser than other soft tissues due to lymphomas' hypercellularity and high nuclear-to-cytoplasmic ratio. When lymphoma involves an organ, such as the spleen or kidney, it often shows less enhancement than the normal portions of the organ. Enhancement in lymphoma is usually homogeneous, but with increasing tumor size, central necrosis can lead to a heterogeneous pattern. With ultrasonography, masses may appear homogenous and hypoechoic but, because they are solid, lack the posterior acoustic enhancement characteristic of a cyst.

While CT and MR imaging may be used to detect lymphadenopathy and the pattern of nodal involvement, further investigation may be necessary with functional imaging, such as positron emission tomography (PET) with [18F] fluorodeoxyglucose (FDG) for comprehensive assessment of the extent of disease (**Fig. 6.47**).

Fig. 6.47a–f
a,b Hodgkin lymphoma. Enlarged, homogenous, mildly hyperdense para-aortic and left inguinal lymph nodes.
c,d Gastric lymphoma. Fixed indentation of the greater gastric curvature on upper gastrointestinal examination. CT shows markedly thickened gastric wall.
e,f B-cell lymphoma in HIV-positive patient. Mediastinal and portocaval conglomerate adenopathy, pericardial effusion, and multiple intrahepatic lesions. The hepatic lesions are lower in attenuation then the surrounding normally enhanced liver parenchyma.

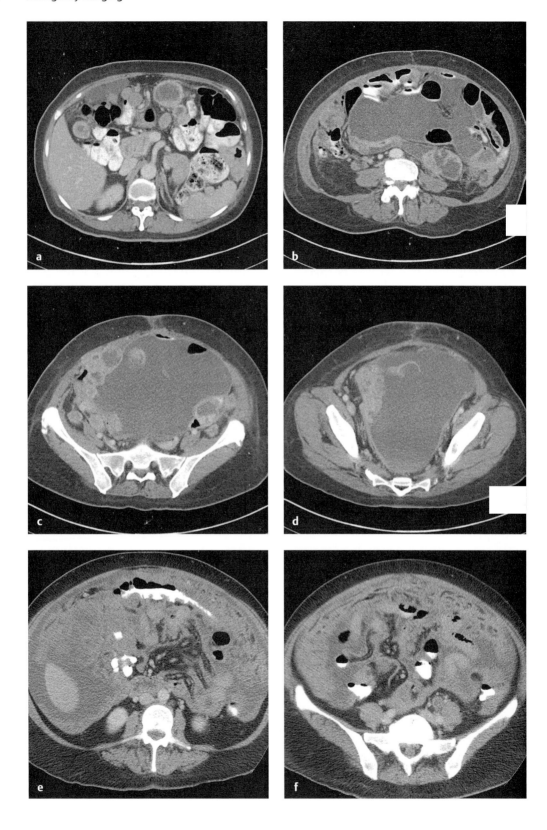

◆ Peritoneal Carcinomatosis

Peritoneal metastases can complicate primary abdominal and pelvic malignancies, the most common of which are ovarian, gastric, colorectal, and pancreatic carcinoma. Hematogenous spread with peritoneal or intra-abdominal seeding may also be seen with breast cancer, lung cancer, and malignant melanoma.

Patients with peritoneal carcinomatosis typically have abdominal distention and diffuse nonspecific abdominal pain related to ascites. Abnormal bowel motility may result in nausea, bloating, and bowel obstruction.

Although peritoneal metastases may be visible on ultrasound as omental matting and thickening of mesentery, CT is generally more effective at both detecting and documenting the extent of peritoneal disease. Metastatic disease can be microscopic, nodular, or masslike. Thickening and enhancement of peritoneal reflections, the omentum ("omental cake"), mesenteric stranding, and ascites are other manifestations.

Treatment is multimodal and depends on the primary tumor; usually a combination of surgical cytoreduction, intraperitoneal perioperative chemotherapy, and systemic chemotherapy are employed. Generally, peritoneal carcinomatosis implies a poor prognosis (**Fig. 6.48**).

Fig. 6.48a–f
a–d Peritoneal carcinomatosis due to uterine sarcoma. Malignant ascites with multiple intraperitoneal metastases.
e,f Omental caking due to ovarian carcinoma. Ascites, peritoneal nodules, and omental thickening.

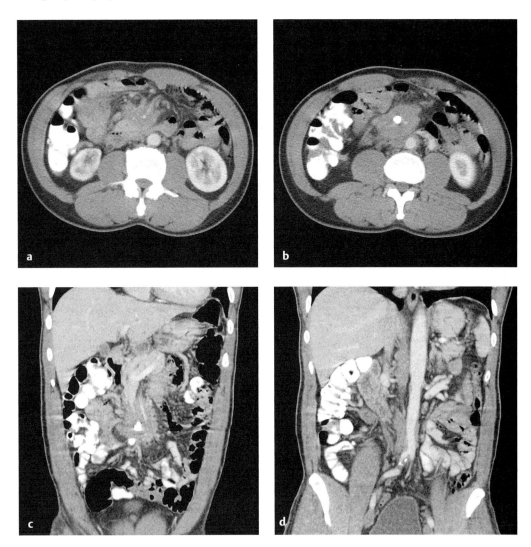

◆ Sclerosing Mesenteritis

Sclerosing mesenteritis is an idiopathic disorder that causes inflammation and fibrosis of the adipose tissue of the bowel mesentery, seen in older adults between the fifth and seventh decades. When symptomatic, sclerosing mesenteritis presents with abdominal pain, altered bowel habits, and weight loss. A firm left upper quadrant or epigastric mass is sometimes palpated on physical exam. Sclerosing mesenteritis is also one of the many incidental findings discovered on emergency CT for various abdominal complaints.

CT shows a soft tissue mass in the mesentery that compresses surrounding structures. Traversing vessels may be surrounded by low-attenuation halos within the generally hyperdense mass, sometimes referred to as the "fat ring sign." Calcifications and small lymph nodes may also be seen. In some cases, sclerosing mesenteritis appears only as "misty mesentery," a nonspecific finding due to various causes of mesenteric inflammation or venolymphatic engorgement.

Management is primarily supportive, with most cases following a benign and self-limited course. Persistent or severe inflammation may respond to corticosteroid, cyclophosphamide, or azathioprine treatment. Surgical biopsy may be necessary to exclude clinical and radiological mimics such as lymphoma, carcinoid syndrome, and peritoneal carcinomatosis (**Fig. 6.49**).

Fig. 6.49a–d Sclerosing mesenteritis. Central mesenteric soft tissue mass with central calcification and adjacent retroperitoneal and periaortic inflammatory stranding.

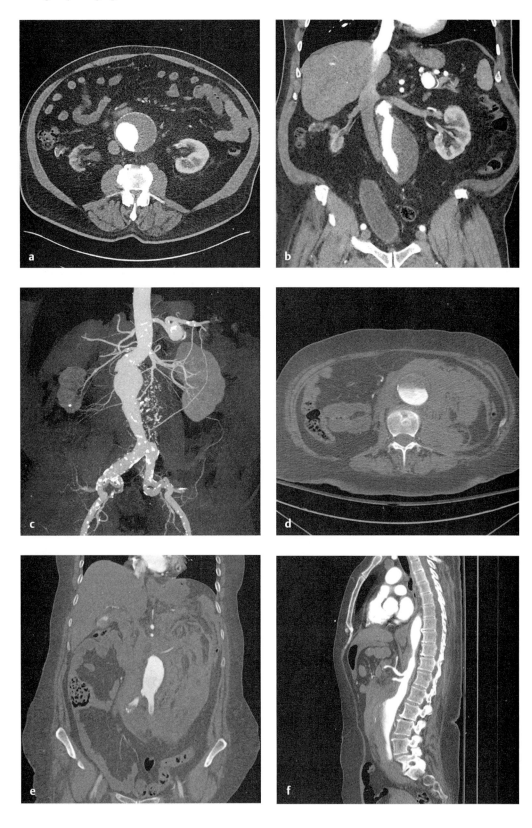

◆ Abdominal Aortic Aneurysm

Abdominal aortic aneurysm (AAA) is defined by focal aortic dilatation greater than 3 cm and results from degeneration of the medial layer of the aortic wall. Risk factors and associated conditions include smoking, atherosclerosis, vasculitis, and collagen-vascular disorders, such as Marfan or Ehlers-Danlos syndrome. Abdominal aneurysms generally progress over time, enlarging by approximately 0.4 cm per year. Smoking predisposes to more rapid expansion.

Most unruptured aneurysms are asymptomatic. Hematuria or flank pain may be present if the renal arteries are compromised. Acute, severe abdominal or back pain with a pulsatile abdominal mass indicates acute rupture. Acutely ruptured AAA typically presents with severe abdominal or back pain, severe hypotension, and a pulsatile abdominal mass. Many patients die before surgery can be performed.

Ultrasound permits rapid assessment of patients with suspected ruptured aneurysm. The normal abdominal aorta is less than 3 cm in diameter, measured from outer wall to outer wall, with the iliac arteries less than 1.5 cm. Fluid surrounding the aorta or in the hepatorenal space (the Morison pouch) indicates possible leak or rupture.

Abdominal CT (noncontrast followed by arterial-phase imaging) is the most accurate method for diagnosis and evaluation. Smaller unruptured aneurysms are often managed conservatively depending on comorbidities. Ruptured AAA is diagnosed by detecting an indistinct or discontinuous aortic wall, retroperitoneal hematoma or stranding, or extravasation of intravenous contrast. Large or acutely ruptured aneurysms are usually treated with endoluminal stent grafts. CT allows the surgeon to determine which aortic branches are involved (renal arteries, celiac trunk, superior mesenteric artery) and provides the measurements necessary to plan any needed interventional or surgical management (**Fig. 6.50**).

Fig. 6.50a–f
a–c Abdominal aortic aneurysm. 7-cm infrarenal aortic aneurysm with large mural thrombus. Extensive atherosclerotic calcification. Hypoplastic right kidney.
d–f Ruptured abdominal aortic aneurysm. Infrarenal aortic aneurysm with extensive periaortic hematoma.

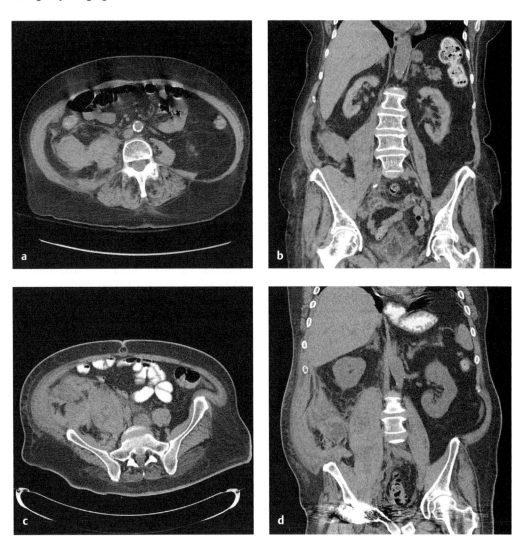

◆ Retroperitoneal Hematoma

Spontaneous retroperitoneal hematoma (RPH) should be suspected in the patient with clinical and laboratory evidence of significant blood loss, but without signs of external or gastrointestinal hemorrhage. Trauma, ruptured abdominal aortic or iliac artery aneurysm, underlying renal or adrenal disease, complications of surgery, blood dyscrasias, pancreatitis, malignancy, and supratherapeutic anticoagulation can all cause retroperitoneal hemorrhage.

The clinical presentation depends on the volume of hemorrhage, rapidity of onset, and the ability of surrounding soft tissue to contain or tamponade the blood. Acute abdominal or flank pain, hypotension, and anemia or progressive decrease in hematocrit usually prompt CT investigation. The Grey Turner sign—bruising over the flanks that appears 24 to 48 hours after hemorrhage—is not useful in early diagnosis.

Retroperitoneal hematoma can sometimes be detected with bedside ultrasonography as an anechoic or heterogenous hypoechoic mass. A complex fluid collection located between the kidney and the pararenal fascia is typical of RPH and should be discriminated from intraperitoneal hemorrhage. Plain abdominal films are insensitive for detection of RPH but may show loss of the psoas muscle border, displaced bowel loops, or other indirect evidence of displacement of retroperitoneal structures.

Noncontrast CT is usually adequate for diagnosis of RPH. Acute and subacute hematomas typically appear as a heterogenous high-attenuation mass with surrounding soft tissue stranding, while clot density decreases as the hematoma ages, eventually becoming hypointense to muscle.

Many RPH can be observed. Rapid or continuing bleeding or hemodynamic instability are indications for angiographic study and possible embolization (**Fig. 6.51**).

Fig. 6.51a–d Retroperitoneal hemorrhage. Large right intrapsoas and retroperitoneal soft tissue mass with adjacent fat stranding.

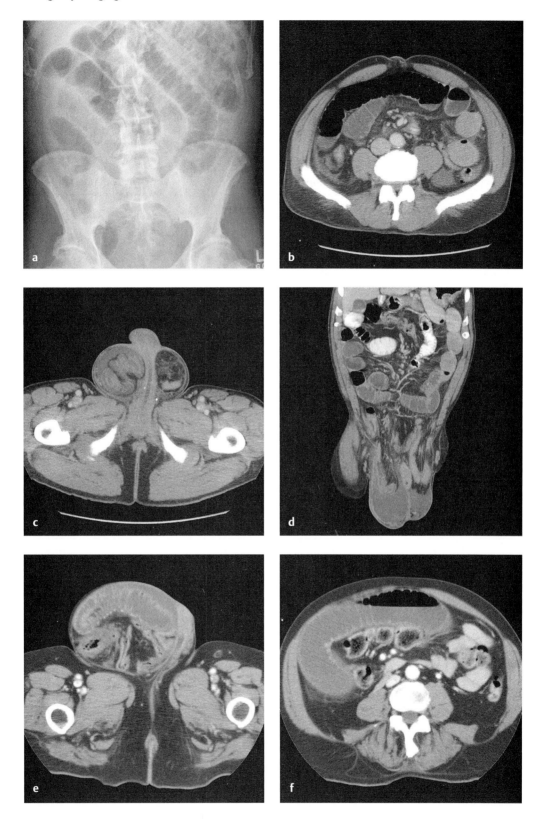

◆ Incarcerated Inguinal Hernia

An indirect inguinal hernia is a defect in the lower abdominal wall that permits fat, and sometimes omentum and bowel, to herniate through the internal inguinal ring along the course of the spermatic cord in males and the round ligament in females. Direct hernias are less common and occur medial to the inferior epigastric artery. The primary clinical significance of hernias lies in their potential for bowel incarceration and infarction. In this situation, patients present clinically with acute scrotal pain or symptoms of small-bowel obstruction. Clinical findings are usually obvious; a tender mass or swelling in the groin or scrotum. Inguinal hernias may or may not be easily reducible.

Ultrasound can be used as a preliminary imaging modality in the emergency department, and an inguinal hernia is diagnosed if fat or peristalsing bowel can be identified in the scrotum or inguinal canal. CT with intravenous and, if possible, oral contrast is reserved for the patient with a nonreducible, potentially incarcerated, hernia. Small bowel obstruction and urgent surgical management are indicated by dilated bowel, bowel-wall thickening or hypoenhancement, and associated ascites. (**Fig. 6.52**).

Fig. 6.52a–f
a–d Incarcerated right inguinal hernia causing small bowel obstruction. Plain radiograph with multiple air-filled dilated loops of small bowel consistent with small-bowel obstruction. CT shows small amount of ascites in both paracolic gutters. Right inguinal hernia containing dilated and thick-walled small bowel with adjacent ascites. A left inguinal hernia, also present, contains fat, nonobstructed small bowel, and ascites.
e,f Coincident left inguinal hernia causing small-bowel obstruction. Large right inguinal hernia containing both dilated and nondilated loops of small bowel. The dilated loop extends into the abdominal cavity and is thick-walled and fluid-filled.

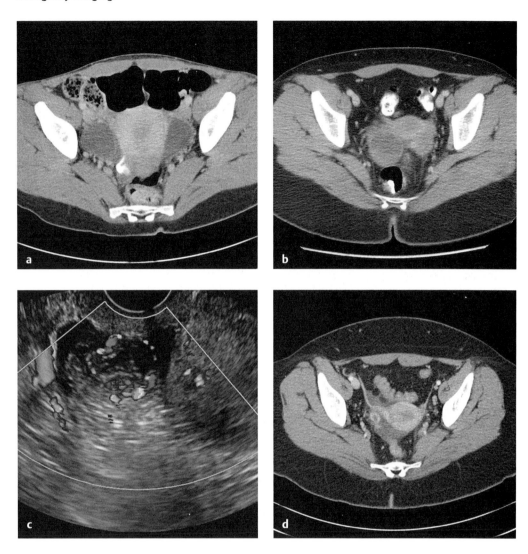

◆ Benign and Indeterminate Ovarian Cysts

In women of reproductive age, dominant ovarian follicles or simple cysts can measure up to 3 cm in diameter. After ovulation, the dominant follicle becomes a corpus luteum, which has a characteristically thick vascular wall. These are also typically 3 cm or less in diameter. Consensus recommendations for follow-up of incidentally discovered ovarian cysts have been proposed by the Society of Radiologists in Ultrasound. The following recommendations are based on sonographic appearance and depend upon whether the patient is pre- or postmenopausal:

Benign-appearing cysts are typically round or oval, anechoic with smooth walls, no solid component, septa, or internal vascularity.

- In women of reproductive age:
  - < 3 cm are normal and should not be mentioned.
  - 3–5 cm should be described in a report but are almost certainly benign and do not need follow-up.
  - 5–7 cm should be described in a report, are almost certainly benign, but should be followed yearly.
  - > 7 cm should be evaluated by MR for more accurate characterization.
- In postmenopausal women:
  - < 1 cm are clinically inconsequential and do not need follow-up.
  - 1–7 cm should be described in a report, are almost certainly benign, but should be followed yearly.
  - > 7 cm should be evaluated by MR for more accurate characterization.

Hemorrhagic cysts have weblike internal echoes due to fibrin strands, a solid-appearing area with concave margins in the cyst, no internal color flow, circumferential arterial flow in cyst wall.

- In women of reproductive age:
  - < 3 cm are normal and need not be mentioned.
  - 3–5 cm should be described in a report but do not need follow-up.
  - > 5 cm should be described in a report and should be followed up in 6–12 weeks to ensure resolution.
- In late postmenopausal women:
  - Hemorrhagic cysts are likely neoplastic and surgical evaluation should be considered.

Indeterminate but probably benign cysts: Thin-walled cysts with a single septum or focal calcification can be managed as simple cysts. Suspected hemorrhagic cyst, endometriomas, or dermoids should be followed up in 6–12 weeks if the appearance is not definitive. If an apparently hemorrhagic cyst does not resolve, further imaging should be undertaken, and if the cyst cannot be diagnosed as an endometrioma or dermoid, the patient should be referred for surgical evaluation (**Fig. 6.53**).

Fig. 6.53a–d
a Simple bilateral adnexal ovarian cysts.
b–d Hemorrhagic ovarian cysts. (**b**) Simple cyst containing dependent hemorrhage. (**c**) Hemorrhagic corpus luteum cyst with surrounding hyperemia and internal lacy echoes on endovaginal sonography. (**d**) Hemorrhagic involuting corpus luteum with associated hemoperitoneum.

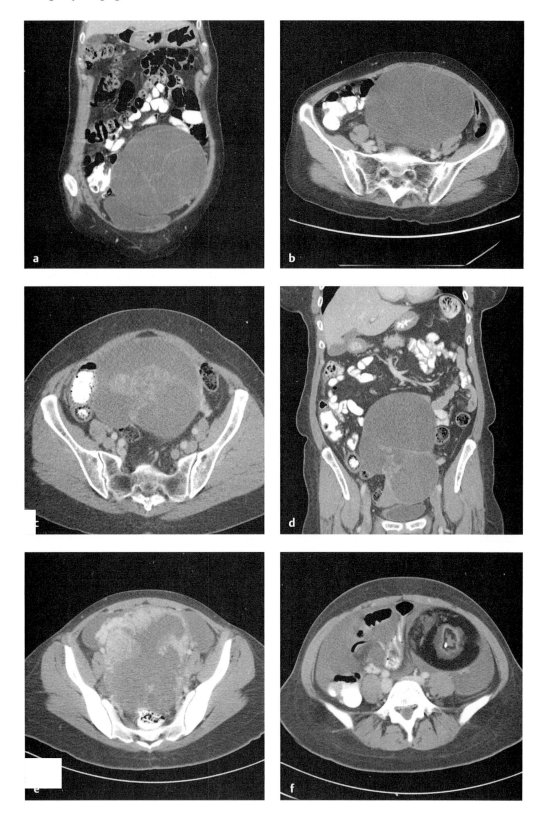

◆ Cystic Ovarian Neoplasms and Ovarian Carcinoma

Ovarian neoplasms comprise a diverse group of benign and malignant tumors that arise from the different tissues present in the ovaries. These include benign serous and mucinous epithelial neoplasms, ovarian carcinoma, germ cell tumors, and sex-cord stromal tumors. The ovaries are also a preferential site of metastatic disease from primary endometrial, breast, colon, stomach, and cervical cancers.

The symptoms of early ovarian cancer are either nonexistent or limited to vague and nonspecific abdominal discomfort. Not uncommonly, the diagnosis is made in the emergency department when a CT is performed to evaluate abdominal pain. Unfortunately, many patients with ovarian carcinoma come to medical attention with advanced disease and a consequently poor prognosis.

Risk factors include age, nulliparity, and close relatives with ovarian carcinoma; 5 to 13% of ovarian carcinomas are associated with mutations in the *BRCA1* and *BRCA2* genes. Fifty percent of patients with early-stage ovarian carcinoma will have elevated CA-125 antigen, which can be helpful if imaging findings are equivocal. Unfortunately this marker is also elevated in other conditions, including cirrhosis, early pregnancy, pelvic inflammatory disease, and nonovarian abdominal malignancies.

Ultrasound, CT, and MRI can all evaluate adnexal tumors for features of malignancy and can identify benign masses with characteristic appearances such as endometriomas, teratomas, and simple cysts. Ovarian neoplasms can be cystic, solid, or mixed and may contain serous or mucinous secretions. Up to 20% are bilateral.

Benign cystic ovarian neoplasms are characterized by multiple thin (< 3 mm) septations, nonhyperechoic nodules without vascular flow on ultrasound, and no ascites. Patients with these findings should be evaluated further with MRI or referred for surgical evaluation.

Malignant cystic ovarian neoplasms are characterized by thick, irregular (> 3 mm) septations, nodules with vascular flow on ultrasound, and moderate or large abdominal ascites. Patients with one or more of these findings should be referred for surgical evaluation (**Fig. 6.54**).

Ovarian carcinoma staging can be seen in **Table 6.7**.

Table 6.7 Ovarian carcinoma staging

Stage 0	Carcinoma in situ (common in cervical, vaginal, and vulvar cancers)
Stage I	Confined to the organ of origin
Stage II	Invasion of surrounding organs or tissues
Stage III	Spread to distant nodes or tissues within the pelvis
Stage IV	Distant metastases

Fig. 6.54a–f
a,b Benign mucinous cystadenoma. Large cyst with multiple thin septa. No nodule or ascites.
c,d Ovarian carcinoma. Multicystic mass with thick enhancing septa. Enlarged bilateral iliac chain lymph nodes. No ascites.
e,f Ovarian carcinoma and synchronous teratoma. Cystic pelvic mass with thick septa, nodular wall, and large-volume ascites. A second, predominantly fat-density, mass contains a small central calcification and is pathognomonic for a teratoma (dermoid cyst).

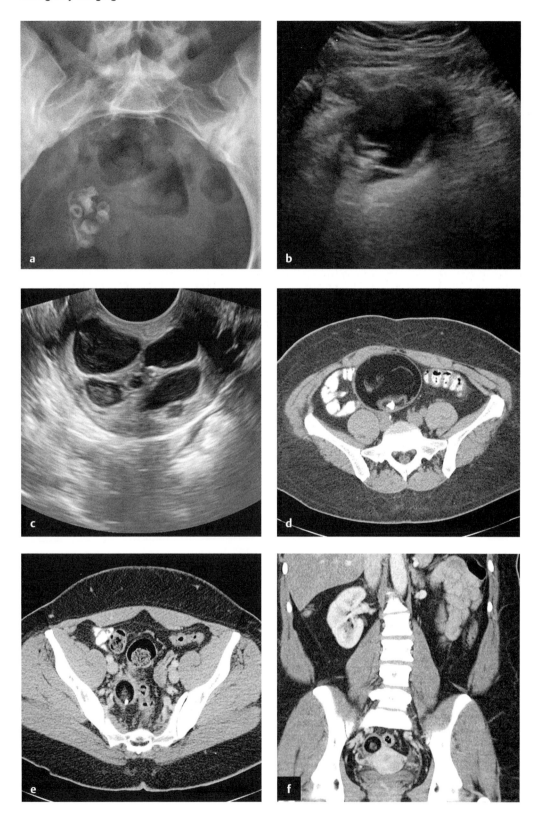

◆ Ovarian Teratoma

Ovarian teratomas, or dermoid cysts, are the most common group of ovarian germ cell tumors and may be divided into three main subtypes: mature, immature, and monodermal teratomas (i.e., struma ovarii tumor). Teratomas can range dramatically in size and contain differentiated tissues including hair, teeth, bone, and neural tissue. Uncomplicated ovarian dermoids tend to be asymptomatic and are often an incidental finding on ultrasound or CT obtained for other reasons. Mature ovarian teratomas are predisposed to torse and may present with acute pelvic pain.

When visible on plain radiographs, mature teratomas appear as fat-containing cysts or toothlike calcifications within the pelvis. On ultrasound, mature teratomas are typically echogenic with reduced distal sound transmission and reveal a mixture of sonographic patterns reflecting the cyst contents, including shadowing echogenic calcifications, linear reflections corresponding to hair within sebaceous material, or fat-fluid levels. CT usually shows a well-defined, fat-filled cyst often containing a soft tissue element and an eccentric calcification (Rokitansky nodule), sometimes identifiable as a tooth. MR can confirm the presence of fat within an adnexal mass, which is diagnostic of teratoma.

Most teratomas are slow-growing and benign and enlarge at a rate of less than 2 mm a year. Immature teratomas are malignant and are characterized by large-size (> 10 cm), irregular borders, and a dominant solid component often containing small foci of fat and calcification (**Fig. 6.55**).

Fig. 6.55a–f
a,b   Mature teratoma. Intrapelvic cluster of calcifications forming vestigial teeth and mandible. Ultrasound shows echogenic structures corresponding to calcification with adjacent cyst containing internal echoes (hair).
c,d   Mature teratoma. Large, heterogeneous, predominantly fat-containing, mass with internal soft tissue and mural calcification (Rokitansky nodule).
e,f   Mature teratoma. Small, heterogeneous, right adnexal mass containing fat, calcification, and soft tissue.

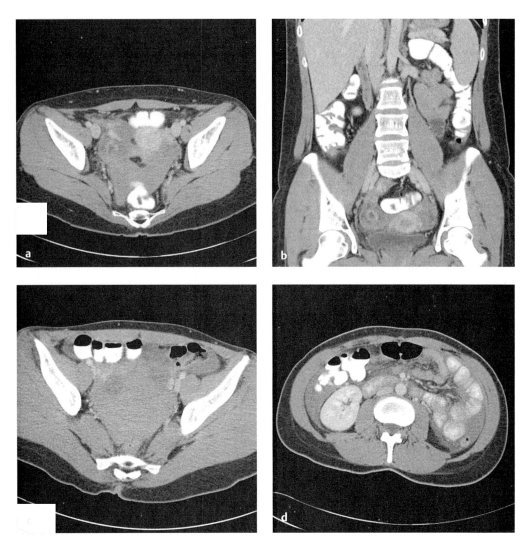

◆ Ruptured Ovarian Cysts

Ruptured ovarian cysts present clinically with abrupt-onset adnexal or lower abdominal pain in adolescent and young adult women, usually in the mid to late menstrual cycle. Vessels surrounding corpus luteum cysts can rupture into the cyst or externally into the pelvic peritoneal cavity. Ovarian follicular and corpus luteum cysts are physiologic, are commonly identified in gynecologic imaging, and should be considered normal unless the patient is prepubertal, postmenopausal, or pregnant or if the cyst diameter exceeds 2.5 cm.

On ultrasound, hemorrhagic cysts typically measure 3 cm, have a thin outer wall, and demonstrate posterior acoustic through-transmission. Complex cysts may display thin, reticular septations corresponding to fibrin strands in the retracting clot.

A ruptured corpus luteum cyst appears as an enhancing round or crenellated mass on CT. On ultrasound with Doppler flow imaging it may be surrounded by a hypervascular ring ("ring of fire"). If the cyst has ruptured into the peritoneum, a moderate amount of echogenic fluid (30–45 HU) and clot (45–100 HU) will be evident in the pelvis. Hemoperitoneum from cyst rupture can be massive and even life-threatening. Control of bleeding may require laparoscopic or, rarely, open surgery.

Other causes of acute or subacute adnexal pain include tubo-ovarian abscess, ectopic pregnancy, appendicitis, and pelvic inflammatory disease. Human chorionic gonadotropin levels should be obtained and interpreted (preferably before imaging) to exclude ectopic pregnancy, another important cause of acute pelvic pain and hemoperitoneum (**Fig. 6.56**).

Fig. 6.56a–d
a,b Ruptured corpus luteum cyst. Hemoperitoneum limited to the pelvis with a small right adnexal cyst that demonstrates thick, crenellated, irregular walls (corpus luteum).
c,d Hemoperitoneum due to ruptured ovarian cyst. Extensive intrapelvic clot and large volume of high-attenuation intraperitoneal fluid within the pelvis and paracolic gutters.

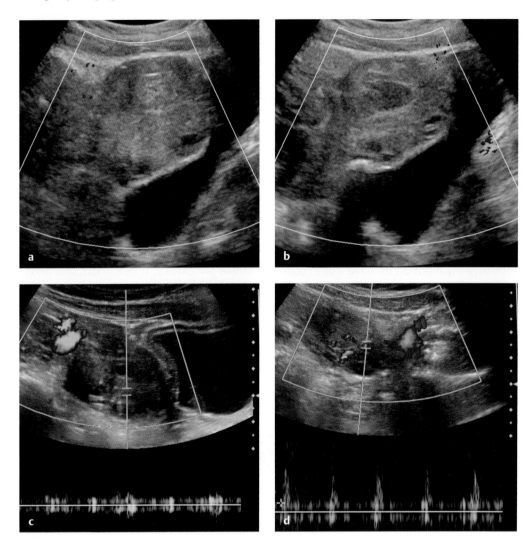

◆ Ovarian Torsion

Abnormal rotation of an ovary, fallopian tube, and vascular pedicle can compromise arterial, venous, and lymphatic flow. It is a relatively uncommon cause of acute lower abdominal pain in women and is a gynecological emergency requiring urgent surgical intervention to prevent hemorrhagic infarction and necrosis. Ovarian torsion has a bimodal age distribution with peaks in reproductive age and in postmenopausal women. It may reflect excessive mobility of the adnexa or may be associated with adnexal masses.

Lower abdominal pain in ovarian torsion may be colicky or constant and is often out of proportion to the other exam findings. Fever, nausea, and vomiting may accompany pain, and intermittent torsion/detorsion sometimes occurs.

Transvaginal ultrasound is diagnostic. Initially lymphatic and venous obstruction leads to ovarian engorgement and edema. Over time, arterial flow to the ovary is compromised, and color Doppler will show reduced or absent vascularity. Secondary imaging findings include free pelvic fluid, an underlying ovarian mass, and a "whirlpool sign," reflecting the twisted vascular pedicle. Ovarian torsion is usually unilateral, with a slight predilection for the right side. The contralateral ovary should show normal size and vascularity.

If CT is obtained, it will show an enlarged ovary and distended pedicle, sometimes with inflammatory stranding and variable pelvic fluid. These findings are nonspecific, however, and CT cannot accurately evaluate vascular flow. If ovarian torsion is to be excluded, ultrasound is mandatory.

Most ovaries are not salvageable, and consequently a salpingo-oophorectomy is usually performed. There is no established length of time from onset of pain to irreversible ovarian loss, and spontaneous detorsion has been reported (**Fig. 6.57**).

Fig. 6.57a–d
a,b Torsed ovary in a 30 year old. Enlarged adnexal mass containing several peripheral follicles but with no vascular flow on color Doppler interrogation.
c,d Torsed ovary in a 10 year old. The right ovary measures 3.8 × 2.5 × 2.2 cm and has no detectable color or Doppler flow. The left ovary measures 2.2 × 1.3 × 1.2 cm with normal arterial flow on both color and Doppler interrogation.

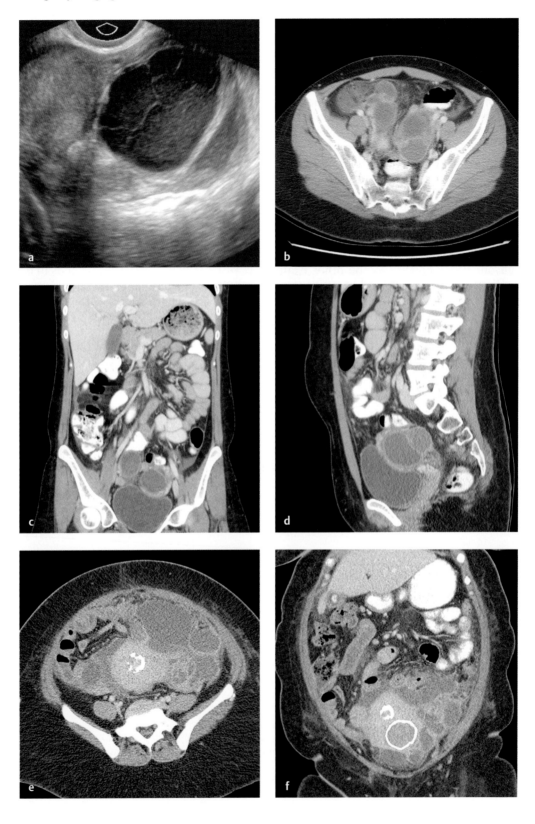

◆ Tubo-Ovarian Abscess

Tubo-ovarian abscess (TOA) is an infection of the fallopian tube, ovary, and adjacent structures. It is usually a complication of pelvic inflammatory disease (PID), an infection of the upper genital tract secondary to *Chlamydia trachomatis* or *Neisseria gonorrhoeae*. TOA presents with acute pelvic pain, fever, and leukocytosis.

Pelvic ultrasound is normally the first imaging study performed and will show a complex adnexal cystic/solid mass. Pressure on the mass using the transvaginal ultrasound probe will be exquisitely painful but helpful in differentiating from other pelvic pathology, which should not cause discomfort. The ipsilateral fallopian tube is often dilated, thick-walled, and fluid-filled, reflecting an associated pyosalpinx or hydrosalpinx. Increased echogenicity of the pelvic fat indicates inflammatory edema. The tubo-ovarian abscess itself will have thick walls and may contain fluid with or without solid components.

Contrast-enhanced CT shows multiple adnexal thick-walled cysts or tubular fluid collections corresponding to the distended fallopian tube as well as adjacent inflammatory change in the mesenteric/abdominal fat.

Treatment includes broad-spectrum antibiotics to cover primarily anaerobic organisms. Consultation with interventional radiology or surgery may be necessary for appropriate drainage of the abscess from a transvaginal, transgluteal, or transabdominal approach if conservative treatment is not effective (**Fig. 6.58**).

Fig. 6.58a–f
a–d Tubo-ovarian abscess. A hypoechoic intrapelvic mass with multiple septations. CT shows tubular intrapelvic low-attenuation fluid collections with thick, enhancing margins. None contain contrast, which is present in the rectum and sigmoid.
e,f Tubo-ovarian abscess. Large multicystic mass surrounding the uterus, with mural enhancement and adjacent inflammatory changes. The uterus contains several calcified myomas.

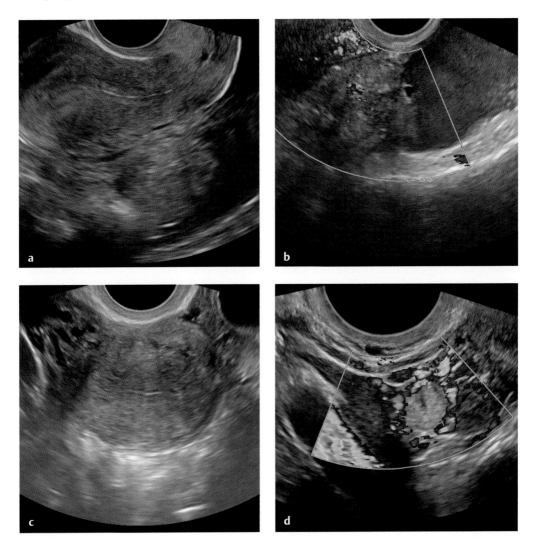

◆ Ruptured Ectopic Pregnancy

Ectopic pregnancy is the implantation of a fertilized ovum outside of the uterine cavity, and while 95% are found in the fallopian tube, unusual locations include the uterine myometrium, uterine scar from prior Cesarean section, the ovary, cervix, or peritoneum. Ruptured ectopic pregnancy is the leading cause of death in the first trimester of pregnancy and should be suspected in any woman with vaginal bleeding and cramping pelvic pain 6 to 8 weeks after her last menstrual period. Symptom onset may be delayed if the pregnancy is not located in the fallopian tube. Predisposing factors include a previous ectopic pregnancy, tubal surgery, pelvic infection, and patients using an intrauterine device for contraception. Ectopic pregnancy rupture can be associated with a temporary relief of pain, but intraperitoneal hemorrhage with hypovolemic shock may ensue.

Bedside ultrasound should be performed for any pregnant patient with pelvic pain or vaginal bleeding regardless of the quantitative beta-hCG level. An early intrauterine pregnancy is often not visualized in patients with a beta-hCG less than 1,500 IU, and in this case a repeat beta-hCG and ultrasound in 48 hours should be performed. Transvaginal ultrasound should identify an intrauterine pregnancy at beta-hCG levels > 2,000 IU, and a yolk sac and fetal pole should be detected by transabdominal ultrasound at beta-hCG levels greater than 6,000 IU. Nonvisualization of an intrauterine pregnancy should prompt a careful search for an adnexal mass separate from the ovary; ectopic gestations may show a thick echogenic ring or surrounding hypervascularity. In up to a fourth of patients, an ectopic gestation is not definitely identified. Hemoperitoneum should be evident in the uterine cul-de-sac in ruptured ectopic pregnancy.

Methotrexate therapy is reserved for patients with a beta-hCG < 3,000 and a mean gestational sac < 3 cm or who present less than 3 weeks after their missed menses. Surgery is indicated for patients who present later or in whom an ectopic pregnancy has ruptured (**Fig. 6.59**).

Fig. 6.59a–d
a,b Ruptured ectopic pregnancy. Normal uterus without identifiable intrauterine gestational sac. Vascular adnexal mass with large amount of fluid in the rectovaginal pouch.
c,d Ruptured ectopic pregnancy. Normal uterus without identifiable intrauterine gestational sac. Adnexal mass with hypervascular ring.

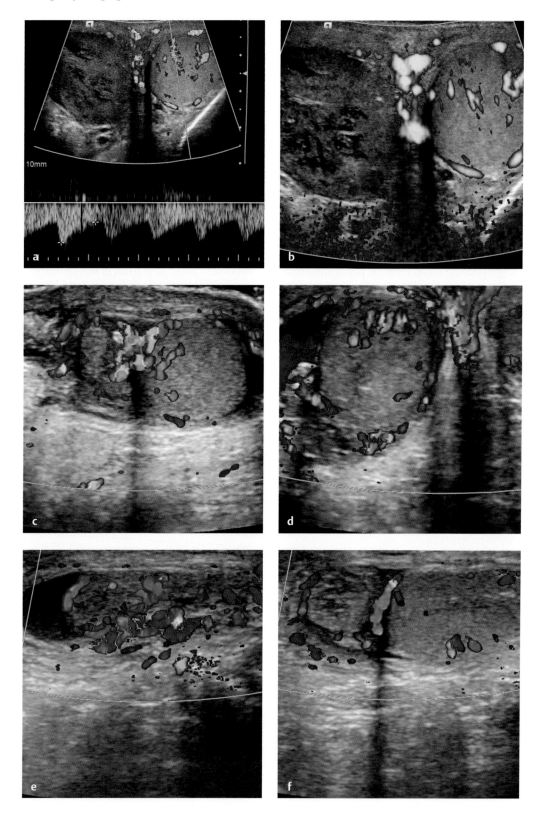

◆ Testicular Torsion and Torsed Appendix Testis

Testicular torsion, in which the testis twists within the scrotum due to an insufficiently broad posterior attachment, can occur at any age but is most commonly seen in adolescent boys. With torsion, draining veins are obstructed, with consequent testicular edema and pain. Continued rotation compromises arterial inflow. Unrelieved torsion, in the absence of spontaneous detorsion, results in testicular ischemia and infarct. Testicular salvage is possible if surgery is performed within 10 hours of pain onset (ideally, within 6 hours).

Symptoms include acute scrotal pain and swelling, nausea, vomiting, and low-grade fever. The affected hemiscrotum may appear swollen, tender, and inflamed. Because these findings are indistinguishable from acute epididymo-orchitis, which does not require surgical management, testicular ultrasound is frequently indicated to exclude torsion as a cause of acute testicular/scrotal pain.

The diagnosis is based on Doppler ultrasound imaging of the affected testis, which, if torsed, will not demonstrate intratesticular vascular flow. Images of the testicular parenchyma may be normal or show mild edema or increased echogenicity. False-negative examinations can occur in patients with early torsion or transient torsion/detorsion. In these cases, the testis can appear hyperemic, mimicking epididymo-orchitis. A heterogeneous, hypoechoic testis in a patient with prolonged symptoms indicates infarction and/or hemorrhage.

Torsion of the appendix testis is the most common cause of acute scrotal pain in boys and is much more common than true testicular torsion. The testicular appendix, a remnant of the müllerian duct, is located at the upper pole of the testis between the testis and the head of the epididymis. Like testicular torsion and epididymitis, appendix testis torsion presents with acute or subacute scrotal pain. Clinically, a small firm blue nodule may be palpable over the superior aspect of the affected testis (the "blue dot sign"). Pain is usually more gradual in onset than with testicular torsion and may be localized to the upper aspect of the testis. Urinary and systemic symptoms are absent.

Ultrasound shows an enlarged appendix testis (> 5 mm) with variable periappendiceal hyperemia and normal intratesticular flow. Appendiceal torsion may be accompanied by hydrocele, scrotal wall thickening, and enlargement of the epididymal head.

Patients are treated supportively with NSAIDs and scrotal support. Pain usually resolves within 5 to 10 days (**Fig. 6.60**).

Fig. 6.60a–f
a,b   Testicular torsion in an adult. (**a**) Normal vascularity and flow in the left testicle compared with absent vascularity in the right testicle. (**b**) Completely absent flow in the right testicle with areas of hypoechogenicity despite color Doppler at maximum sensitivity.
c,d   Torsed appendix testis in a child. Enlarged appendix testis with surrounding hyperemia and absent internal doppler flow. Normal flow in the adjacent testicle.
e,f   Torsed appendix testis. Similar findings in another child who also has a small reactive hydrocele adjacent to the torsed appendix.

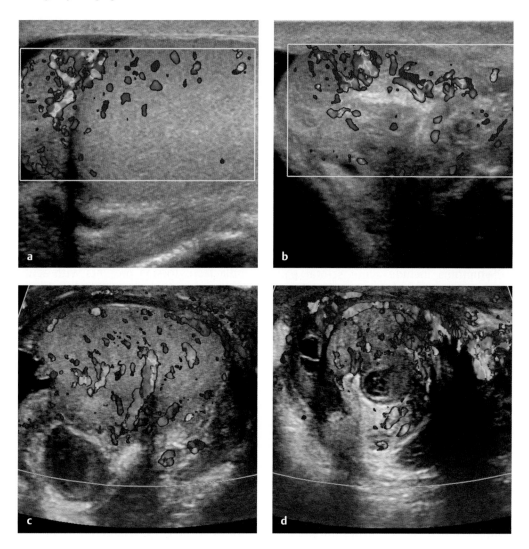

◆ Epididymitis and Epididymo-orchitis

Epididymitis is a common cause of acute-onset unilateral scrotal pain. It may be associated with inflammation of the testis (epididymo-orchitis). The clinical presentation ranges from mild swelling and tenderness to fever, dysuria, and urethral discharge. Infection usually originates in the bladder or prostate gland and is transmitted via lymphatics to the epididymis and testis. Common causative organisms are *Chlamydia trachomatis, Neisseria gonorrhoeae*, and *Escherichia coli*. Peak incidences are in the 20s and 60s, reflecting sexually transmitted infection in younger men and obstructive uropathy in older age. Pain associated with epididymitis is typically relieved when the testes are elevated over the pubis symphysis; pain associated with testicular torsion is not relieved by this maneuver.

Epididymitis is often diagnosed clinically, but ultrasound is frequently requested in the emergency setting to exclude testicular torsion. Subacute testicular pain can be seen in tumor, chronic epididymitis, and varicocele. Findings include epididymal enlargement, decreased echogenicity and increased epididymal/testicular blood flow with a low resistive index.

Untreated epididymis may progress to epididymo-orchitis, scrotal abscess, or, ultimately, testicular infarction. Follow-up ultrasounds are usually indicated at 4 to 6 weeks to ensure complete resolution of the infection (**Fig. 6.61**).

Fig. 6.61a–d
a,b Epididymitis. Increased blood flow to the right epididymis. Normal testicular flow.
c,d Epididymo-orchitis with abscess. Increased blood flow to right epididymis and testis. A complex, 1-cm round fluid collection with internal echoes is a small, adjacent intrascrotal abscess.

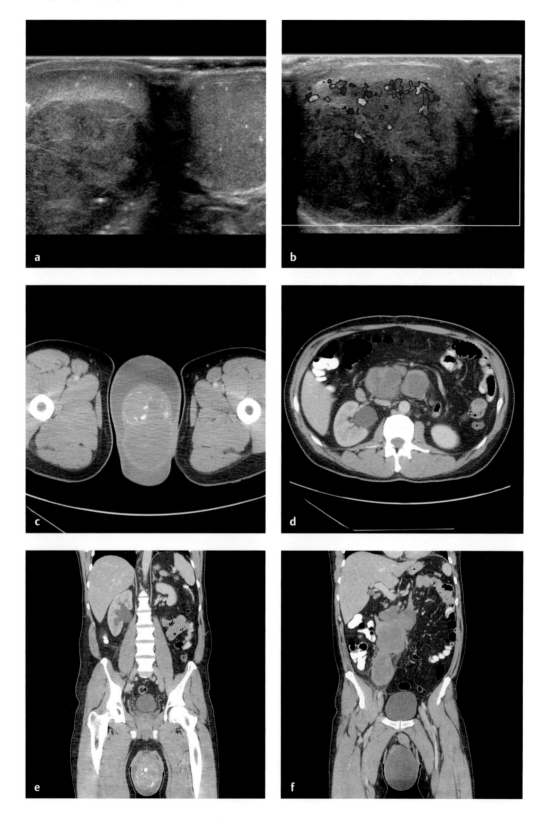

◆ Testicular Carcinoma

Primary testicular carcinoma is the most common solid malignancy in young men, with most cases occurring between ages 10 and 35. Testicular neoplasms are divided into primary germ cell tumors (GCT), which comprise the majority, and non–germ cell tumors, which account for less than 10% of testicular cancers. The most common pure cell histology is a seminoma, but mixed GCT are more common overall.

Patients present with a painless scrotal mass or incidentally detected testicular enlargement on physical examination. When small, testicular neoplasms are most frequently located on the posterior aspect of the testicle and are nontender. Some patients will report a dull ache or sense of heaviness in the scrotum. Many patients are initially misdiagnosed clinically with epididymitis, orchitis, or hydrocele.

Testicular microlithiasis (five or more calcific foci) is commonly seen in normal patients and in up to half of patients with germ cell tumor. It has been associated with an increased risk of testicular cancer in patients with other risk factors such as cryptorchidism. In otherwise asymptomatic individuals its association is dubious and generally does not merit imaging surveillance.

Sonographic imaging of the testis is the primary diagnostic study. Testicular neoplasms are typically well-defined and hypoechoic with respect to normal testicular tissue, but they may be heterogeneous and contain calcifications or cysts. Increased vascularity is not typically seen, and more characteristic of orchitis/epididymitis. CT imaging is employed for staging and detection of retroperitoneal lymphadenopathy, which is usually the first site of extratesticular disease.

Radical orchiectomy is the primary treatment of testicular carcinoma, with adjuvant chemotherapy and radiation therapy depending on type and extent of disease. Many testicular cancers are very responsive to chemotherapy, and prognosis is usually good even when metastatic disease is present (**Fig. 6.62**).

Fig. 6.62a–f
a,b Mixed germ cell tumor. Heterogeneous right testis with areas of low attenuation, reduced flow within the abnormal portion of the testis, and microlithiasis.
c–f Metastatic testicular carcinoma. Large, heterogenous testicular mass containing numerous calcifications. Right iliac and para-aortic adenopathy with associated ureteral compression and hydronephrosis.

7
Musculoskeletal

◆ Approach

Most musculoskeletal examinations obtained in the emergency department are requested for characterization of fractures, evaluation of joint effusions, exclusion of osteomyelitis in patients with cellulitis, and detection of foreign bodies in lacerations and puncture wounds. For most osseous injuries, plain radiographs are sufficient for diagnosis, and CT is reserved for more precise characterization of complex fractures (including tibial plateau and calcaneal fractures), localization of intra-articular bone fragments, and detection of soft tissue abscess or gas. MRI is often the best choice for evaluation of cartilaginous, meniscal, and ligamentous injuries, but it is usually not necessary (or even available) in the emergency department.

While one should always evaluate every bone included on a radiograph, it is very helpful to know the exact location of the patient's pain as well as the mechanism of injury. Fractures can be extremely subtle, and degenerative changes or remote injuries can simulate acute fractures. Accurate clinical information reduces perceptual failures and allows more accurate assessment of a borderline finding.

"Satisfaction of search" is a well-known cause of error among radiologists; after identifying one fracture, it is important to make sure that no other fractures are present. Another common cause of diagnostic error in interpreting bone radiographs is failing to obtain adequate orthogonal and (if necessary) supplemental views, either because the patient was unable to cooperate or incorrectly positioned, or because the optimal study for the clinical problem was not ordered.

Finding an area of focal soft tissue swelling or poor subcutaneous fat definition should increase suspicion for an adjacent subtle fracture. A joint effusion, particularly in the knee or elbow, is another important indirect sign of a fracture.

Long-bone fractures should be described concisely, using consistent descriptive and anatomic terms and addressing fracture location, configuration, and alignment. Although exact classification and most measurements are usually best left to the treating clinician, the radiologic interpretation should provide all descriptive information necessary to categorize a fracture for accurate orthopedic diagnosis and management.

Location

- Proximal
- Diaphyseal
- Metaphyseal
- Distal
- Intra-articular

Configuration

- Compound (open)
- Simple (transverse, oblique, or spiral)
- Segmental
- Comminuted
- Avulsed
- Impacted
- Osteochondral
- Torus (buckle)
- Incomplete (greenstick)

Alignment

- Displacement
- Distraction
- Override
- Angulation

Radiographs are often obtained in patients with cellulitis or skin ulcer in order to exclude osteomyelitis. Most bone radiographs obtained in this setting are normal or show sequelae of underlying diabetes mellitus such as vascular calcification or neuropathic arthropathy. Radiographic findings that indicate bone infection include focal cortal loss, periosteal new bone formation, and, less commonly, sclerosis or an endosteal lytic lesion. MRI and radionuclide bone scan are more sensitive for detection of bone infection but need not be urgently obtained.

In patients with lacerations and puncture wounds, ultrasound or radiographs can localize foreign bodies. Sensitivity for detection depends on the size and density of the object. Metal, glass, stone, and bone fragments are usually radio-opaque and often localizable by radiographs or CT. In contrast, wood splinters and plastic are usually not seen on plain radiographs but, if large enough, can be found using high-frequency ultrasound. Dry wood (as in a pencil) may be visible on CT as a linear body with the approximate attenuation of air.

◆ Imaging

Shoulder

Radiographs

- AP internal rotation
- AP external rotation
- Axillary and/or trans-scapular

Checklist

- Scapula body
- Acromion
- Coracoid process
- Clavicle
- Humeral head
- Glenohumeral, acromioclavicular, and coracoclavicular articulations

Common Injuries

- Anterior dislocation
- Posterior dislocation
- Acromioclavicular separation
- Clavicle fracture
- Humeral head/neck fractures

Elbow

Radiographs

- AP
- Lateral
- *Angled oblique (Greenspan)*

Checklist

- Humerus
- Ulna
- Radius
- Effusion (anterior and posterior fat pad signs)
- Position and appearance of ossification centers (in children)
- Radiocapitallar and anterior humeral line alignment (in children)

Common Injuries

- Dislocation
- Radial head fracture
- Coronoid process fracture
- Olecranon fracture
- Humeral supracondylar fracture
- Humeral epicondylar avulsion

Hand and Wrist

Radiographs

- AP
- Lateral
- Oblique
- Scaphoid (wrist)

Checklist

- Soft tissues
- Distal radius and ulna
- Carpal bones
- Metacarpals
- Phalanges

- Carpal arch alignment (AP)
- Lunate-capitate alignment (lateral)

Common Injuries

- Distal radius/ulnar styloid fracture
- Scaphoid fracture
- Lunate and perilunate dislocation
- Triquetral fracture
- Metacarpal fracture
- Dorsal and volar plate avulsion fractures
- Amputations

Pelvis

Radiographs

- AP
- *Judet (bilateral oblique)*
- *Inlet and outlet*

Checklist

- Pubic rami, pubic symphysis, and ischial tuberosities
- Acetabula
- Femoral heads and necks
- Iliac bones
- Sacral alae and sacroiliac articulations
- Lower lumbar vertebrae/transverse processes
- Pelvic soft tissues

Common Injuries

- Lateral compression fracture
- Anterior-posterior compression fracture/open-book fracture
- Windswept pelvis
- Vertical shear fracture
- Pubic ramus fracture
- Acetabular fracture

Hip

Radiographs

- AP
- *Cross-table lateral*
- *Frog-leg lateral*

Checklist

- Pubic rami, pubic symphysis, and ischial tuberosities
- Acetabula
- Femoral heads and necks
- Iliac bones
- Pelvic soft tissues

Common Injuries

- Subcapital, transcervical, and basicervical femoral neck fracture
- Intertrochanteric or subtrochanteric fracture
- Greater or lesser trochanter avulsion
- Dislocation
- Pubic ramus fracture
- Acetabular fracture
- Slipped capital femoral epiphysis (children)

Knee

Radiographs

- AP
- Cross-table lateral
- *Oblique*
- *Patellar (sunrise)*

Checklist

- Soft tissues
- Patella
- Quadriceps and patellar tendons
- Effusion or lipohemarthrosis
- Femoral condyles
- Tibial plateau and spines
- Fibular head

Common Injuries

- Patellar fracture
- Quadriceps or patellar tendon rupture
- Anterior cruciate ligament injury (look for lateral condylar notch sign)
- Tibial plateau fracture
- Tibial spine avulsion
- Segond fracture (associated with ACL tear)

- Proximal fibular avulsion fracture (arcuate sign, associated with posterolateral ligamentous injury)

Ankle and Foot

Radiographs

- AP
- Lateral
- Oblique
- *Calcaneus*

Checklist

- Soft tissues
- Distal fibula
- Medial tibial malleolus
- Cortex of distal tibia and talar dome (look for osteochondral fractures)
- Posterior tibia (lateral view)
- Tibiotalar interval and ankle mortise congruity
- Talus
- Calcaneus and midfoot (navicular, cuboid, cuneiforms)
- Base of fifth metatarsal
- Alignment of metatarsals with respect to cuneiforms
- Metatarsal shafts (stress fractures)
- Phalanges

Common Injuries

- Rotational ankle injuries (distal fibular, bimalleolar, and trimalleolar fractures)
- Axial load (pilon) fractures of the distal tibia
- Salter Harris fractures in children and adolescents (triplane fracture, Tillaux fracture)
- Calcaneal fractures
- Lisfranc fracture dislocations
- Metatarsal stress fractures
- Fifth metatarsal fractures (Jones, Pseudo-Jones)

Extremity Computed Tomography

Indications: Complex fractures involving the elbow, tibial plateau, ankle, and calcaneus. Exclusion of intra-articular fracture fragments.

Technique: 150 mA, 120 kV

Images: 2.5-mm axial with 0.6-mm reconstruction and 2-mm coronal and sagittal reformations, optional 3D reformations

Lower Extremity CT Angiography

Indications: Suspected lower extremity vascular injury.

Technique: 150 mA, 120 kV

IV contrast: 1.5 mL/kg at 5 mL/sec with 30 mL saline chaser. Timing bolus (20 mL) plus 5 sec or empiric 25-second delay

Images: 2.5-mm axial with 0.6-mm reconstruction and 2-mm coronal and sagittal reformations, optional 3D reformations. Image both lower extremities.

Upper Extremity CT Angiography

Indications: Suspected upper extremity vascular injury.

Technique: 150 mA, 120 kV

IV contrast: 1.5 mL/kg at 5 mL/sec with 30 mL saline chaser. Timing bolus (20 mL) plus 5–8 second delay

Images: 2.5-mm axial with 0.6-mm reconstruction and 2-mm coronal and sagittal reformations, optional 3D reformations. The arm may be positioned on the side, which results in less motion but more noise, or above the head, which has less noise but more motion.

◆ Orthopedic Hardware

While the variety of orthopedic screws, plates, prostheses, and other appliances is broad and may be daunting, it is helpful to be able to describe the more commonly seen hardware (**Fig. 7.1**).

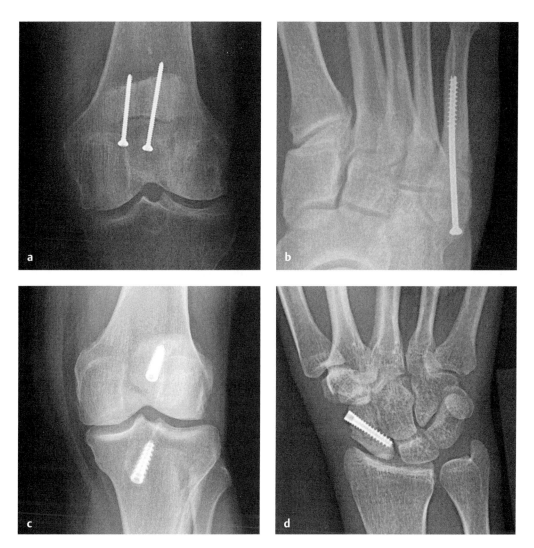

Fig. 7.1a–v

a Cortical screws are designed to affix dense cortical bone and have narrow, shallow threads. They usually traverse both near and far cortices.

b Cancellous screws have wider and deeper threads to grip porous cancellous bone. If the proximal part of the screw is smooth, they are termed partially threaded screws. When a partially threaded screw traverses two bone fragments, it will pull the distal bone fragment toward the proximal one as it is tightened. When a screw is used in this manner, it is sometimes called a lag screw. Cannulated screws (**b**) have a flat distal end and hollow core, for placement over a guide wire. Cancellous screws are frequently also cannulated as seen here.

c Interference screws are bullet-shaped screws for affixing a tendon graft in cruciate ligament repair.

d Headless variable compression screws (Acutrak or Herbert) have wide threads at one end and narrow threads at the other. They function as lag screws to compress two fragments against each other and are used in repair of scaphoid waist and some osteochondral fractures. (*Continued on page 406*)

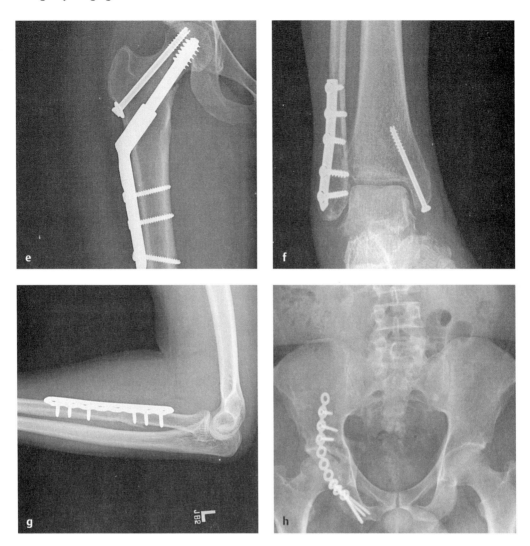

Fig. 7.1a–v (*Continued*)

e   Dynamic hip screws are partially threaded cancellous screws used to affix some femoral neck fractures. The screw telescopes into a sleeve fixed to the femoral shaft as the patient begins to bear weight and the femoral neck compacts under normal stress.

f   Ankle fracture fixation. Cortical plate and screws affix a distal fibular fracture. Partially threaded, cannulated, cancellous screw affixes a medial malleolar fracture.

f,g   (**f,g**) Cortical plates are used to appose fractured bone and come in several varieties. They are often contoured for use in specific locations and usually affixed with screws that traverse both the near and far cortex of the bone to which they are attached. (**f,g**) Compression plates are used for simple diaphyseal fractures in otherwise healthy bone. Oval holes with sloped margins allow screws and bone on either side of a fracture to move toward each other as the screws are tightened. (**g**) Low-contact plates have an undulating appearance along their juxtacortical surface that improves vascular supply adjacent to the plate by limiting periosteal compression to the points of screw fixation.

h   Reconstruction plates have notches along the sides that allow them to be contoured in the operating room. They are often used in fixation of pelvic fractures.

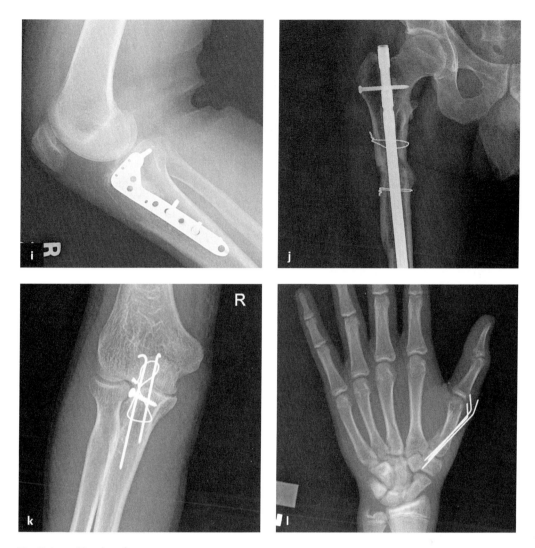

Fig. 7.1a–v (*Continued*)
i Buttress plates are wide or flared plates that provide additional support for fixation of comminuted fractures. They are usually used at the distal radius, distal tibia, distal femur, and proximal tibia.
j Cerclage wires support circumferential apposition of fractures in tubular bones.
k Tension band wires are used commonly at the patella and elbow to affix a portion of bone so that the attached muscles act to force fragments together rather than pull them apart.
l Kirschner wires (K-wires) are thin wires, used in fracture stabilization in small bones and in comminuted fractures with multiple fragments. (*Continued on page 408*)

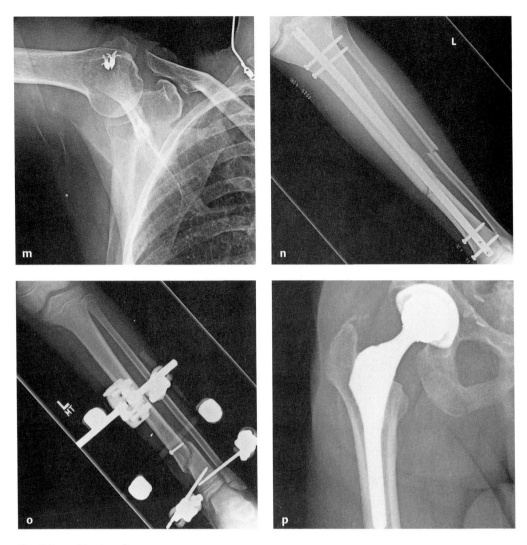

Fig. 7.1a–v (*Continued*)

m   Suture anchors are small screws that insert into bone and contain an eyelet through which a suture is threaded. They are commonly used in repair of shoulder rotator cuff injuries.

n   Intramedullary nails are rods placed through the intramedullary cavity of a long bone. If supported by affixing screws, they are termed interlocking nails.

o   External fixators are used for open fractures, fractures associated with infected wounds, and for rapid fixation of unstable fractures in polytrauma.

p   Hip arthroplasties that involve acetabular and femoral head replacement are termed total hip arthroplasty. In hemiarthroplasty, the femoral head is replaced but the acetabulum is preserved.

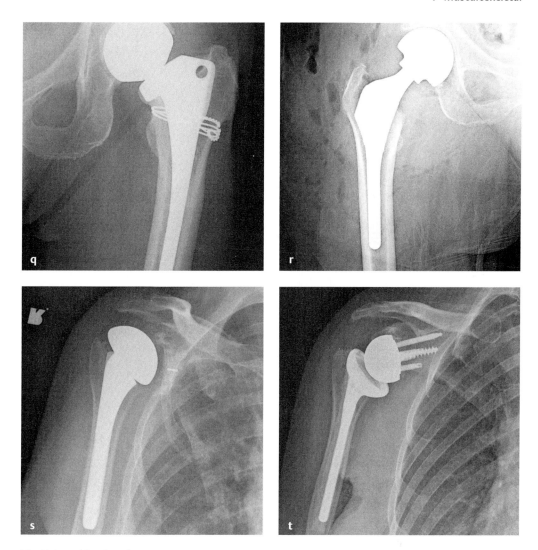

Fig. 7.1a–v (*Continued*)

q Unipolar hemiarthroplasties have a single component.

r Bipolar hemiarthroplasties have a smaller internal sphere within the larger femoral head prosthesis. Prostheses can be cemented or noncemented and are often supported by acetabular screws.

s,t Shoulder prostheses can be manufactured either with the socket replacing the glenoid or with the socket replacing the humeral head. The latter is termed a reverse shoulder arthroplasty. (*Continued on page 410*)

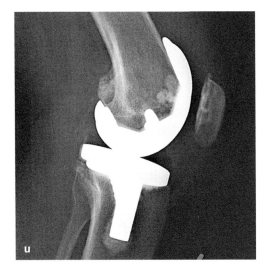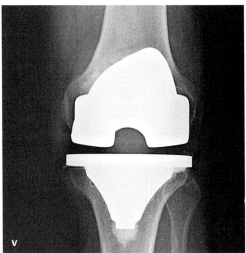

Fig. 7.1a–v (*Continued*)
u,v   Knee prostheses include femoral, tibial, and dorsal patellar components.

◆ Clinical Presentation and Differential Diagnosis

Clinical Presentations and Appropriate Initial Studies

Soft Tissue Swelling

- Radiograph
- Ultrasound
- CT for detection of subtle air if necrotizing fasciitis is considered
  - Cellulitis
  - Soft tissue abscess
  - Necrotizing fasciitis
  - Deep venous thrombosis
  - Foreign body

Atraumatic Pain

- Radiograph
  - Primary bone malignancy
  - Metastasis
  - Osteomyelitis
  - Osteoid osteoma
  - Stress fracture
  - Hardware failure or loosening

Arthropathy

- Radiograph
  - Inflammatory arthritis
  - Septic arthritis
  - Degenerative arthropathy
  - Gout or other crystal-induced disease
  - Posttraumatic arthropathy
  - Neuropathic arthropathy

Differential Diagnosis

Multiple Lytic Lesions

- Metastases
- Multiple myeloma
- Lymphoma

Destructive Bone Lesion

- Metastasis
- Primary bone tumor
- Lymphoma
- Plasmacytoma
- Eosinophilic granuloma
- Osteomyelitis

Intramedullary Lesion with Chondroid Matrix

- Enchondroma
- Bone infarct
- Chondrosarcoma
- Sclerotic bone lesion
- Osteoblastic metastasis (breast, prostate)
- Bone island
- Paget disease
- Lymphoma

Benign-Appearing Expansile Lesion

- Fibrous dysplasia
- Solitary bone cyst
- Aneurysmal bone cyst
- Giant cell tumor

Monoarthropathy

- Osteoarthritis
- Gout
- Rheumatoid arthritis
- Septic arthritis
- Tuberculosis
- Trauma

Arthritis with Osteopenia

- Rheumatoid arthritis
- Juvenile rheumatoid arthritis
- Lupus
- Septic arthritis
- Tuberculosis

Arthritis with Normal Bone Density

- Osteoarthritis
- Gout
- Calcium pyrophosphate deposition (CPPD)
- Psoriatic
- Ankylosing spondylitis
- Neuropathic arthropathy

Destructive Arthropathy

- Rheumatoid arthritis
- Juvenile rheumatoid arthritis
- Psoriatic arthritis
- Neuropathic arthropathy

Sacroiliitis

- Ankylosing spondylitis
- Inflammatory bowel disease
- Psoriatic arthritis
- Reiter syndrome (asymmetric)

Arthritis—Hands and Feet

- Osteoarthritis
- Erosive osteoarthritis
- Rheumatoid arthritis
- Psoriatic arthritis
- Gout (foot)

Arthritis—Shoulders and Hips

- Rheumatoid
- Crystal arthropathy
- Collagen vascular disease

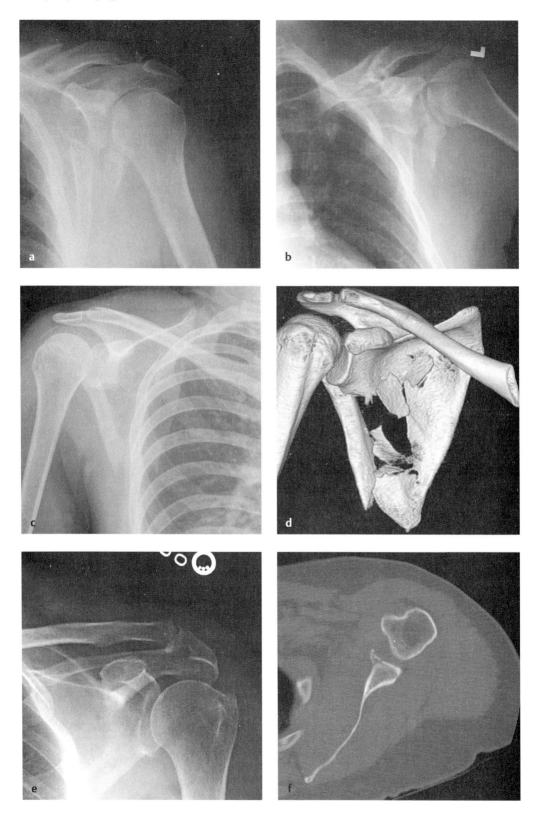

◆ Scapular Fracture

Scapular fractures result from direct impact to the shoulder and are usually associated with high-energy mechanisms. Patients with a scapular fracture are consequently likely to have associated torso injuries including pneumothorax, pulmonary contusion, rib or vertebral compression fractures, upper and lower extremity fractures, and upper extremity neurovascular structures (axillary artery and nerve, brachial plexus).

Scapular fractures may be difficult to diagnose on conventional radiographs but are easily appreciated on chest CT obtained in polytrauma. They are described as body, spine, acromion, coracoid, scapular neck, and glenoid fractures. Fragment displacement is usually minimal due to the supporting muscles and periosteum. Unless the glenoid fossa is involved, most scapular fractures are managed nonoperatively with a sling and outpatient orthopedic evaluation. Fractures that extend to the articular surface may require operative reconstruction (**Fig. 7.2**).

Fig. 7.2a–f
a,b Comminuted scapular body fracture with extension to glenoid articular surface and associated midclavicular fracture. Normal glenohumeral, acromioclavicular, and coracoclavicular relationships.
c,d Scapular body fracture. The inferior scapular body cortex is not well seen on frontal radiograph. CT with 3D reformation shows the complex fracture to advantage.
e,f Inferior glenoid rim fracture in a patient who fell on an outstretched hand without dislocating the shoulder. The radiograph shows subtle cortical discontinuity and a small bone fragment separate from the inferior glenoid. CT confirms an anterior/inferior glenoid rim fracture similar to the bony Bankhart lesion seen following anterior shoulder dislocations.

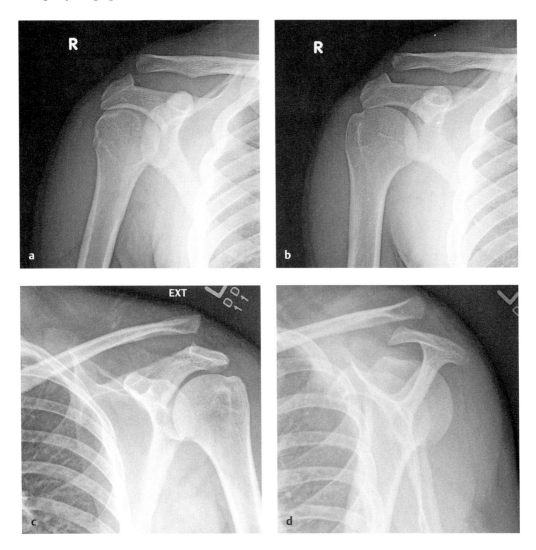

◆ Acromioclavicular Separation

Acromioclavicular separation can result from a direct blow to the shoulder or a fall onto the shoulder with the arm adducted. These mechanisms force the scapula inferiorly and medially with respect to the distal clavicle. In the case of a fall on the outstretched hand, the scapula is transiently displaced superiorly from the clavicle, injuring the acromioclavicular ligament.

The inferior cortex of the acromion and distal clavicle should normally align on the AP view. The distance between the acromion and distal clavicle is variable but usually less than 8–10 mm. Weight-bearing views with comparison to the uninjured shoulder may be necessary to demonstrate subluxation.

- Grade I: Normal or slight acromioclavicular subluxation. Acromioclavicular ligament sprain with intact coracoclavicular ligament.

- Grade II: Acromioclavicular ligament tear with acromioclavicular widening or distal clavicular elevation. Coracoclavicular ligament injury without widening of the normal coracoclavicular distance (< 1.3 cm).

- Grade III: Disruption of both acromioclavicular and coracoclavicular ligaments. Acromioclavicular subluxation with elevation of distal clavicle relative to the acromion. Coracoclavicular distance > 1.3 cm or a side-to-side difference of > 5 mm on bilateral AP views. Weight-bearing radiographs may be necessary to reveal these findings.

Grade I and II injuries are usually treated conservatively. Grade III injuries may benefit from operative stabilization (**Fig. 7.3**).

Fig. 7.3a–d
a,b   Grade II acromioclavicular separation. The distal clavicle is separated from the acromion by 1 shaft's width and is elevated 1.2 cm with respect to the coracoid.
c,d   Grade III acromioclavicular separation. The distal clavicle is separated from the acromion by 1.5 shafts' width and is elevated 3 cm with respect to the coracoid.

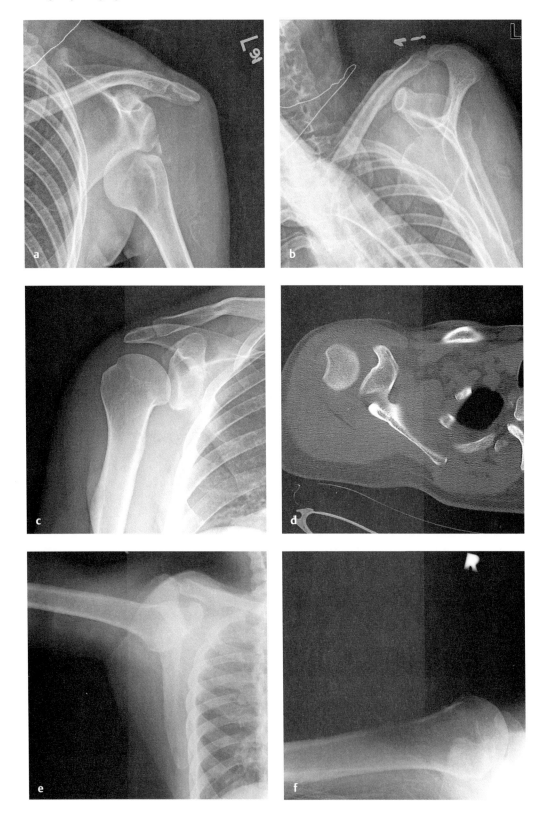

◆ Anterior Shoulder Dislocation and Luxatio Erecta

Anterior shoulder dislocation is the most common type of shoulder dislocation (~ 95%) and occurs with forced arm abduction, external rotation, and extension. The humeral head is displaced anterior, medial, and inferior to its normal location, and its posterolateral surface strikes the anteroinferior surface of the scapular glenoid. In anterior dislocation, impaction fractures of the posterolateral humeral head (Hill-Sachs lesion) and anteroinferior glenoid labrum avulsion (Bankart lesion) commonly occur. An osseous glenoid rim fracture, when present, is referred to as a bony Bankart lesion.

Pain and muscle spasm are the rule, and patients typically hold the affected arm in slight abduction and external rotation.

Anterior shoulder dislocations are well characterized using a standard trauma series consisting of AP views in internal and external rotation, the scapular-y view, and the axillary view. CT or MR may be useful for evaluation of osteocartilaginous fractures or intra-articular fragments. MR, in particular, is superior for identification of rotator cuff, capsular, and glenoid labral injuries.

Luxatio erecta (inferior dislocation) is an uncommon variant of anterior dislocation and tends to occur in elderly individuals. The mechanism of injury is forceful hyperabduction with impingement of the humeral neck on the acromion. In this injury the arm is held upward or behind the head. The displaced humeral head is often palpable on the lateral chest wall.

The AP radiograph is diagnostic; the humeral head is inferiorly displaced with the humeral shaft directed superolaterally along the glenoid margin. The humeral articular surface is directed inferiorly and is no longer in contact with the inferior glenoid rim.

Luxatio erecta is almost always accompanied by detachment of the rotator cuff and neurovascular compression. Associated fractures are also common but difficult to detect clinically because of severe shoulder pain. Early reduction should be attempted in an effort to prevent any neurologic or vascular damage. In most cases, reduction is not difficult and may be accomplished by the use of traction-countertraction maneuvers (**Fig. 7.4**).

Fig. 7.4a–f
a,b Anterior shoulder dislocation. The humeral head is dislocated inferiorly and anteriorly with respect to the scapular glenoid. Several small bony fragments adjacent to the glenoid reflect an associated bony Bankart lesion.
c,d Hill-Sachs lesion. Radiograph and CT after reduction of anterior shoulder dislocation; lateral humeral head impaction fracture.
e,f Luxatio erecta. Anterior-inferior right humeral head dislocation with fixed adduction of the humerus. Normal acromioclavicular and coracoclavicular relationships.

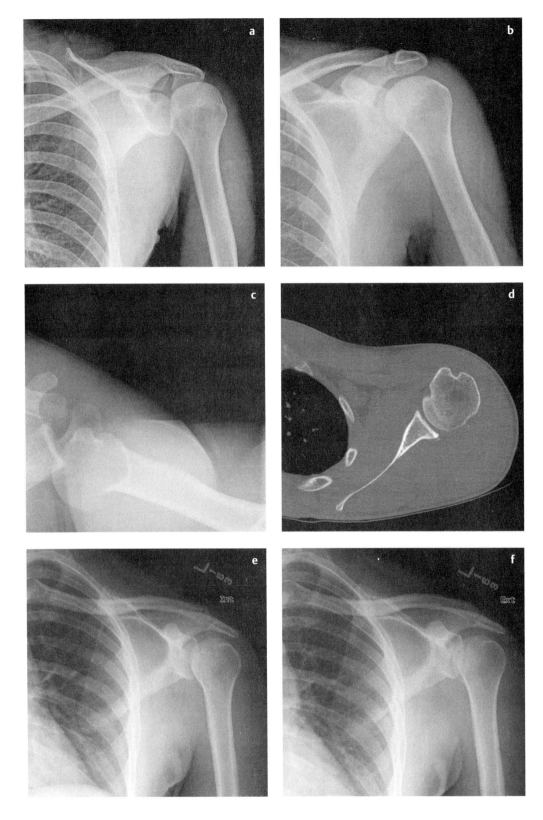

◆ Posterior Shoulder Dislocation

Posterior shoulder dislocation is much less common than anterior shoulder dislocation (~ 5%) and can be a difficult diagnosis both clinically and radiographically. Posterior dislocations follow seizures, electrocution, or a blow to the back of the shoulder with the arm internally rotated and abducted. Patients are usually unable to rotate their arm externally but do not present with striking deformity, and these injuries can be missed if axillary or scapular-y views are not obtained.

On frontal radiographs, the normal superposition of humeral head on the glenoid and the humeral profile in external rotation, which demonstrates the greater tuberosity, is lost. Because the humeral head is held in internal rotation, it appears rounded (the "lightbulb" sign). Most patients cannot externally rotate the affected arm, and standard internally and externally rotated AP radiographs appear identical. A fracture of the anterior humeral head, known as the trough line or reverse Hill-Sachs lesion, reflects impaction of the anterior humeral head against the posterior glenoid rim. The corresponding fracture of the posterior glenoid (when present) is called a reverse Bankart lesion.

Reducing a posterior shoulder dislocation is generally more difficult than reducing an anterior dislocation; if available, orthopedic consultation is indicated prior to reduction, as is adequate sedation, analgesia, and muscle relaxation (**Fig. 7.5**).

Fig. 7.5a–f
a–d Posterior shoulder dislocation. (**a**) Frontal radiograph shows lateral displacement of the humeral head with little overlap of the glenoid fossa. (**b**) Postreduction radiograph for comparison; the humerus now articulates normally with the glenoid. (**c**) Axillary view confirms posterior dislocation and impaction on the anterior humeral head. (**d**) Postreduction axial CT shows impaction at 10 o'clock, consistent with "reverse" Hill-Sachs lesion, and small avulsion of posterior glenoid, corresponding to reverse Bankart lesion.
e,f Subtle posterior shoulder dislocation. The orientation of the humeral head is unchanged on internal and external rotation radiographs and demonstrates the "lightbulb" sign. A subtle, vertically oriented crescentic lucency is superimposed on the mid-humeral head (trough sign).

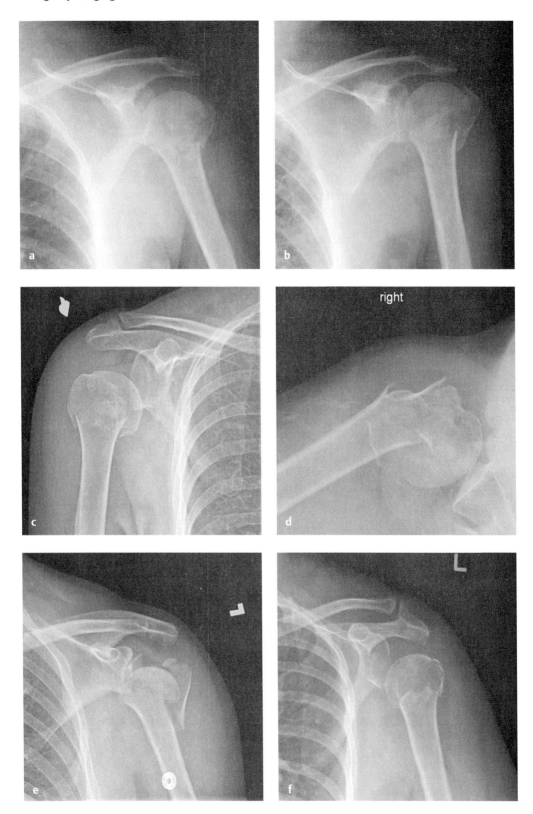

◆ Humeral Head Fracture

Humeral head and neck fractures are typically seen in elderly women after a fall on an outstretched hand. In younger patients, this injury is a consequence of high-energy trauma and is usually associated with other significant injuries. Patients present with shoulder pain, swelling, and tenderness; crepitus; and ecchymosis. Sensory disturbance, paresthesia, and diminished pulses indicate associated axillary nerve or artery injury.

Radiographs should be obtained in AP, transscapular, and (if possible) axillary views. Articular surface fractures may be associated with a hemarthrosis that displaces the humeral head inferiorly (pseudosubluxation).

The Neer classification system divides the proximal humerus into four parts, which are located between the epiphyseal lines where fractures primarily occur: the anatomic neck, the surgical neck, and the greater and lesser tuberosities. Fragments are considered displaced if separated by more than 1 cm or > 45° angulation. A one-part fracture contains no displaced fragments, regardless of the number of fracture lines. Two-part, three-part, and more severely comminuted fractures are characterized by progressively greater displacement and angulation of the small fragments.

One-part fractures are treated with immobilization and analgesics, but all other proximal humeral fractures require urgent orthopedic consultation in the emergency department because of the high risk of complications. Closed reduction, operative fixation, or a combination of the two may be necessary (**Fig. 7.6**).

Fig. 7.6a–f
a,b   One-part humeral head fracture. Transverse, slightly impacted fracture of the surgical humeral neck with separation and minimal displacement of the greater tuberosity. No fragments are separated by more than 1 cm, nor is there significant angulation of any fragment.
c,d   Two-part humeral head fracture. Impacted fracture of the surgical humeral neck with ~ 90° angulation of the humeral head with respect to the shaft.
e   Three-part humeral head fracture. Displaced fractures with separation and displacement of the diaphysis, medial humeral head, and greater tuberosity.
f   Pseudosubluxation. Nondisplaced (one-part) fractures of the humeral neck and greater tuberosity. The humeral head is inferiorly subluxed due to an associated hemarthrosis. Because none of the fragments are separated by more than 1 cm, this is considered a one-part fracture.

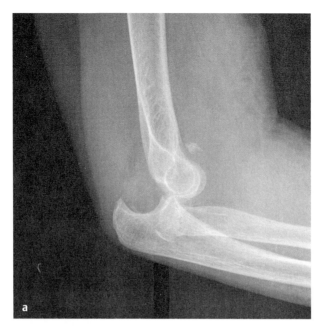

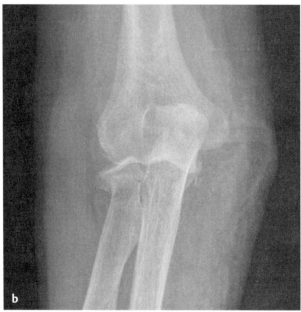

◆ Elbow Dislocation

Elbow dislocations are common, second in frequency only to shoulder and finger dislocations. Ninety percent are posterior and due to a fall on an extended, abducted arm. Clinically, the elbow is flexed at 45° with associated swelling, and the posteriorly dislocated olecranon process is easily palpated in its abnormal position.

Simple dislocations are treated with closed reduction and brief immobilization. Postreduction images should be carefully evaluated for radial head fracture, coronoid process fracture, or intra-articular fragments; CT may be helpful for complex or comminuted injuries. Complex fracture-dislocations and unstable dislocations require operative treatment.

The "terrible triad" refers to elbow dislocation, usually under varus stress, with associated fractures of the ulnar coronoid process and radial head. In this injury, the lateral collateral ligament is almost always disrupted, resulting in an unstable elbow. It is generally managed surgically by reattaching the ulnar coronoid process and affixing the radial head fracture (or replacing the radial head).

Complex fracture/dislocations of the elbow are more likely to be complicated by osteoarthritis, range of motion limitation, instability, and recurrent dislocation (**Fig. 7.7**).

Fig. 7.7a,b Posterior elbow dislocation. The ulna is dorsally dislocated with respect to the humerus, and the trochlea contacts the base of the coronoid process. A triangular fragment anterior to the distal humeral metaphysis corresponds to the fractured coronoid process tip. The radial neck is impacted, and the radial head is fractured and volarly angulated. A large joint effusion and marked soft tissue swelling are present. These findings correspond to a "terrible triad injury."

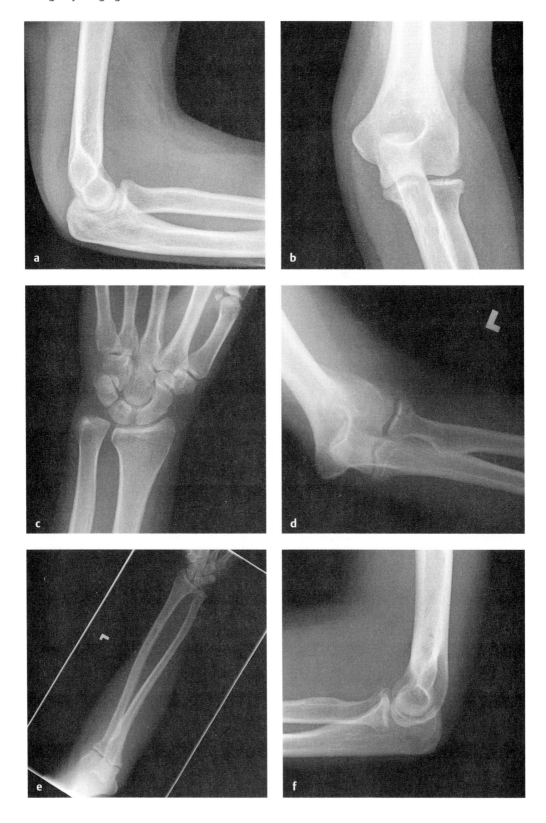

◆ Radial Head Fracture and Essex-Lopresti Fracture-Dislocation

Radial head fractures, the most common of the adult elbow fractures, are due to falls on an outstretched hand in which the radial head is driven into the humeral capitellum. Associated injuries are common and include coronoid fracture, elbow dislocation, medial collateral ligament injury, interosseous membrane injury, and damage to the triangular fibrocartilage complex at the wrist.

Passive pronation and supination of the forearm are painful, especially over the lateral elbow. Most fractures are subtle and reflect impaction at the radial neck. In the setting of acute trauma, a joint effusion, even if there is no cortical disruption or contour deformity, indicates a nondisplaced radial head fracture and should be treated accordingly. Signs of an effusion include elevation of the anterior elbow fat pad (sail sign) and visibility of the posterior olecranon fat pad.

The Mason classification is summarized in **Table 7.1**.

Type I (nondisplaced) fractures are treated conservatively with brief immobilization and analgesia. Displaced or otherwise complicated fractures, and those with restricted range of movement, should be referred to an orthopedic surgeon. Type II injuries are treated with open reduction and internal fixation. Type III injuries often require excision of the radial head and prosthetic replacement.

The Essex-Lopresti fracture-dislocation is defined by interosseous ligament disruption, usually accompanied by a fracture of the radial head and disruption of the triangular fibrocartilage of the wrist. The result is a dislocation of the distal radioulnar joint, causing pain in the wrist and forearm, with pronation and supination, and swelling and tenderness over the fractured radial head.

On standard elbow radiographs, radial head fractures may be subtle, and the Essex-Lopresti fracture-dislocation is especially difficult to diagnose. The radio-capitellar line should transect both the radial head and the capitellum on lateral view. Lateral projection is also best for assessment of any distal radioulnar dislocation.

Prompt consultation with orthopedic surgery should be arranged for assessment of both the elbow and distal radioulnar joint. Treatment consists of repair or replacement of the radial head (**Fig. 7.8**).

Table 7.1 Mason classification of radial head fractures

Type I	Nondisplaced fracture
Type II	Marginal fracture with displacement (impaction, depression, angulation)
Type III	Comminuted fracture involving entire head
Type IV	Associated with dislocation of the elbow

Fig. 7.8a–f
a,b Intra-articular radial head fracture. Nondisplaced, mildly impacted, intra-articular radial head fracture. Elevation of the anterior and posterior elbow fat pads (elbow effusion). The ulna and distal humerus are normal.
c–f Essex-Lopresti fracture-dislocation. Impacted intra-articular radial head fracture with associated widening of the distal radioulnar articulation and subluxation of the distal ulna.

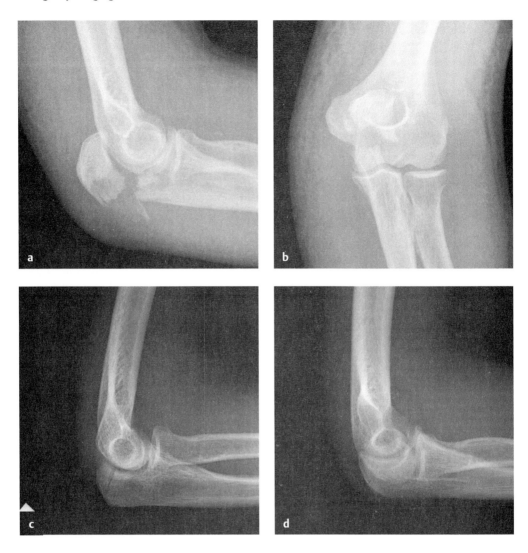

◆ Ulnar Olecranon Fracture

Olecranon fractures are common in the elderly, but they can occur at any age. Distal humeral fractures and radial head fractures may be associated with and result in the grossly unstable "floating elbow."

Best seen on lateral view, the fracture appears as a defect extending from the dorsal olecranon cortex to the articular surface of the trochlea. In most cases, the fracture fragments are widely distracted by the unopposed action of the triceps muscle, which inserts on the olecranon (**Table 7.2**).

In most cases, olecranon fractures require open reduction and internal fixation to restore the articular surface and preserve the elbow extensor mechanism. Nondisplaced fractures can be managed conservatively (**Fig. 7.9**).

Table 7.2 AO classification

Type A	Extra-articular
Type B	Intra-articular
Type C	Intra-articular fracture involving both the olecranon and radial head

Fig. 7.9a–d
a,b Displaced intra-articular olecranon fracture. Minimally comminuted intra-articular olecranon fracture with extension to the trochlear joint surface. Approximately 8 mm fragment displacement; marked soft tissue swelling.
c,d Nondisplaced olecranon fracture. Subtle, nondisplaced intra-articular fracture.

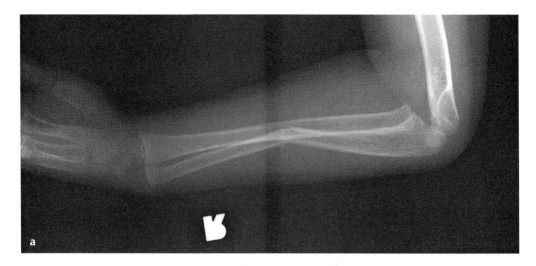

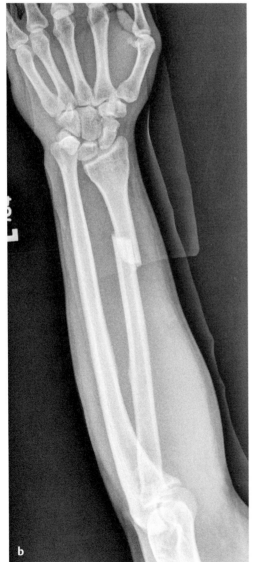

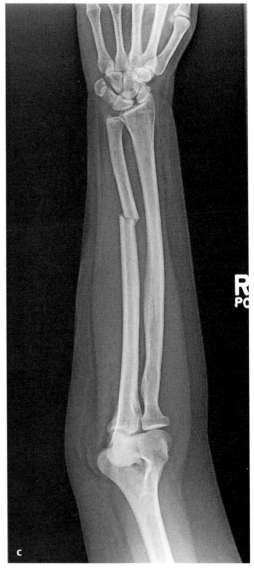

◆ Forearm Fractures

The Monteggia fracture (or fracture-dislocation) is a proximal ulnar fracture accompanied by radial head dislocation. It can be caused by a direct blow or a fall on an outstretched hand and results in elbow deformity, swelling, and pain with supination or pronation. Radial head dislocation may be subtle; in the normal elbow, a line drawn through the center of the radial head and shaft should intersect the capitellum on all views. Suspect dislocation if this is not the case.

Most pediatric fractures can be managed by closed reduction. Adult fractures usually require operative fixation.

The Galeazzi fracture is a distal radial diaphysis fracture with dislocation of the distal radioulnar joint (DRUJ). Galeazzi fractures are three times as common as Monteggia fractures. The mnemonic MUGR, which stands for "Monteggia—ulna, Galeazzi—radius," aids in recalling which bone is fractured in these injuries.

Galeazzi fractures are usually seen in children between 9 and 12 years of age and result from impact to the dorsolateral wrist or a fall onto an outstretched hand.

Radiographic findings include a transverse or oblique distal radial diaphysis fracture, widened DRUJ, and distal subluxation of the ulna relative to the radius.

Urgent operative fixation is normally required for adults with Galeazzi fractures in order to stabilize the fracture and DRUJ. Children younger than 10 years may be treated with closed reduction and splinting, but they should have prompt follow-up orthopedic evaluation.

A nightstick fracture is an isolated midshaft ulnar fracture that results from direct trauma to the ulna along its subcutaneous border. In cases of assault, it is a defensive fracture that occurs when a victim attempts to protect his face from an overhead blow. In contrast to the similar-appearing Monteggia fracture, the radiocapitellar relationship is normal.

Nondisplaced fractures are treated with splint immobilization. Open reduction and internal fixation is usually necessary when displacement is greater than 50% or angulation is greater than 10° in any plane (**Fig. 7.10**).

Fig. 7.10a–c
a Monteggia fracture (pediatric). Midulnar incomplete fracture with apex volar angulation and volar dislocation of the distal radius relative to the capitellum.
b Galeazzi fracture (adult). Transverse distal radius fracture with 2-cm override and disruption of the DRUJ with dislocation of the distal ulna. Carpal alignment is normal.
c Nightstick fracture. Transverse fracture at the junction of the mid- and distal ulnar thirds with slight radial displacement and ulnar angulation of the distal fragment. Marked forearm soft tissue swelling.

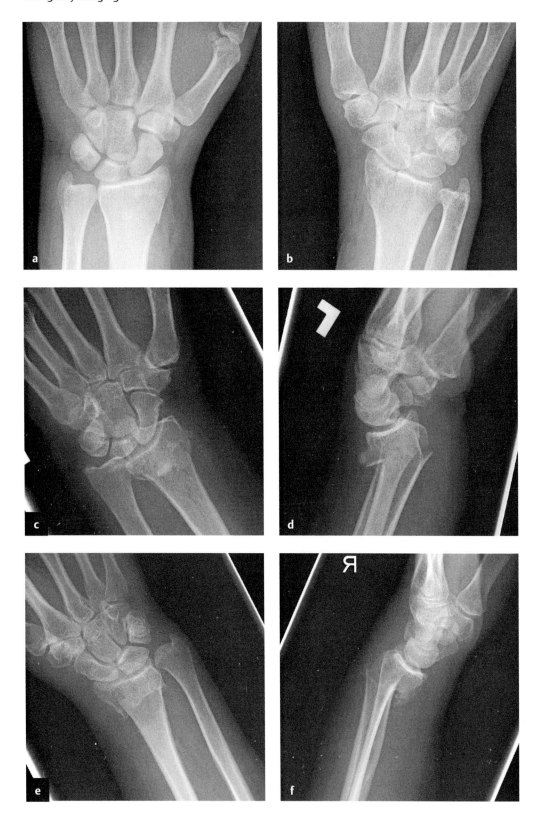

◆ Distal Radius Fractures

Hutchinson fracture is an oblique fracture of the radial styloid that extends into the radiocarpal joint. It is also sometimes called a chauffeur's fracture, recalling the historical mechanism of injury: a kickback of an early model automobile's crank handle striking the chauffeur's wrist.

The fracture is due to axial compression of the scaphoid into the distal radius with radial styloid fracture and radial collateral ligament avulsion. Hutchinson fractures are often associated with scapholunate injury and perilunate dislocation. It is an unstable fracture and requires operative fixation and immobilization.

Colles fracture is an intra- or extra-articular transverse fracture of the distal radius with dorsal displacement and dorsal angulation (apex volar) of the distal fragment, and it is usually due to a fall onto a hyperextended wrist. Clinically, the hand appears to have a "dinner fork" deformity. Colles fractures are more common in elderly women, reflecting demineralization. Most can be managed with closed reduction and cast immobilization with the wrist held in neural to slight flexion.

In contrast to the Colles fracture, the Smith fracture is characterized by volar angulation of the distal fragment. These extra-articular injuries are sometimes called a reverse Colles fracture, reverse Barton, or Goyrand fracture. Smith fractures result from either a direct blow to the back of the wrist or a fall onto a flexed wrist with the forearm in supination. The hand is palmarly displaced with respect to the forearm, resulting in a "garden spade" deformity on physical examination. Less common than Colles fractures, they are usually seen in younger patients with high-energy trauma. Because of its location, the median nerve is susceptible to injury and should be evaluated before and after closed reduction. Smith fractures are unstable and often require open reduction and internal fixation, particularly if there is intra-articular involvement or if the wrist remains grossly unstable after attempted closed reduction.

Plain radiographs (AP, lateral, oblique) of the wrist are sufficient for diagnosis. Distal radius fractures are classified according to (1) extension into the radiocarpal joint, (2) extension to the distal radioulnar articulation, and (3) the presence of an associated ulnar styloid fracture. These features should be included in a description to facilitate the orthopedic surgeon's ability to make optimal management decisions (**Fig. 7.11**).

Fig. 7.11a–f
a,b Hutchinson fracture. Nondisplaced oblique fractures of the radial aspect of the distal radii in two patients. Visible carpal and metacarpal bones are normal.
c,d Colles fracture. Comminuted, dorsally angulated distal radius fracture with associated ulnar styloid fracture but without involvement of the radiocarpal or distal radioulnar joints.
e,f Smith fracture. Transverse distal radius fracture without radiocarpal extension, radioulnar extension, or associated ulnar styloid fracture. Moderate volar angulation of the distal fragment.

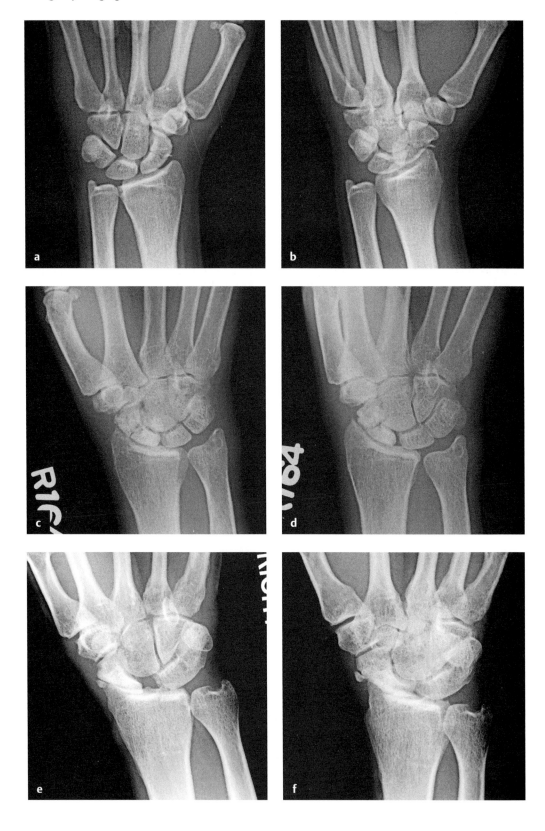

◆ Scaphoid Fracture and Scapholunate Dissociation

Scaphoid fracture is the most common of the carpal fractures and is usually due to a fall on an outstretched hand. Patients present with wrist pain with tenderness over the "anatomic snuffbox," or dorso-radial aspect of the wrist near the base of the thumb.

The standard wrist radiographic series (PA, lateral, and oblique) may not be diagnostic. The scaphoid view, a frontal radiograph with the wrist in ulnar deviation, elongates the scaphoid and should be obtained if scaphoid injury is suspected. While radiographs with scaphoid view are the best initial examination and will detect most acute fractures, CT and MRI are also highly sensitive studies and can detect subtle fractures and bone contusions in the patient with a negative wrist radiograph. Immobilization with radiographs obtained 1 to 2 weeks after the injury will also sometimes reveal a previously occult fracture.

Scaphoid fractures can be located at the distal pole (10%), waist (70%), or proximal pole (20%). The primary vascular supply to the scaphoid is via the radial artery, two branches of which supply the distal pole and waist of the scaphoid. With no direct arterial supply, the proximal pole depends on fracture union for revascularization. De-layed diagnosis or nonunited fracture may lead to proximal scaphoid avascular necrosis, which appears as sclerosis, fragmentation, and collapse.

Primary treatment is nonoperative with wrist immobilization in slight flexion and radial deviation. Time to union can vary based on location of the fracture and may be as long as 24 weeks for proximal scaphoid fractures. Surgical intervention is reserved for nonunion, displaced, or unstable fractures.

Scapholunate dissociation is the most common ligamentous disruption of the carpus and is often associated with scaphoid fracture. In trauma, the scapholunate ligament fails under high-energy loading of the extended, ulnar-deviated wrist. Scapholunate ligamentous disruption can also be related to chronic arthritis.

On PA radiographs, the normal scapholunate interval should be less than 2 mm. In scapholunate dislocation it is greater than 3 mm.

Pain is localized over the dorsal scapholunate region and exacerbated by dorsiflexion. Scapholunate ligament reconstruction may be required to prevent persistent instability (**Fig. 7.12**).

Fig. 7.12a–f
a,b   Scaphoid waist fracture. Acute, nondisplaced, transverse scaphoid waist fracture.
c,d   Scaphoid avascular necrosis. Remote, ununited, scaphoid waist fracture with dense sclerosis and fragmentation of the proximal and distal fragments.
e,f   Scapholunate dislocation with remote scaphoid fracture and avascular necrosis. The scapholunate interval is 6 mm. The proximal scaphoid pole is sclerotic with slight fragmentation at the scaphoid waist. Marked radiocarpal narrowing and subchondral sclerosis.

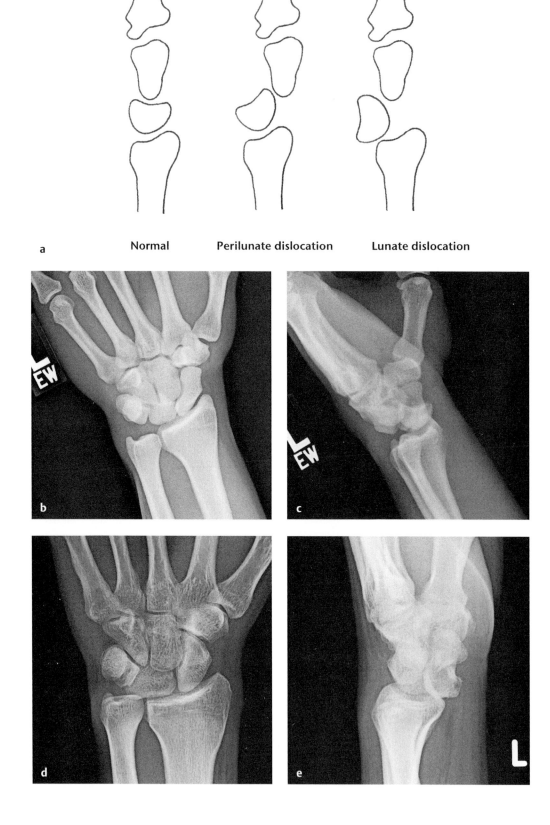

a   Normal   Perilunate dislocation   Lunate dislocation

◆ Perilunate and Lunate Dislocation

Perilunate and lunate dislocations occur after a fall on an outstretched arm with the wrist dorsiflexed; they present clinically with swelling, decreased mobility, and dorsal wrist pain. The median nerve is at risk for injury, and its function should be carefully assessed.

In perilunate dislocation, the lunate articulates normally with the distal radius, but the capitate is dorsally displaced with respect to the lunate. On the lateral radiograph, the capitate appears dorsally displaced with respect to the lunate. When a carpal fracture is also present, the term "trans" is applied to the name followed by the site of fracture; for example, transtriquetral or transscaphoid perilunate fracture-dislocation.

Lunate dislocation is an uncommon injury due to high-energy axial loading of the wrist in dorsiflexion. It results in volar displacement and rotation of the lunate relative to the distal radius.

On the lateral radiograph, the lunate does not articulate normally with either the capitate or the distal radius. In contrast to perilunate dislocation, in which the radiolunate articulation is preserved and the remainder of the carpus is displaced dorsally, the capitate remains aligned with the long axis of the radius.

In both perilunate and lunate dislocation, the dislocated lunate appears as a triangle with its apex superimposed on the proximal carpal row on PA radiographs.

All lunate and perilunate dislocations should be immobilized and referred to an orthopedic surgeon for reduction and definitive management (**Fig. 7.13**).

Fig. 7.13a–e
a,b Perilunate versus lunate dislocation. In perilunate dislocation, the lunate retains its normal articulation with the radius and the scaphoid is superimposed on the lunate on the lateral view. In lunate dislocation, both the lunate–capitate and lunate–radius articulations are disrupted. The scaphoid is visible dorsal to the lunate, which is displaced and rotated toward the palm.
b,c Perilunate dislocation. The proximal carpal row is dorsally displaced with respect to the lunate. The lunate is volarly rotated and the lunatocapitate articulation is disrupted. The lunate articulates normally with the distal radius. On the AP radiograph, the rotated lunate assumes a triangular appearance.
d,e Lunate dislocation. The proximal carpal row is dorsally displaced with respect to the lunate. The lunate is volarly rotated and dislocated with respect to both the capitate and the distal radius. On the AP radiograph, the lunate assumes a triangular appearance.

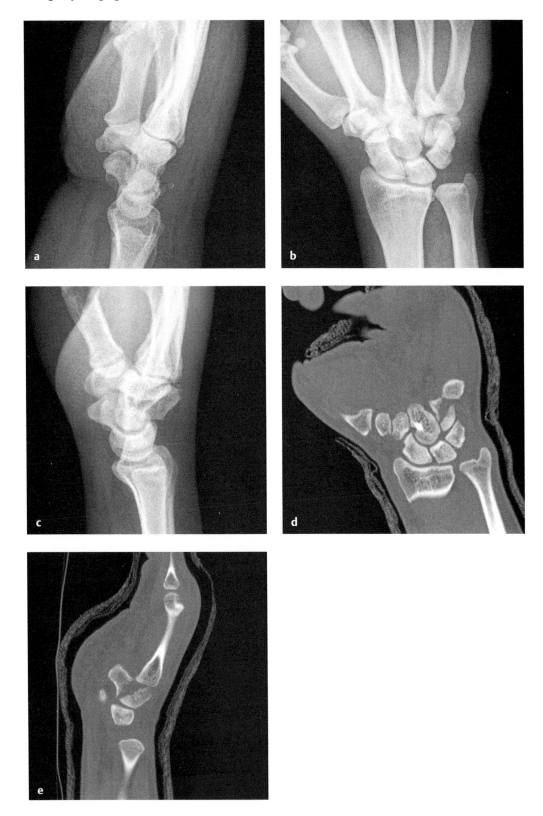

◆ Nonscaphoid Carpal Fractures

Triquetral fractures are the second most common carpal fracture, usually involve the dorsal surface of the triquetrum and are due to falls on an extended wrist in ulnar deviation. The ulnar styloid or the hamate impinges on the dorsal triquetrum and shears off a small fragment, which is visible dorsal to the wrist on the lateral view. Triquetral fractures may be associated with ligamentous damage.

Any dorsal fragment on the lateral view is presumed to be a triquetral fracture in the setting of trauma. PA radiographs may show an uncommon transverse fracture but are usually normal.

Patients present with motion-related pain and tenderness on the dorsoulnar aspect of the wrist, superficial to the pisiform. Management is nonoperative, with 6 weeks immobilization. Surgical intervention is rarely required but may be indicated to excise a persistently symptomatic dorsal chip fracture.

Hamate fractures are classified into four types based on their location and mechanism of injury: fractures of the distal articular surface, hook fractures, comminuted body fractures, and proximal-pole articular surface fractures. Patients complain of pain and tenderness over the palm of the hand. Because of their proximity to the hamate as they traverse the wrist, branches of the ulnar nerve or artery are at risk for injury.

A distal articular fracture is often accompanied by fifth-metacarpal subluxation and may occur when an axial force is transmitted down the shaft of the metacarpal, such as with a fist strike or fall.

Fractures of the hook of the hamate are most common in athletes involved in sports with repetitive swinging (e.g., baseball, golf, hockey). These fractures may result from repeated microtrauma or a direct trauma, such as when the force of a swing is transmitted directly to the palm of the hand, fracturing the hook at its base.

Visualization of a hamate fracture can be difficult on standard wrist radiographs; CT is generally more sensitive in detecting and evaluating radiographically occult carpal fractures when clinically suspected.

Nondisplaced hook fractures are immobilized for 6 to 8 weeks. Patients with displaced fractures should be referred to an orthopedic surgeon for operative fixation (**Fig. 7.14**).

Fig. 7.14a–e
a Triquetral fracture. A tiny osseous fragment lies dorsal to the lunatocapitate articulation on lateral view.
b–e (**b,c**) Hamate fracture. The proximal carpal row appears distorted with superposition of the hamate, pisiform, and triquetrum on plain radiographs. A tiny dorsal fragment lies adjacent to the dorsal carpometacarpal articulation on lateral view. (**d,e**) CT shows that the hamate body is transected at the base of the hook. There is a small bone island within the adjacent capitate.

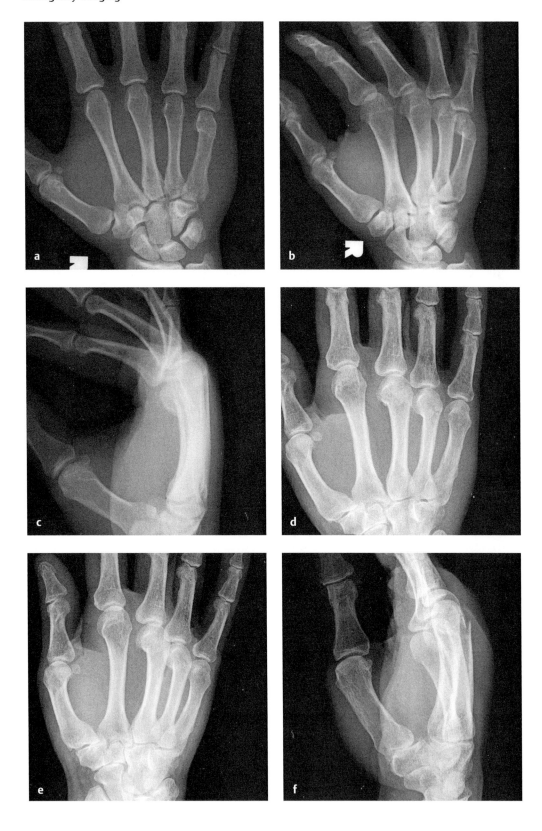

Metacarpal Neck Fractures

Fractures of the distal metacarpal metaphyses (metacarpal neck), especially of the fourth and fifth metacarpals, are commonly referred to as boxer's fractures. A direct impaction injury sustained while punching with a clenched fist, they account for 20% of all hand fractures. Patients present with tenderness and swelling over the dorsum of the hand.

Metacarpal neck fractures are easily diagnosed on oblique and lateral views of a standard wrist radiograph series. They may be mildly comminuted and are almost always volarly angulated.

Fractures are inherently unstable, and volar angulation and rotation of the distal fragment is common. Any rotation, identi-

fied as angulation toward the radial aspect of the hand on the AP radiograph, must be reduced. The degree of acceptable volar angulation varies according to the metacarpal injured. In the fourth and fifth metacarpals, for example, less than 30–40° angulation is acceptable without limitation in function. In contrast, fractures of the second and third metacarpals require a more accurate anatomical reduction to less than 10° in order to restore normal function. For fractures with smaller degrees of angulation, immobilization with flexion of the metacarpophalangeal joint for 2 to 3 weeks is followed by buddy-taping. Unstable fractures may require operative intervention with either K-wire or plate fixation (**Fig. 7.15**).

Fig. 7.15a–f
a–c   Fifth metacarpal neck (boxer's) fracture. Undisplaced fifth metacarpal neck fracture with volar angulation and mild dorsolateral soft tissue swelling. No distal fragment rotation on PA view.
d–f   Third and fourth metacarpal neck fractures. Undisplaced third and fourth metacarpal neck fractures with mild volar angulation and radial angulation of the distal fragments. The fifth metacarpal is intact. Moderate dorsolateral soft tissue swelling.

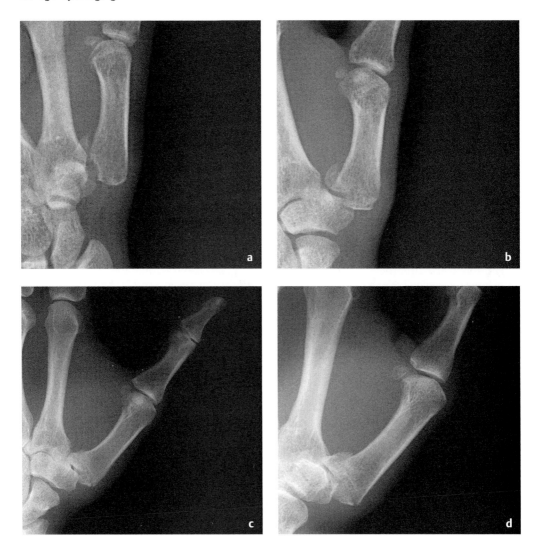

◆ Base of Thumb Fractures

A Bennett fracture is a noncomminuted intra-articular fracture-dislocation at the base of the first (thumb) metacarpal. Associated dorsolateral subluxation or dislocation of the metacarpal shaft is due to proximal tension exerted by the abductor pollicis longus. A smaller fragment of the ulnar aspect of the first metacarpal base articulates with the trapezium and index metacarpal. The most common mechanism is a longitudinal force upon a partially flexed thumb.

The diagnosis is usually obvious on standard radiographs. CT may be required to fully characterize the carpometacarpal injury for operative planning.

The Rolando fracture is a comminuted fracture-dislocation of the first metacarpal base. Similar in appearance to the Bennett fracture, it indicates greater applied force and complete articular disruption. Standard radiographs are usually adequate for diagnosis. Rolando fractures often require CT to fully characterize the intra-articular component and carpometacarpal injury.

Rolando fractures are unstable, have a poor prognosis, and may be complicated by posttraumatic arthritis despite optimum management.

Emergent treatment for these fractures includes ice, elevation, and immobilization in a thumb splint. They require referral to an orthopedist for definitive treatment with internal or external fixation depending on the type of fracture and degree of osseous displacement (**Fig. 7.16**).

Fig. 7.16a–d
a,b   Bennett fracture. Simple intra-articular fracture involving the ulnar base of the first metacarpal. Mild proximal subluxation of the metacarpal shaft.
c,d   Rolando fracture. T-shaped, mildly comminuted intra-articular fracture of the first metacarpal base. Slight radial and proximal subluxation of the metacarpal shaft.

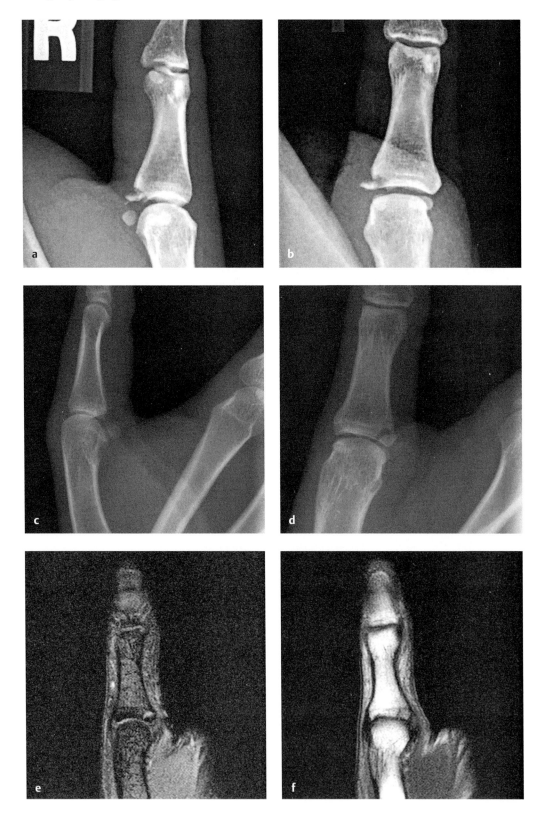

◆ Gamekeeper's Thumb

Gamekeeper's thumb, also known as skier's thumb, is an avulsion or tear of the ulnar collateral ligament (UCL) of the (thumb) metacarpophalangeal joint. Historically, the injury was seen among gamekeepers who broke the necks of ducks and geese after pinning the bird's neck between their thumb and forefinger, causing a repetitive strain injury. This mechanism is now rare, and gamekeeper's thumb is seen in skiers who forcibly abduct the thumb during a fall or aggressive pole-plant.

The diagnosis is based on history and clinical examination. The goal of emergency imaging is to identify and characterize any radiographically visible osseous avulsion fracture. Specialized imaging, including ultrasound and MRI, can be used to identify a Stener lesion, in which the avulsed ligament is displaced below the adductor pollicis aponeurosis. This is present in most complete tears, prevents normal healing, and normally requires surgical management.

Immobilization is the primary initial treatment for nondisplaced avulsion fractures and ligament strains without major instability; a thumb spica cast or splint should be placed for 6 weeks. Surgery is usually indicated for ligamentous injuries with significant thumb instability and for displaced fractures (**Fig. 7.17**).

Fig. 7.17a–f
a,b Gamekeeper's thumb. Minimally displaced avulsion of the ulnar base of the first proximal phalanx (oblique and PA radiographs).
c–f (**c**) Nondisplaced avulsion of the ulnar base of the first proximal phalanx, nearly invisible on oblique radiograph. (**e**) STIR MRI shows increased signal at the avulsion site. (**f**) T1-weighted image shows the radial and ulnar collateral ligaments at the first carpometacarpal joint.

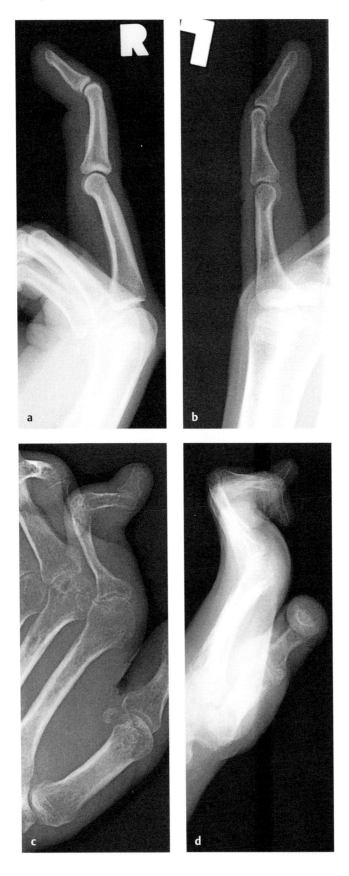

◆ Finger Deformities

Mallet finger is the consequence of either an extensor tendon stretching injury (soft tissue mallet finger) or an intra-articular avulsion fracture of the dorsal distal phalanx (bony mallet finger). It is due to a jammed finger—forced flexion of the distal phalanx with the distal interphalangeal (DIP) joint in extension—and commonly occurs in sports injuries in which a baseball or basketball strikes the fingertip. Patients present with dorsal pain and swelling with inability to actively extend the DIP joint.

For bony mallet finger injuries, lateral radiographs show the avulsed fragment, any degree of displacement, and the extent of articular surface involvement. In the reliable patient, treatment is conservative, with a dorsal splint that maintains the DIP joint in extension for 6 to 8 weeks. If the fracture is displaced or involves more than 25% of the articular surface, closed reduction and internal fixation with K-wires is usually necessary.

Swan neck deformity is extension of the proximal interphalangeal (PIP) joint and flexion of the DIP joint, either as a compli-cation of trauma or as a result of inflammatory arthropathy. The deformity reflects an imbalance between the forces acting on the joint following injury with impaired flexion at the PIP joint and impaired extension at the DIP joint. In most traumatic cases, a volar plate avulsion of the proximal middle phalanx or dorsal plate avulsion of the distal phalanx is identified.

Boutonnière deformity is characterized by flexion of the PIP joint and hyperextension of the metacarpophalangeal (MCP) and DIP joints. It is seen after PIP dislocations, with a jammed finger, and in patients with inflammatory arthropathies.

The proximal flexion deformity is due to weakening or laxity of the central portion of the extensor tendon at the PIP joint. With laxity or disruption, the lateral bands migrate palmar to the axis of rotation of the PIP joint and become flexors of the PIP joint. The head of the proximal phalanx pops through the gap in the central slip like a finger through a button hole, giving rise to the name "boutonnière" (**Fig. 7.18**).

Fig. 7.18a–d
a   Mallet finger. The distal phalanx is abnormally flexed with respect to the middle phalanx. No acute fracture.
b   Swan neck deformity. The finger is hyperextended at the PIP articulation and flexed at the DIP articulation. No fracture.
c,d   Boutonnière deformity in rheumatoid arthritis. The second through fourth proximal phalanges are hyperextended at the MCP and DIP joints and flexed at the PIP joint. The second proximal and middle phalanges are gracile. Marginal MCP and PIP erosions with near complete obliteration of the joint spaces.

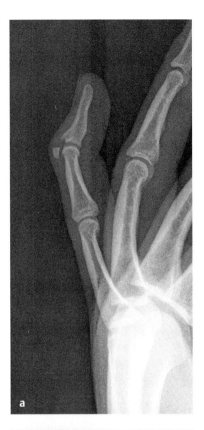

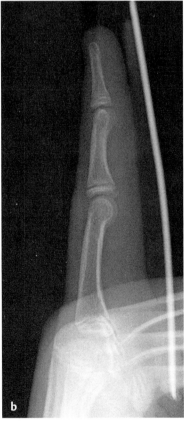

◆ Dorsal and Volar Plate Avulsion Fractures

Abrupt stress on the extensor digitorum tendon can avulse a fragment of bone from its insertion site on the dorsal base of the distal phalanx. This is referred to as a dorsal plate avulsion fracture, and it results from forced flexion of an extended DIP joint (jammed finger), which can result in mallet-finger deformity if not successfully managed. Patients are unable to actively extend the DIP joint fully. Primary treatment consists of splinting in extension for 6 to 8 weeks.

Volar plate avulsions are due to hyperextension at the PIP joint. The volar plate forms the floor of the PIP joint and can rupture at its insertion onto the middle phalanx. Subluxation or dislocation of the PIP joint is often seen with this injury as a result of associated collateral ligament disruption.

With volar plate avulsion, middle phalanx extension is not limited by the volar ligaments. In this case unopposed contraction of the flexor digitorum profundus can lead to an associated flexion deformity at the DIP joint that resembles a swan's neck; the finger is extended at the PIP and flexed at the DIP.

Radiographs show a small fragment of bone avulsed from the volar base of the middle phalanx.

Small fractures can be splinted in flexion. If the small fragment comprises greater than 30% of the articular surface, surgical fixation is often necessary (**Fig. 7.19**).

Fig. 7.19a,b
a Dorsal plate avulsion. A 2-mm triangular fragment comprising the proximal dorsal margin of the distal phalanx base is displaced 5 mm from the remainder of the phalanx. The distal phalanx is flexed (mallet finger deformity).
b Middle phalanx volar plate avulsion. Skeletally immature. A tiny fragment at the volar base of the middle phalanx is separated from the epiphysis by 2 mm. The fracture extends to the articular surface.

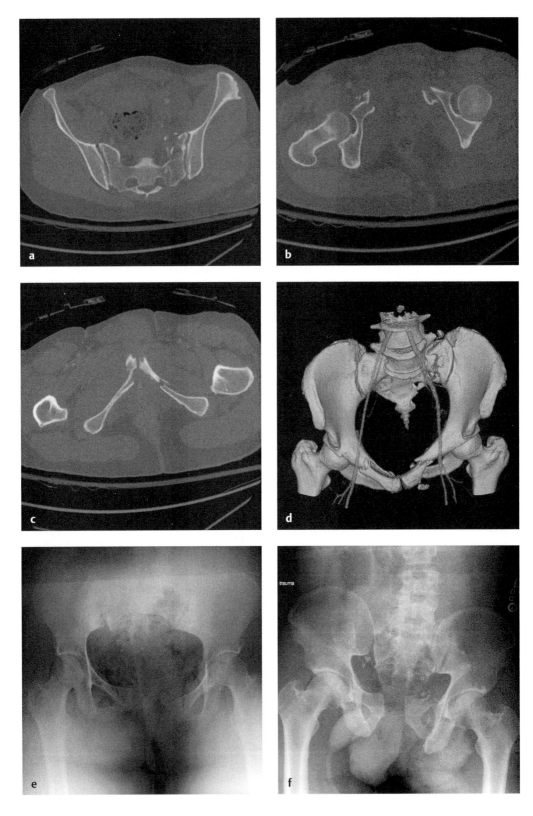

◆ Pelvis Fractures

Lateral compression (LC) pelvic fractures result from lateral impact, usually from landing on one's side in a fall or as a consequence of a broadside motor vehicle collision. They are characterized by iliac or sacral compression and superior and inferior pubic ramus disruption.

Clinical and CT evaluation should address potential associated injury to the urethra, vagina, and bladder. Although life-threatening pelvic bleeding is less common with LC fractures than with other pelvic disruptions, these fractures are frequently due to a high-energy impact and are associated with craniocervical, thoraco-abdominal, and extremity injuries.

Anterior-posterior compression (APC), or "open book," fractures are due to frontal or dorsal pelvic impact with compression and failure of the pelvic ring. Pubic symphysis diastasis or bilateral superior and inferior pubic ramus fractures separate the anterior pelvis in the midline. The sacroiliac articulations, sacrum, and iliac bones may be intact in minor injuries but often fail posteriorly in severe trauma, widening the pelvis like an opened book. APC fractures are frequently seen in front-end collision or motorcycle accidents.

Type I APC injuries, in which symphyseal diastasis is < 2.5 cm and no posterior pelvic fracture or sacroiliac injury is evident, are mechanically and hemodynamically stable. APC type II and III injuries are characterized by anterior and posterior pelvic ring disruption, are unstable, and generally require operative repair.

Vertical shear fractures result from vertical or longitudinal forces after a fall onto an extended lower extremity or in head-on motor vehicle accidents. Force transmitted along the axis of one leg to the ipsilateral hemipelvis usually disrupts the pelvic ring at the pubic symphysis anteriorly and shears the ipsilateral sacroiliac joint posteriorly with craniad displacement of the injured side. In some cases, vertical fractures through the sacrum and ipsilateral pubic rami have an identical effect. If the pubic ramus fractures are located contralateral to the sacroiliac joint diastasis (or sacral fracture), the fracture is described as a bucket-handle fracture. Conversely, if the fractures or diastasis are on the same side, it is termed a Malgaigne fracture. Both are unstable.

Virtually all ligamentous attachments are disrupted in vertical shear fractures, and these are often associated with severe spinal and lower extremity injuries.

Most trauma patients will have a portable AP pelvic radiograph while undergoing primary evaluation/resuscitation; this is generally adequate for identification and preliminary characterization of most fractures. Abdominopelvic CT imaging, performed in major trauma, permits more precise fracture evaluation as well as exclusion of visceral injury or active hemorrhage. The latter is emergently evaluated angiographically and, if necessary, embolized (**Fig. 7.20**).

Fig. 7.20a–f
a–d Type I lateral compression pelvic fracture. The superior and inferior pubic rami are fractured and mildly displaced. The left sacral ala is buckled and comminuted.
e Anterior-posterior compression-type pelvis fracture. The pubic symphysis is grossly diastatic. The right sacroiliac joint is widened. Associated left posterior column acetabular fracture.
f Vertical shear pelvis fracture. Marked diastasis of the pubic symphysis and right sacroiliac articulation with elevation of the right hemipelvis. Associated left superior and inferior pubic ramus fractures. Tiny metallic rings correspond to tacks from prior laparoscopic hernia repair.

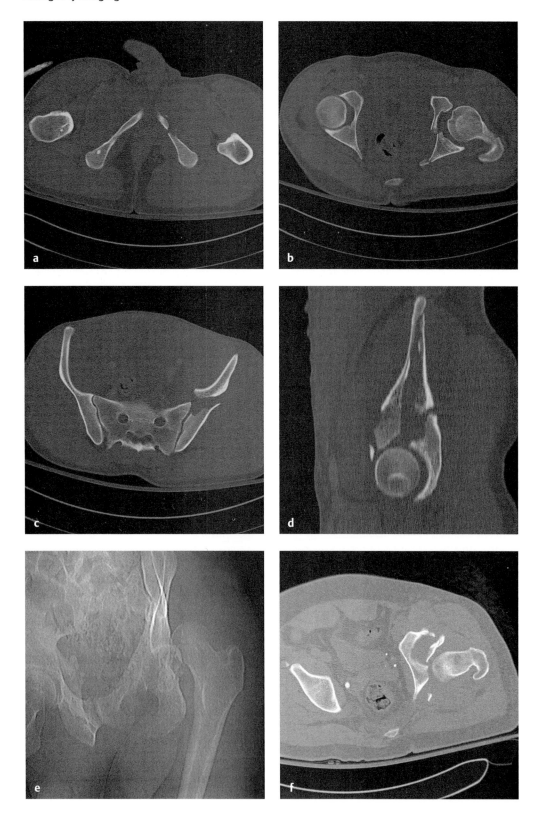

◆ Acetabular Fracture

Acetabular fractures are high-energy injuries, often caused by motor vehicle accidents and falls, in which the femoral head is driven into the acetabulum. A number of complex fracture patterns can result depending on the direction and magnitude of the impacting force. When viewed from the side, a line drawn from the lower sacroiliac articulation through the middle of the inferior pubic ramus divides the acetabulum into two "columns," and the integrity of one or both is the basis of classification and surgical management. Associated sciatic nerve injuries are common given the proximity of the posterior column to the sciatic notch at the inferior sacroiliac articulation. Isolated posterior wall fractures are often the result of posterior hip dislocation.

On the frontal radiograph, the anterior column is identified by the iliopectineal line (sciatic notch to upper symphysis pubis). The posterior column is identified by the ilioischial line (sciatic notch to inferior pubic ramus). Bilateral oblique (Judet) views are often obtained as part of plain radiographic evaluation. The "obturator" oblique, in which the obturator foramen (the oval space bounded by the pubic rami, symphysis, and acetabulum) is visible, shows the anterior column and acetabular wall to advantage. The contralateral "iliac" oblique best shows the posterior column and acetabular wall.

Pelvic CT, generally performed as part of comprehensive abdominal imaging in major trauma, is highly sensitive and specific for acetabular fractures and can identify nondisplaced fractures, intra-articular fracture fragments, and any associated pelvic soft tissue injury. Treatment is often operative, with the surgical aim of restoring a congruent hip joint. Small posterior wall fractures and minimal displacement of the acetabular dome can sometimes be managed with traction (**Fig. 7.21**).

The basic acetabular fracture (Letournel) classification is seen in **Table 7.3**.

Table 7.3 Basic acetabular fracture classification (Letournel)

Obturator ring–involving	
Both-column	Anterior and posterior column fractures with extension to obturator ring and to iliac wing
T-shaped	Transverse acetabular fracture with downward extension to the obturator ring
Obturator ring–sparing	
Transverse	Transverse acetabular fracture without involvement of obturator ring or iliac bone
Transverse and posterior wall	Transverse fracture with triangular posterior wall fragment
Isolated posterior wall	Isolated triangular posterior wall fragment (most common)

Fig. 7.21a–f
a–d Both-column acetabular fracture. The medial wall of the acetabulum, obturator ring, and iliac bone are fractured.
e,f Isolated posterior wall fracture associated with posterior hip dislocation. The posterior acetabular wall is fractured, and fragments are anteriorly displaced into the hip joint.

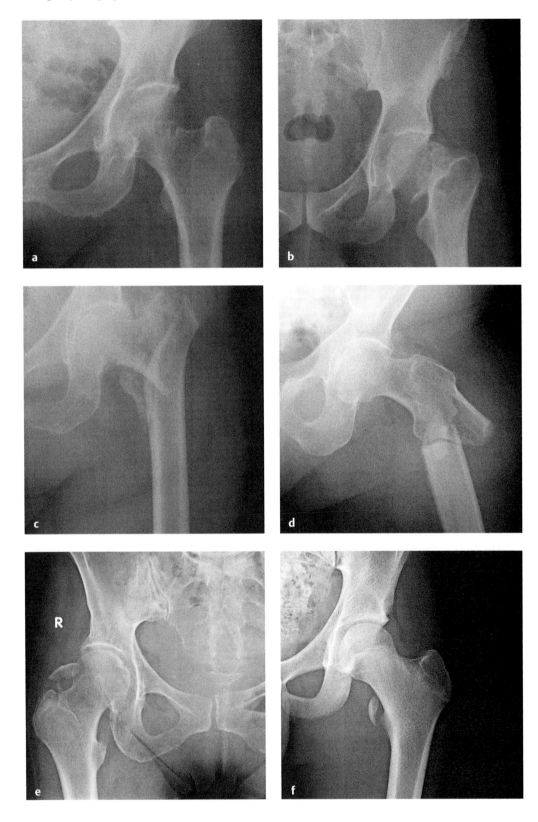

◆ Femoral Neck Fractures

Most femoral neck fractures result from low-energy falls in elderly patients with demineralized bones. They are more common in women, particularly in those with low estrogen levels. Other risk factors include advanced age, poor general health, alcoholism, and frequent falls. Proximal fractures in young patients are usually due to high-energy trauma.

Intracapsular fractures involve the subcapital (most common) and transcervical femoral neck. Most are due either to direct impact upon the greater trochanter or to external rotation of the leg with compression of the femoral neck against the posterior acetabulum. Stress fractures due to repetitive loading are seen in athletes, military recruits, ballet dancers, and patients with underlying osteopenia. Clinical findings include an inability to bear weight and pain on femur rotation.

Plain radiographic signs include discrete cortical or trabecular disruption, a sclerotic line secondary to impaction, angulation of the cortex or trabeculae, and rotation of the femoral head. In severe osteoporosis, minimally displaced fractures may be difficult to identify; MRI and CT detect subtle fractures in the patient who, despite apparently negative radiographs, is unable to bear weight. MRI has the advantage of identifying bone marrow edema and hemorrhage, and it is a better tool for diagnosing acute, nondisplaced fractures.

One-third of femoral neck fractures are extracapsular. Intertrochanteric fractures are the most common type and, like intracapsular fractures, tend to occur in older or osteoporotic patients after a fall from sitting or standing. The fracture is located between the greater and lesser trochanters and may extend to the subtrochanteric femur. Simple intertrochanteric fractures can be stable. Comminuted fractures and those with subtrochanteric extension are usually unstable. Treatment is operative in ambulatory patients. Basicervical fractures are often extracapsular and are treated like intertrochanteric fractures. Subtrochanteric fractures involve the proximal femoral shaft within 5 cm of the trochanters. They are all unstable.

Treatment of most hip fractures is operative, provided that the patient is able to undergo surgery safely, with primary goals of pain control, fracture stabilization, and early ambulation.

Greater trochanter fractures occur in adults following direct impact or forceful muscle contraction. Lesser trochanteric avulsion fractures are uncommon and usually occur in children and adolescents. In lesser trochanter avulsion, the apophyseal injury is due to forceful contraction of the iliopsoas muscle, which inserts on the lesser trochanter. Pain occurs primarily with leg flexion and internal rotation (**Fig. 7.22**).

Fig. 7.22a–f
a   Subcapital fracture. The subcapital lateral femoral neck cortex and trabeculae are disrupted.
b   Basicervical fracture. Mildly displaced fracture at the junction of the femoral neck and trochanters with moderate varus angulation.
c   Intertrochanteric fracture. Comminuted intertrochanteric fracture with mild varus angulation and craniad displacement of the major distal fragment. Slight subtrochanteric extension. Greater and lesser trochanter fragments are separated from the femoral neck and proximal femoral diaphysis.
d   Subtrochanteric fracture with varus angulation, override, and medial displacement of the distal fragment.
e,f   (**e**) Greater and lesser trochanter avulsions. A comminuted fragment arises from the greater trochanter in an adult. (**f**) Lesser tuberosity apophysis avulsion in an adolescent.

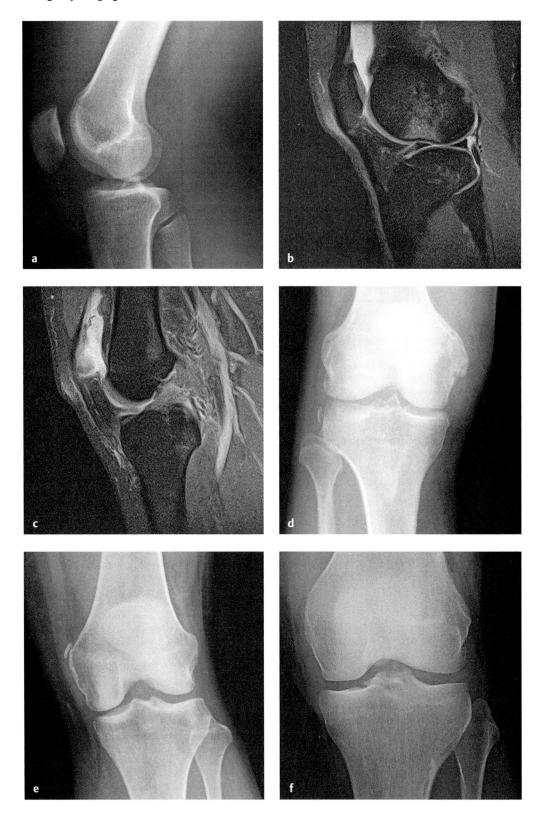

◆ Ligamentous Injuries of the Knee

The function of the anterior cruciate ligament (ACL) is primarily to prevent anterior translation of the tibia with respect to the femur. ACL tears result from twisting, hyperextension, or translation forces usually seen in sports injuries involving jumping or pivoting, or it can occur with impact. An audible pop at the moment of injury is considered pathognomonic. Patients present with severe knee pain, instability, traumatic joint effusion, and hemarthrosis.

The main function of the posterior cruciate ligament (PCL) is to prevent posterior translation of the tibia relative to the femur. PCL injuries are uncommon but are seen in knee dislocations, athletic injuries, and motor vehicle accidents in which the tibia is forcibly displaced posteriorly while the knee is flexed ("dashboard injury").

Although cruciate ligament tears cannot be directly identified on plain radiographs, the lateral femoral notch sign (a depression in the lateral condylopatellar sulcus seen on lateral view), Segond fracture, anterior tibial spine avulsion, and Pellegrini-Stieda disease are fractures that indicate significant ligamentous injury. Bone contusions of the medial aspect of the lateral femoral condyle and the posterior lateral tibial plateau are commonly associated with ACL tear and are usually evident on CT or MRI.

The Segond fracture is a vertical avulsion fracture of the lateral tibial plateau, located immediately distal to the tibial articular surface. It results from lateral capsular ligament traction under internal rotation and varus stress and frequently accompanies ACL disruption and/or meniscal injury.

Pellegrini-Stieda disease is posttraumatic calcification at the tibial collateral ligament bursa following injury to the medial collateral ligament and usually reflects subacute or remote collateral ligament injury.

Tibial spine avulsion fractures are frequently seen in children and adolescents with minor trauma but also occur in adults with significant knee injuries. The intercondylar eminence serves as an attachment point for both the anterior and posterior cruciate ligaments, and avulsions should be considered a marker for associated cruciate ligament injury: CT or MRI will usually identify the cruciate ligament attached to the avulsed fragment (**Fig. 7.23**).

Fig. 7.23a–f
a–c (**a,b**) Anterior cruciate ligament tear. Lateral femoral notch sign. STIR sequence shows corresponding increased T2 signal in the lateral femoral condylar bone marrow; impacted fracture with bone contusion as well as large knee effusion. (**c**) Complete ACL tear with intraligamentous edema visible as high signal on STIR sequence.
d Segond fracture. Vertically oriented crescentic fragment adjacent to the lateral tibial plateau.
e Pellegrini-Stieda disease. A well-defined corticated calcification adjacent to the medial femoral condyle indicates remote ligamentous injury.
f Tibial spine fracture. Broad avulsion of the intercondylar eminence.

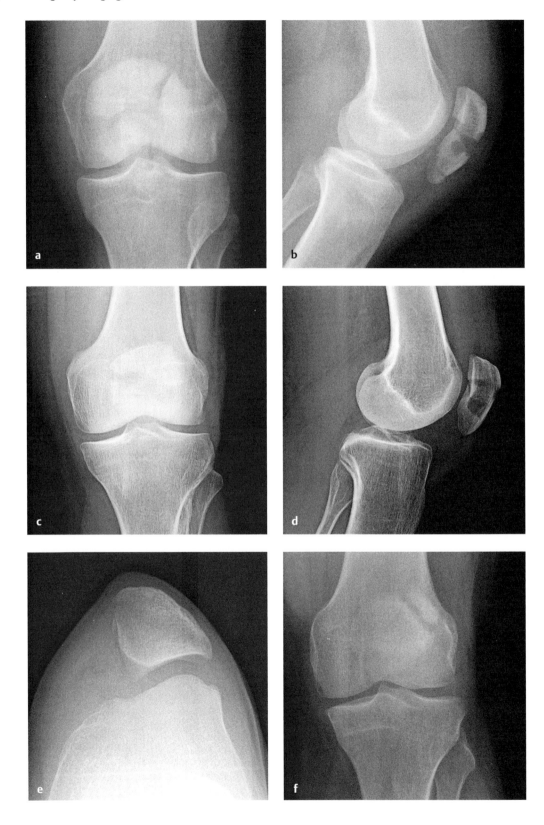

◆ Patellar Fracture

Patellar fractures follow direct impact to the knee or sudden quadriceps contraction during a fall or stumble. Fractures may be transverse, vertical, comminuted (stellate), or osteochondral. Transverse fractures are the most common type and are more likely to be associated with impaired knee extension. Patients typically have severe pain and swelling. Avulsions of the medial patellar ligament are frequently seen following patellar dislocation and may show a small bony fragment arising from the medial patella.

Craniocaudal fragment distraction should be assessed on the lateral view. The sunrise or axial view is advantageous for the identification of osteochondral and vertical marginal fractures. Patella alta, in which the ratio of patellar tendon length to patellar height is > 1.5, may be seen in distal pole fractures or in patients with patellar tendon rupture. MRI may be necessary to delineate the full extent of osseous and soft tissue injuries.

A bipartite or multipartite patella is a normal anatomic variation that can be mistaken for a fracture on AP view. The bipartite patella is often present in both knees, has smooth cortical contours, and is usually located at the the superolateral aspect of the patella.

Open fractures, transverse fractures with more than 3 mm craniocaudal distraction, and patients with compromised knee extension require surgical fixation. Simple nondisplaced fractures can be treated with immobilization of the knee in extension (**Fig. 7.24**).

Fig. 7.24e–f
a,b Comminuted patellar fracture. Stellate fracture with both vertical and transverse components. The superior and inferior fragments are separated by > 10 mm anteriorly. Large associated knee effusion.
c,d Transverse patellar fracture. Transverse fracture with 3–5 mm-fragment separation.
e Medial patellar avulsion following dislocation. A small flake along the medial aspect of the patella indicates avulsion of the medial patellofemoral ligament.
f Bipartite patella. Smoothly marginated superolateral patellar cleft. The smaller part is often irregular.

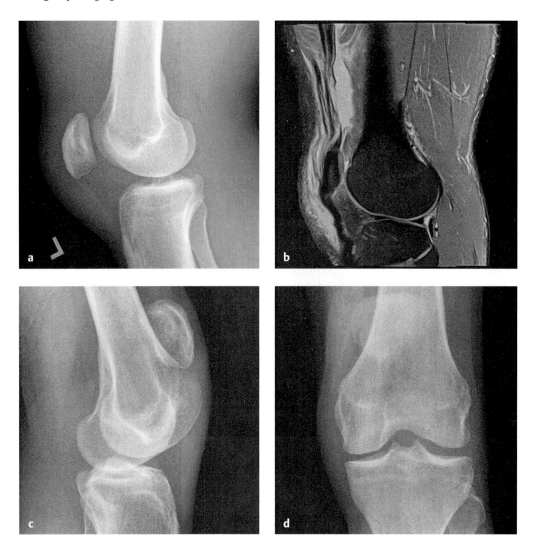

◆ Quadriceps and Patellar Tendon Rupture

Quadriceps tendon rupture follows eccentric quadriceps muscle contraction or a fall onto a flexed knee and usually occurs just proximal to the patellar insertion. It is most commonly seen in patients over 40 and those with predisposing conditions, such as local steroid injection, connective tissue disorders, anabolic steroid use, diabetes mellitus, and chronic renal failure.

Pain, swelling, ecchymosis, and inability to extend the knee against resistance are clinical features. The latter finding depends on whether a tear is partial or complete. The patella is often displaced inferiorly, with a palpable suprapatellar gap in the anterior leg soft tissues. Plain radiographs show edema, effusion, poor definition of the quadriceps tendon, and variable inferior patellar displacement.

Definitive treatment is surgical repair, with the best results obtained in the first 7 to 10 days following injury. MRI can more sensitively define the location and extent of tendon disruption.

Patellar tendon rupture is uncommon. The tendon extends from the tibial tubercle to the inferior pole of the patella and functions as part of the extensor mechanism of the knee. It most commonly ruptures at its patellar attachment and is often associated with a small avulsion fracture.

Risk factors are similar to those of quadriceps tendon rupture and include chronic microtrauma (tendinopathy), degenerative changes (calcifications), rheumatoid arthritis, systemic lupus erythematosus, diabetes, local steroid injection, and chronic renal failure. Mid-substance tears are more common than insertional tears in patients with these predisposing conditions. Patients often report a history of forceful quadriceps contraction against a flexed knee with subsequent impairment of knee extension. Some patients hear an audible "pop" when the tendon ruptures.

Complete rupture is easily identified when the patella has an abnormal craniad position, known as patella alta. In patella alta, the ratio of the patellar tendon length (lower patellar pole to tibial tubercle) to the craniocaudal length of the patella is greater than 1.3 to 1.5. Ultrasonography can also evaluate continuity of the tendon; rupture will be visible as a hypoechoic region, but this modality remains highly operator- and reader-dependent. Early surgical treatment is required for restoration of extensor function (**Fig. 7.25**).

Fig. 7.25a–d
a,b Quadriceps tendon rupture. Marked soft tissue swelling about the distal quadriceps with patella in normal position. STIR MRI shows complete disruption of quadriceps tendon.
c,d Patellar tendon rupture. The patella is grossly displaced proximally and lies anterior to the distal femoral diaphysis. Extensive soft tissue edema anterior to knee joint.

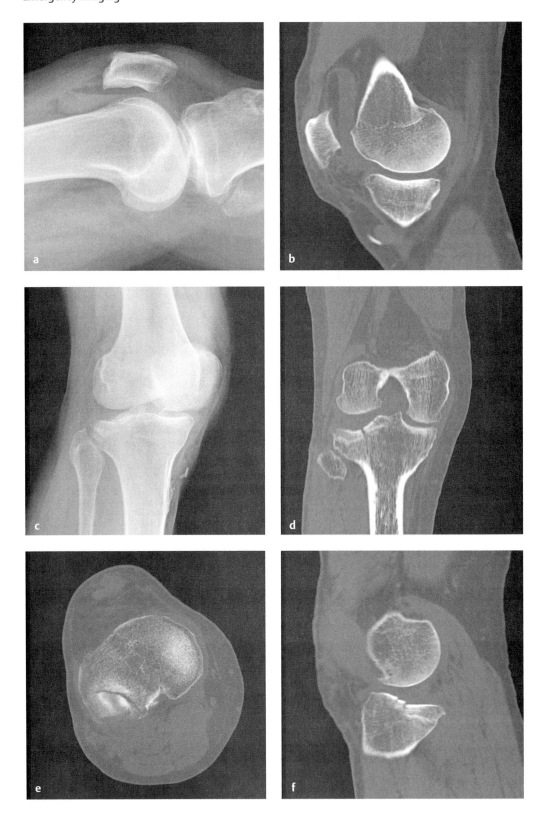

◆ Tibial Plateau Fracture

Tibial plateau fractures result from high-energy axial loading with simultaneous valgus or varus stress upon the knee. In younger individuals, the tibial plateau tends to split, often with cruciate or collateral ligamentous disruption and meniscal tear. Tibial plateau depression fractures occur more frequently in older, osteoporotic patients. Because the mechanism involves impact on the side of the fracture, lateral plateau fractures are more common than medial ones, and ligamentous injury opposite the side of impact is often present. Peroneal nerve and arterial injuries may be associated and should be excluded clinically.

Most tibial plateau fractures are associated with a knee joint hemarthrosis or lipohemarthrosis. Lipohemarthrosis, detected by identifying a fat-fluid level within a joint effusion on horizontal-beam radiograph, is a very specific finding for intra-articular fracture, although in many tibial plateau fractures only a simple hemarthrosis may be seen. For this reason, the lateral knee radiograph in trauma should always be performed using a horizontal X-ray beam. Radiographs obtained using a beam perpendicular to the X-ray table do not detect lipohemarthroses.

AP and lateral views should be obtained along with supplemental 40-degree internal (lateral plateau) and external rotation (medial plateau) oblique projections. CT with coronal and sagittal reformations is indicated in tibial plateau fractures to better delineate the degree of fragmentation or depression of the articular surface, evaluate ligamentous integrity, and aid in operative planning. MRI can be used, if necessary, to assess associated injuries to cruciate and collateral ligaments with greater sensitivity.

Nearly all tibial plateau fractures require open operative reduction and internal fixation (**Fig. 7.26**).

Fig. 7.26a–f
a–f (**a,b**) Tibial plateau fracture. Lipohemarthrosis on horizontal beam radiograph and corresponding sagittal reformation. (**c–f**) Minimally depressed fracture of the posterolateral tibial plateau.

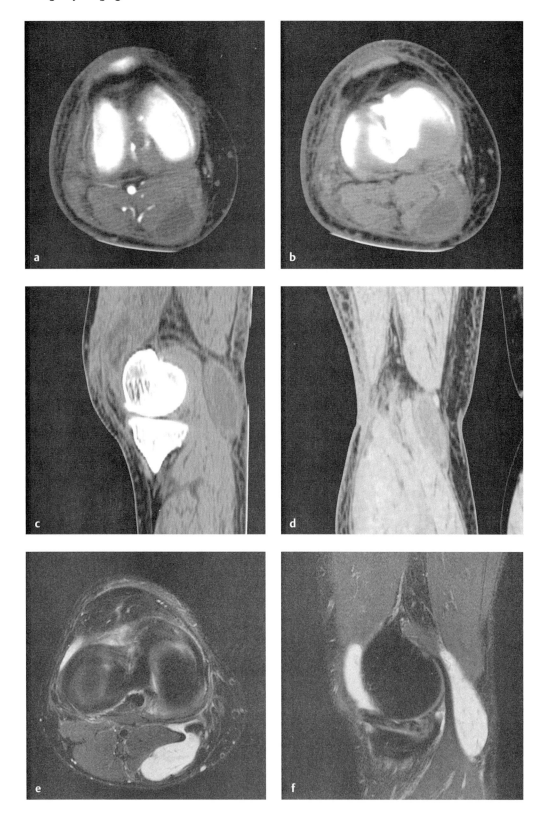

◆ Baker Cyst

A Baker cyst is an enlarged, synovial-lined popliteal fossa bursa that communicates with the knee joint via a stalk interposed between the medial gastrocnemius and the semimembranosus muscle tendon. Patients with rheumatoid arthritis, osteoarthritis, or prior trauma (particularly meniscal tears) are prone to Baker cysts, which are usually evident as a soft mass that tends to enlarge with knee effusion.

Baker cysts can rupture, and symptoms range from minimal to severe, potentially mimicking venous thrombosis or muscle tear. Upper calf warmth, tenderness, edema, and ecchymosis are typical examination findings.

Plain radiographs are somewhat insensitive but may show an apparent soft tissue mass dorsal to the knee. Ultrasound, CT, and MRI are all effective at identifying the cyst as well as adjacent fluid in the case of rupture (**Fig. 7.27**).

Fig. 7.27a–f
a–d   Ruptured Baker cyst. Thick walled fluid collection posterior to the tibia with thin stalk that communicates with the knee joint.
e,f   Baker cyst. T2-weighted MRI showing location of complex cyst between semimembranosus tendon and medial gastrocnemius.

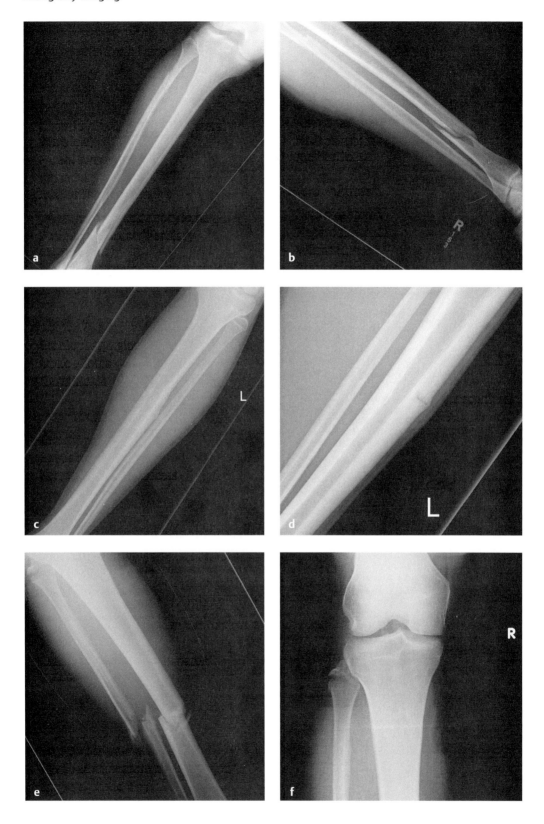

◆ Tibial and Fibular Fractures

Tibial shaft fractures result from high-energy direct impact and often are associated with fibular shaft fractures. The possibility of an acute compartment syndrome with neurovascular compromise should be evaluated and, if detected, treated. Open fractures have a high infection rates and require débridement prior to surgical fixation. Most fractures are repaired by intramedullary nail or cortical plate and screw fixation.

Isolated proximal fibular fractures are common and generally managed nonoperatively.

The Maisonneuve fracture is an unstable spiral fracture of the proximal third of the fibula due to low-energy injury with external rotation about a pronated, everted foot. The distal tibiofibular syndesmosis is disrupted with severe deltoid ligament disruption or medial malleolar fracture. Patients will have proximal fibular and medial malleolar tenderness on examination.

Knee or tibia/fibula radiographs show the proximal tibial fracture. Ankle radiographs may show either a fracture of the distal tibial shaft (the medial malleolus) or widening of the distal tibiofibular syndesmosis (medial clear space > 4 mm). Maisonneuve fractures require surgical fixation to restore ankle joint stability.

Tibial stress fractures are due to repetitive stress, especially with recently initiated activity, and are commonly seen in military recruits, runners, ballet dancers, basketball players, and other athletes. Risk factors include female sex, smoking, and low levels of 25-hydroxyvitamin D. Patients present with pain, swelling, and anterior tenderness. Plain radiographs will show cortical sclerosis disrupted by a lucent cortical fracture. Radiographic findings may be absent, and MRI or radionuclide bone scan are more sensitive diagnostic studies that can be considered.

Fibular avulsion fractures can be seen at the proximal or distal end of the bone. Proximal avulsions reflect injury to the arcuate ligament complex at the posterolateral knee and are frequently associated with anterior cruciate ligament disruption. Distal avulsion fractures indicate a tear of the anterior talofibular ligament, and the avulsed fragment is usually very small in comparison to the larger distal fragments that are seen in rotational injuries (**Fig. 7.28**).

Fig. 7.28a–f
a,b Maisonneuve fracture. Oblique fracture of the distal tibial diaphysis with one cortex-width lateral displacement of the distal fragment. Nondisplaced oblique proximal fibular diaphyseal fracture.
c,d Incomplete anterior tibial stress fracture. Transverse lucency with adjacent cortical thickening/sclerosis.
e,f Comminuted, transverse mid-tibial and fibular shaft fracture with proximal fibular avulsion. High-energy mechanism. One half shaft's-width posterior and lateral displacement of the distal tibial fracture. One shaft's-width posterior and medial displacement of the distal fibular fragment. Proximal fibular avulsion (arcuate sign) indicates posterolateral knee ligamentous disruption and potential associated cruciate ligament injury.

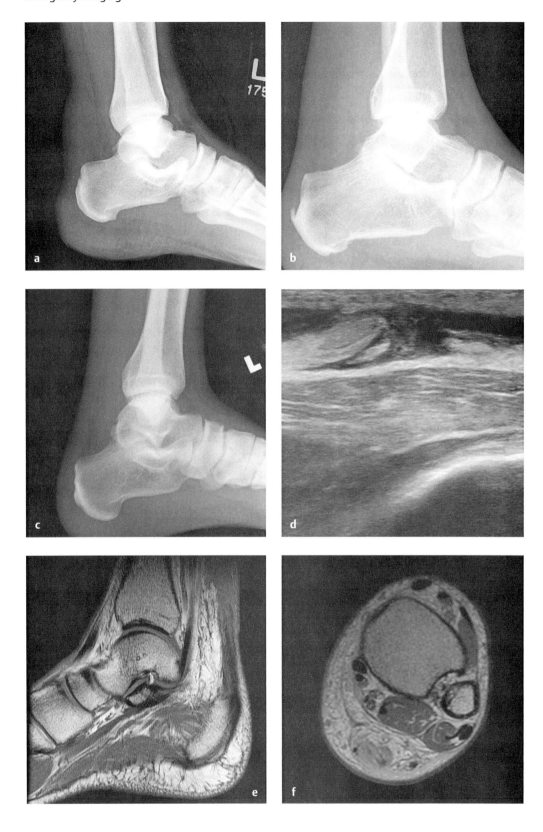

◆ Achilles Tendon Rupture

Achilles tendon rupture is the most common tendinous ankle injury and is seen in both repeated microtrauma and acute injury. Age, fluoroquinolone use, diabetes mellitus, and systemic inflammatory illnesses are predisposing factors. Acute pain and swelling are common presenting symptoms. In complete tears, plantar flexion against resistance will be impaired and a defect in the Achilles tendon may be palpable.

Dorsal ankle soft tissue swelling and fat infiltration of the pre-Achilles fat pad are radiographic findings. Ultrasound reveals an enlarged tendon with areas of hypoechogenicity. Complete tears appear as a discontinuous tendon often with acoustic shadowing at the margins. MRI will show increased T2 signal in the edematous tendon, which is normally similar to cortical bone in signal intensity.

Partial tears are treated conservatively with immobilization. Complete rupture or failure of conservative management usually requires anastomosis or graft for repair (**Fig. 7.29**).

Fig. 7.29a–f
a,b Soft tissue edema in Achilles tendon rupture. Two examples with obscured pre-Achilles fat pads.
c,d Tendon rupture on ultrasound. Radiograph shows poor definition of the pre-Achilles fat pad at the level of the tibiotalar articulation. Ultrasound shows complete tendon tear with fluid/hematoma around the tendon.
e,f MRI of tendon rupture (T1-weighted image). Increase in tendon diameter and loss of normal low T1 signal corresponds to tendon edema.

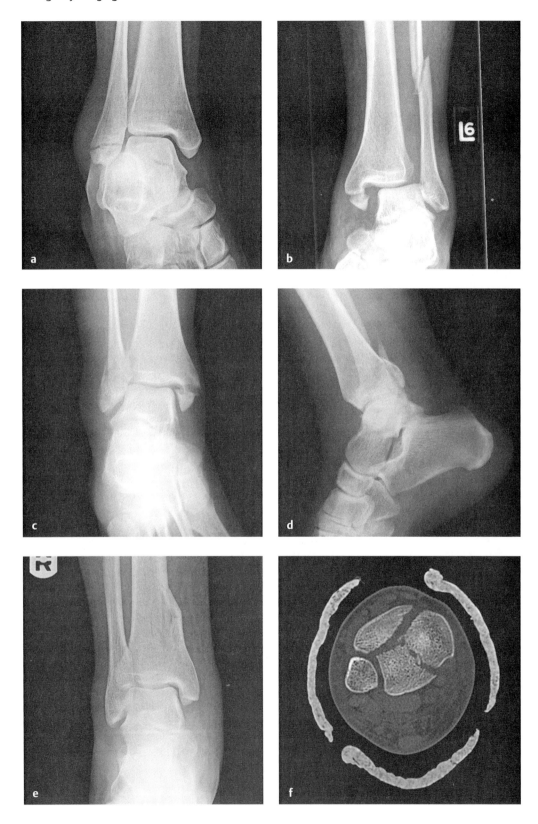

◆ Ankle Fractures

Ankle fractures are common and can be broadly divided into rotational injuries (medial or lateral unimalleolar, bimalleolar, or trimalleolar fractures) and axial loading injuries (pilon fractures). Bimalleolar fractures involve the distal fibula (lateral malleolus) and the medial tibial malleolus. Trimalleolar fractures involve the lateral malleolus and both the medial and posterior tibial malleoli. For bimalleolar and trimalleolar fractures, the Danis-Weber classification is commonly used and assesses stability and need for operative management based on the level of the fibular fracture component. The Danis-Weber classification that refers to level of fibular fracture is seen in **Table 7.4**.

Pilon fractures are due to high-energy axial loading forces. They involve the distal tibial articular surface (tibial plafond), are usually comminuted, and are associated with distal vascular injuries.

Radiographs, consisting of AP, oblique (ankle mortise view), and lateral views, are generally obtained for ankle injuries if the patient is unable to bear weight or is tender over the posterior aspect of the medial or lateral malleolus, the navicular, or the base of the fifth metatarsal. The oblique (mortise) view best shows the relationship between the malleoli and the adjacent talus; the ankle mortise should be symmetrical, and the distal tibiotalar space should be less than 5 mm. Pilon and other complex intra-articular fractures usually require CT for optimal characterization (**Fig. 7.30**).

Table 7.4 Danis-Weber classification of fibular fracture

Classification	Fracture	Notes
Type A	Transverse avulsion fracture, distal to the ibial plafond	The tibiofibular syndesmosis and deltoid ligaments are intact, but may be associated with oblique or vertical medial malleolus fracture. Type A fractures are usually stable and can often be managed with closed reduction.
Type B	Oblique or spiral fracture extending superiorly and laterally up the fibular shaft	The tibiofibular syndesmosis is either intact or only partially torn, but Type B fractures may be associated with medial malleolus fracture or deltoid ligament injury. They are usually unstable.
Type C	Fracture above the level of the tibiofibular syndesmosis	The syndesmosis is disrupted with visible widening of distal tibiofibular articulation. Type C fractures are almost always associated with deltoid ligament injury or medial malleolus fracture. They are unstable and require operative fixation.

Fig. 7.30a–f
a Isolated lateral malleolar fracture (Weber type A). Transverse, nondisplaced fracture through the distal fibula with associated soft tissue swelling. The ankle mortise, tibia, and calcaneus are intact.
b Bimalleolar fracture (Weber type C). Oblique distal fibular diaphysis fracture with one cortex-width lateral displacement of the distal fragment. Widening of the distal tibiofibular space (interosseous membrane). Transverse fracture of the medial tibial malleolus. Gross widening of the ankle mortise with ~ 1.5 cm lateral subluxation of the talus relative to the tibial articular surface. Moderate associated soft tissue swelling.
c,d Trimalleolar fracture (Weber type B). Oblique distal fibular fracture that extends proximal to the tibial plafond. Associated transverse medial malleolar fracture and coronal posterior malleolar fracture. Widened medial tibiotalar distance indicates instability.
e, f Pilon fracture. Comminuted intra-articular distal tibial fracture with three major fragments. Intact fibula.

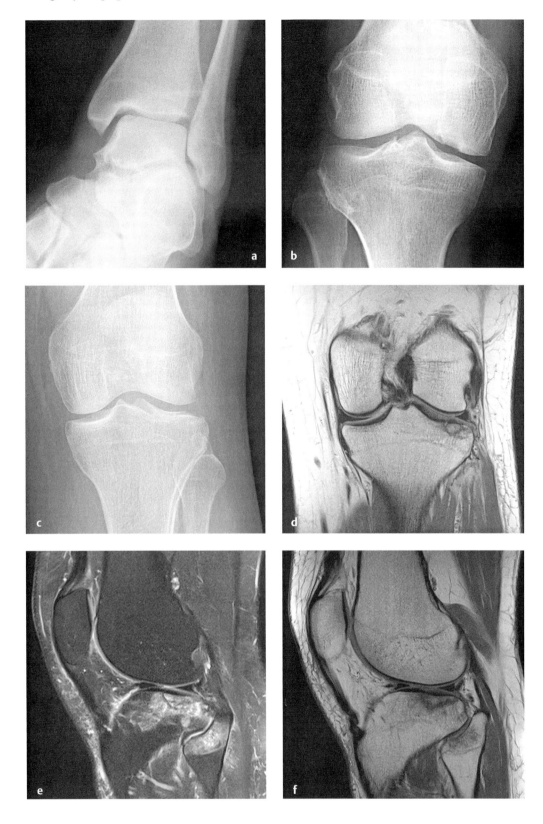

◆ Osteochondral Fracture

An osteochondral fracture separates a fragment made up of bone and articular cartilage from the articular surface. Common locations include the femoral condyle, humeral head, patella, talus, and capitellum of the elbow, and osteochondral fragments are one source of intra-articular loose bodies. Causes include repeated microtrauma, avascular necrosis, arthroscopic surgery complication, and direct impact. The clinical exam is nonspecific, and patients may experience joint pain with locking or may be asymptomatic. Remote fractures are often incidentally discovered on imaging for unrelated reasons.

The radiographic appearance is that of a small osseous fragment separated from the articular surface of a bone by a thin lucent line. The small fragment may be sclerotic. If it has been displaced, a small "divot" may be visible. CT shows similar findings with greater sensitivity. MRI is most sensitive for detecting osteochondral fractures in patients with persistent pain despite normal plain films. The osteochondral fragment is separated from normal marrow by a low-signal-intensity line on T1-weighted images and a high-intensity line on T2-weighted images (**Fig. 7.31**).

Fig. 7.31a–f
a Osteochondral fracture, medial talus. A thin, lucent line separates the osteochondral fragment from the talar dome.
b Osteochondral fracture, medial femoral condyle. A crescentic "divot" corresponds to the location of a remote osteochondral fracture. The small fragment is no longer visible.
c–f Osteochondral fracture, posterolateral tibial plateau. AP radiograph shows a subtle cortical defect in the cortex of the lateral tibial plateau. Coronal T1-weighted and sagittal T1- and T2-weighted images show a fracture involving both bone and cartilage with adjacent marrow edema.

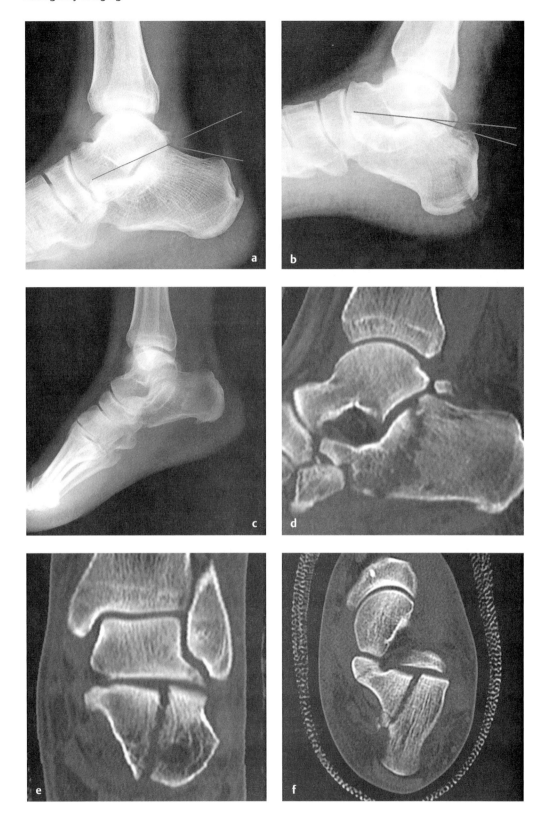

◆ Calcaneal Fracture

Calcaneal fractures result from large axial forces and are seen in patients who fall, landing on their feet. In this case, the entire weight of the body is transmitted to the calcaneus as it decelerates. Fractures are often bilateral and can be associated with thoracolumbar vertebral compression fractures.

Most calcaneal fractures are intra-articular and are defined as such by extension to the subtalar joint. Extra-articular fractures do not involve the subtalar articulation and include fractures of the anterior process, sustentaculum tali, lateral calcaneal process, medial calcaneal process, and Achilles tendon avulsion fractures.

The Boehler angle, a useful normative measurement on lateral foot radiographs, is defined by tangential lines drawn along the anterior upper and posterior upper margins of the calcaneus. Normally 20–40°, the Boehler angle is decreased when the midportion of the bone is fractured and depressed, as it is in most intra-articular fractures.

Lucency and bone condensation are other direct radiographic signs. CT with multiplanar and 3D reformations is invaluable for delineating the full extent of calcaneal deformity, identifying any other associated fractures, and permitting accurate classification and operative planning.

Nondisplaced intra-articular and non-displaced or minimally displaced extra-articular fractures can be managed nonoperatively. Operative aims include restoration of the subtalar and calcaneocuboid articulations, normal dimensions of the calcaneus, and the Boehler angle (**Fig. 7.32**).

Fig. 7.32a–f
a,b (**a**) Boehler angle. Normal calcaneus with angle = 24°. (**b**) Calcaneal fracture with angle = 11°.
c–f Calcaneal fracture. Boehler angle is normal on the lateral radiograph, but a focal area of sclerosis is visible in the body of the calcaneus. CT shows minimally displaced intra-articular calcaneal fracture with three major fragments. The major fracture line extends to the subtalar articulation.

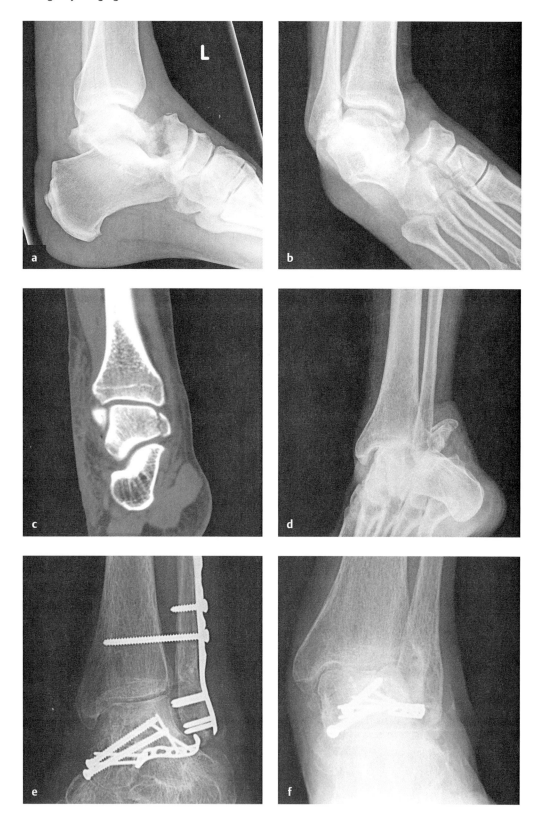

◆ Talar Fracture and Subtalar Dislocation

Talar fractures usually result from hyper-dorsiflexion as a result of falling on the extended foot. The fracture is also sometimes referred to as aviator's astragalus, a historical term describing a common injury seen in World War I pilots; in a crash, the rudder bar would strike the plantar aspect of the pilot's foot.

Talar fractures are classified by anatomic location as head, neck, body, posterior process, or lateral process fractures. The talar neck is the most vulnerable site to injury, as the force is directly transferred from the forefoot to the talus, which impacts the anterior margin of the tibia. The blood supply to the talus is tenuous, and, consequently, capsular disruptions from displaced fractures may result in osteonecrosis. The risk of avascular necrosis increases respectively with the Hawkins classification, shown in **Table 7.5**.

Fractures are often seen in the setting of subtalar dislocation, in which the midfoot is dislocated medially (85%; low energy) or laterally (15%; high energy) with respect to the talus. The more common medial dislocation is due to inversion and results in a foot that is fixed in supination.

Findings on plain radiographs can be subtle, and CT scan may be helpful for detection and characterization of apparently occult fractures (**Fig. 7.33**).

Table 7.5 Hawkins classification of talus fractures

Type I	Nondisplaced fracture
Type II	Displaced fracture with subtalar subluxation or dislocation
Type III	Displaced fracture with subtalar and tibiotalar dislocation

Fig. 7.33a–f
a Talar neck fracture. Comminuted, impacted talar neck fracture due to hyperdorsiflexion.
b,c Medial subtalar dislocation. The cuboid and navicular are medially displaced with respect to the talus. CT shows an associated nondisplaced medial talar fracture.
d–f (**d**) Talar dome avascular necrosis. Complex talar fracture dislocation. (**e**) Radiograph after operative reconstruction shows mild talar dome sclerosis. (**f**) Radiograph 1 year later shows cortical defect and collapse of the talar dome.

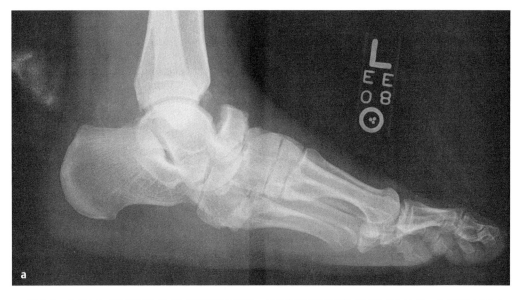

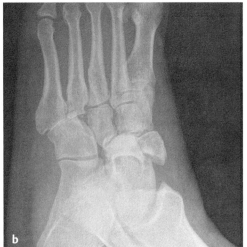

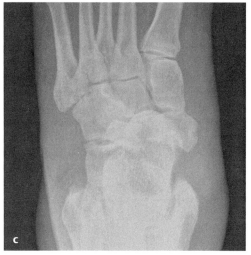

◆ Navicular Fracture

Navicular fractures result either from a direct blow or from indirect axial loading forces. Patients typically present after a fall or a motor vehicle accident with dorsomedial swelling and tenderness. Stress fractures of the navicular result from chronic overuse in runners and other athletes.

The oblique 45° radiograph is best for visualizing tuberosity fractures as well as detecting any associated injury of the navicular poles. Avulsion-type fractures, which tend to result from excessive flexion or eversion of the midfoot, often have associated talonavicular or naviculocuneiform ligamentous injury.

Nondisplaced fractures and stress fractures may be treated nonoperatively; other patterns of navicular fracture may need surgical intervention (**Fig. 7.34**).

Fig. 7.34a–c Navicular fracture. Sagittal fracture through the mid portion of the navicular with dorsal displacement of the lateral fragment and medial displacement of the medial fragment.

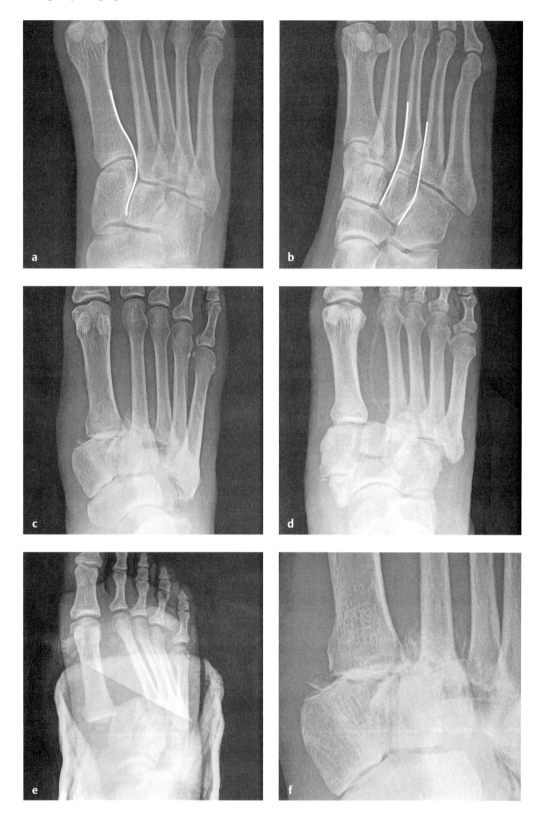

◆ Lisfranc Fracture-Dislocation

The Lisfranc joint is composed of the five tarsometatarsal joints and the Lisfranc ligament, which attaches the base of the second metatarsal to the medial cuneiform. These articulations are susceptible to injury with severe plantar flexion of the foot and direct crushing impact. A Lisfranc fracture (or fracture-dislocation) is a midfoot injury in which one or all of the metatarsals are displaced with respect to the cuboid and cuneiforms. Lisfranc fractures are easily missed, particularly on non-weight-bearing views and in the setting of polytrauma, and delay in diagnosis can lead to chronic arthritis and disability.

Lisfranc injuries may be homolateral or divergent. In homolateral injuries, all metatarsals are laterally displaced with respect to the cuboid and cuneiforms, or the second through fifth metatarsals are displaced while the first metatarsal remains normally aligned with the medial cuneiform. In divergent dislocations, the first metatarsal is medially displaced with respect to the medial cuneiform, while the second through fifth metatarsals are laterally displaced with respect to the middle cuneiform, lateral cuneiform, and cuboid.

On AP view, the medial border of the second metatarsal normally aligns with the medial border of the middle cuneiform. Any separation of more than 2 mm between the bases of the metatarsals suggests a Lisfranc injury. The fleck sign—tiny osseous flakes between the first and second metatarsal bases—indicates an avulsion of the Lisfranc ligament. On the lateral view, the superior border of the first metatarsal base should align with the superior border of the medial cuneiform. On the oblique view, the medial border of the fourth metatarsal should align with the medial border of the cuboid. Associated fractures may also be seen in the third metatarsal, first or second cuneiform, or navicular bones (**Fig. 7.35**).

Fig. 7.35a–f
a,b Normal tarsometatarsal alignment. The first metatarsal should align with the medial cuneiform on the AP radiograph. The second and third metatarsals should align with the middle and lateral cuneiforms on the oblique radiograph.
c,d (**c**) Homolateral Lisfranc fracture-dislocation. All of the metatarsals are laterally displaced with respect to the cuneiforms and cuboid. Several small bony flakes are located adjacent to the medial cuneiform and between the first and second metatarsals. (**d**) Homolateral Lisfranc fracture-dislocation with distraction of the first and second metatarsals. This is also a homolateral dislocation, rather than a divergent one. In this case, the first metatarsal remains aligned with the medial cuneiform, while the second through fourth metatarsals are laterally displaced.
e Divergent Lisfranc fracture-dislocation. The second through fourth metatarsals are laterally displaced with respect to the middle and lateral cuneiforms and the cuboid. The first metatarsal is medially displaced with respect to the medial cuneiform.
f Fleck sign. Multiple small bony flakes are located adjacent to the medial cuneiform and between the first and second metatarsals.

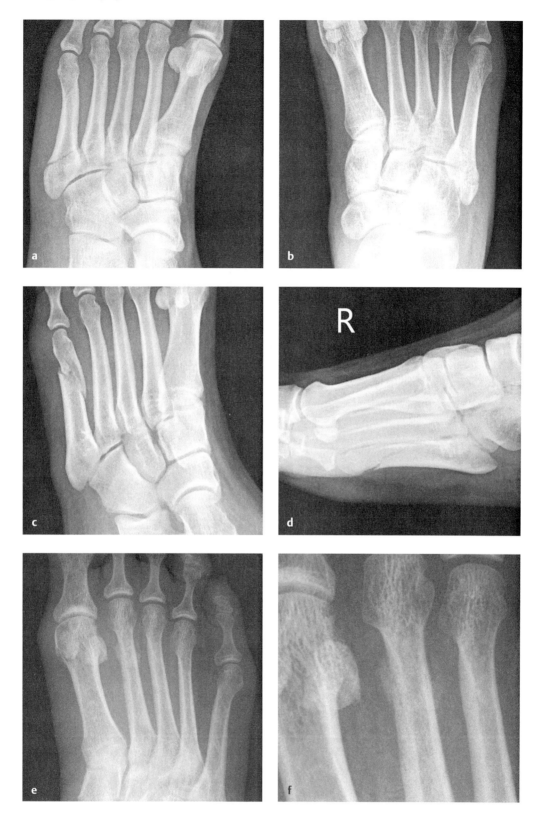

◆ Metatarsal Fractures

Metatarsal fractures are common, and most involve the fifth digit. Metatarsal fractures may be due to impact from an object falling on the foot, landing from a jump, twisting injury, or repetitive stress of marching or dancing. Fifth-metatarsal fractures can be categorized as avulsion fractures of the metatarsal base (pseudo-Jones fractures), transverse extra-articular fractures of the proximal diaphysis (Jones fractures), and distal spiral or oblique fractures. The latter (and often any fifth-metatarsal fracture) are sometimes referred to as dancer's fractures.

The pseudo-Jones fracture is due to avulsion of the lateral plantar aponeurosis or the peroneus brevis tendon, both of which insert on the base. Most are extra-articular and have a good prognosis.

The Jones fracture is an extra-articular transverse fracture of the proximal metatarsal diaphysis. The mechanism is indirect, from forcible adduction or inversion of the forefoot. Unlike avulsion fractures, Jones fractures are predisposed to nonunion.

Metatarsal stress fractures commonly occur at the neck of the second and third metatarsals and at the proximal fifth metatarsal diaphysis. Stress fractures are seen in high-level athletes and military recruits as well as in patients with rheumatoid arthritis, metabolic bone disease, and other neuropathic conditions. Pain often precedes radiographically detectable transcortical fracture.

In the setting of an acute ankle or foot injury, radiographs should be obtained if the patient is unable to bear weight on the foot or has focal tenderness over the proximal fifth metatarsal. Radiographic findings may be absent in early stress fractures; when evident, they include intramedullary sclerosis, periosteal new bone formation, or a nondisplaced transcortical fracture. In patients with suggestive symptoms and negative plain radiographs, radionuclide bone imaging and MRI are highly sensitive studies (**Fig. 7.36**).

Fig. 7.36a–f
a   Jones fracture. Nondisplaced transverse, extra-articular fracture through the proximal fifth metatarsal diaphysis.
b   Pseudo-Jones fracture. Nondisplaced avulsion fracture at the base of the fifth metatarsal limited to the lateral metatarsal tuberosity.
c,d   Spiral proximal fifth metatarsal diaphysis fracture with slight medial displacement of the distal fragment.
e,f   Metatarsal stress fracture. Focal periosteal new bone formation about the distal third of the second metatarsal diaphysis. No discrete transcortical fracture.

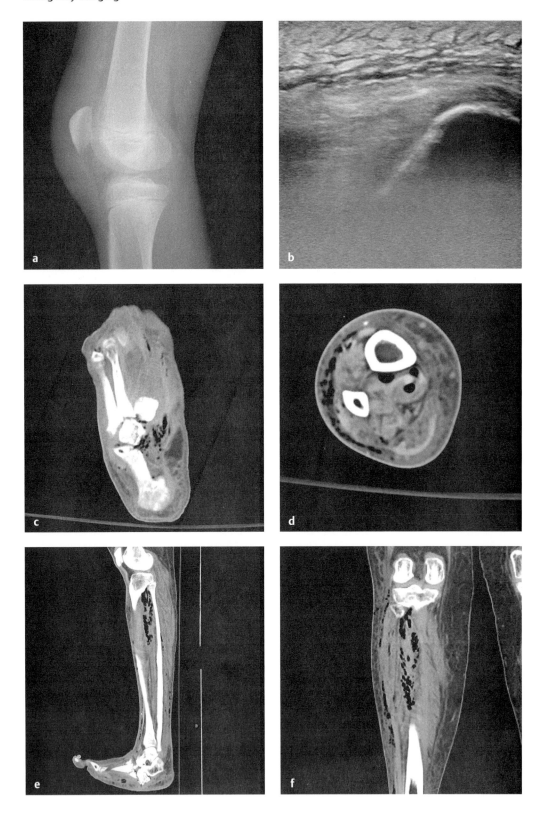

◆ Cellulitis and Necrotizing Fasciitis

Cellulitis is a soft tissue infection that follows epidermal injury and bacterial invasion with clinical features of pain, erythema, edema, and warmth. Patients with peripheral vascular disease, diabetes, or compromised immune systems are at increased risk. Lymphangitis and lymphadenitis may accompany cellulitis and are seen in more severe infections.

Ultrasound is often performed to identify or exclude an abscess. In uncomplicated cellulitis, the subcutaneous tissue appears diffusely echogenic and thickened; if severe, the tissue may show a cobblestone-like appearance. An abscess will appear as a hypoechoic collection with increased through-transmission against this background. CT can confirm the typical findings of cellulitis, dermal thickening, subdermal edema, and prominent subcutaneous lymphatics and can identify significant complications: abscess, myositis, osteomyelitis, and necrotizing fasciitis. Radiographs are generally obtained if there is a question of underlying osteomyelitis, foreign body, or fracture.

Simple cellulitis is treated conservatively with antibiotics and locally supportive measures. If the infection is severe or refractory to prior oral antibiotic treatment, or if an abscess or other complication is detected, intravenous antibiotics may be necessary. Abscesses, unless extremely small, should be aspirated or drained.

Necrotizing fasciitis is a rapidly progressive infection of the fascia characterized by widespread necrosis of the underlying subcutaneous tissues.

Patients often have a recent history of a trivial wound or abrasion, and most are immunocompromised by diabetes, alcoholism, HIV, organ transplants, or other conditions. Infections can be polymicrobial or due to group A streptococci or clostridial species. Swelling, erythema, disproportionately severe pain, blister formation, and ecchymosis are common clinical findings. Crepitus indicates subcutaneous gas and occurs in clostridial and other gas-forming organism infections. Fournier gangrene is one form of necrotizing fasciitis that affects the penis, scrotum, or perineum.

Early diagnosis is important, as effective treatment requires both intravenous antibiotics and surgical débridement. Contrast-enhanced CT is helpful in identifying inflammatory changes in deep muscle or fascia, soft tissue gas, and abscesses. Treatment is by fasciotomy with surgical débridement of necrotic tissue (**Fig. 7.37**).

Fig. 7.37a–f
a,b Cellulitis. Soft tissue swelling about the knee with poor definition of subcutaneous fat. Ultrasound shows "cobblestone" appearance of subcutaneous edema.
c–f Necrotizing fasciitis in a diabetic patient. Extensive deep-tissue edema and emphysema involving the foot and extending proximally along the interosseous membrane. Marked subcutaneous edema of the foot, with subcutaneous fat stranding extending superiorly along the posterior and lateral lower leg. Osseous destruction of the midfoot and hindfoot bones reflects neuropathic arthropathy.

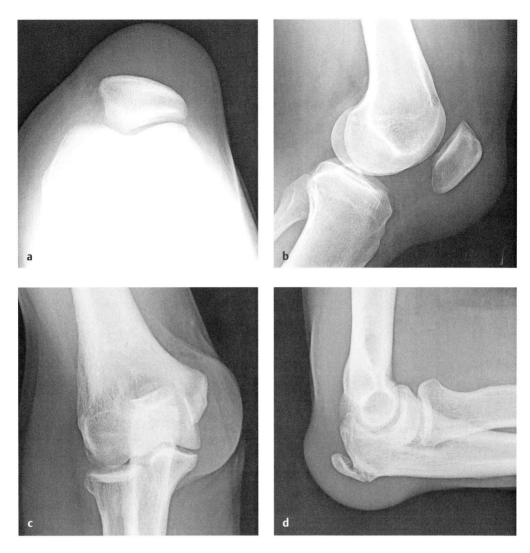

◆ Bursitis

Bursae are small synovial-lined fluid-filled sacs that reduce friction and allow smooth movement around a joint. Irritation or inflammation of a bursa frequently results from repetitive movement, with the most common locations being the shoulder, elbow, knee, and hip. Juxta-articular soft tissue swelling, pain, tenderness, redness, and limited range of motion are typical symptoms.

Ultrasound can identify the distended bursa as an anechoic or hypoechoic fluid collection, sometimes containing nodular debris or calcifications. Doppler imaging may show hyperemia, indicating acute inflammation. Radiographs are obtained if there is a question of underlying bone injury, but they are generally not helpful in evaluating bursitis itself.

Treatment is conservative with rest and NSAIDs; occasionally, antibiotics and aspiration of infected joint fluid may be needed. Acute bursitis may require splinting and surgical removal of foreign bodies within the bursa (**Fig. 7.38**).

Fig. 7.38a–d
a,b Knee bursitis. The patellar bursa is distended with marked associated prepatellar soft tissue swelling.
c,d Elbow bursitis. The olecranon bursa is enlarged superficial to a large enthesophyte at the triceps tendon attachment.

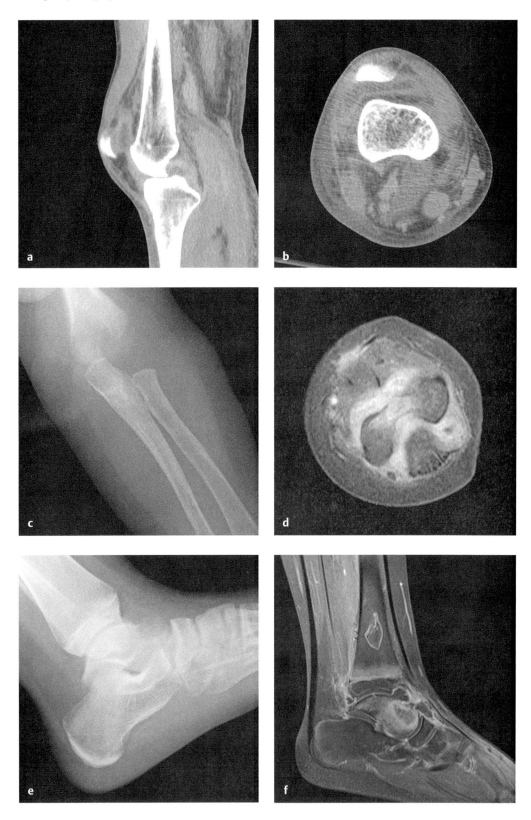

◆ Septic Arthritis

Septic arthritis is an intra-articular infection most commonly seen in intravenous drug users, diabetics, and other immunosuppressed patients. Joint infection can follow hematogenous spread from a distant source or direct extension from adjacent infected soft tissue or bone. Large joints with abundant metaphyseal blood supply are more commonly affected and include the shoulder, hip, and knee. Most patients present with a painful, erythematous joint, soft tissue swelling, decreased range of motion, and, sometimes, fever or systemic malaise.

In the absence of traumatic injury or recent instrumentation, monoarticular septic arthritis is most frequently due to *Staphylococcus aureus* infection, whereas gonococcal infections are most often responsible for polyarticular arthritis. *Neisseria gonorrhoeae* may be difficult to identify and culture from joint fluid aspirate, but it is often associated with pustular skin lesions and tenosynovitis. Among intravenous drug users and immunocompromised patients, nongonococcal gram-negative and anaerobic organisms are other causes of septic arthritis.

Aspiration and culture of joint fluid is required for diagnosis. Radiography and CT imaging serves only an adjunct role in identifying underlying osteomyelitis or soft tissue abscess and in guiding joint aspiration when necessary. Radiographic findings compatible with septic arthropathy include subchondral bone erosion, joint effusion, osteopenia, joint space narrowing, and periarticular soft tissue or muscle edema. MRI with contrast is more sensitive for early cartilaginous damage and may demonstrate synovial enhancement, periarticular soft tissue edema, and effusion.

If not promptly treated, septic arthritis can lead to destruction of articular cartilage and bone, osteonecrosis, osteomyelitis, secondary osteoarthritis, and joint ankylosis. Irreversible damage can occur as early as 48 hours after the onset of symptoms (**Fig. 7.39**).

Fig. 7.39a–f
a,b   Septic knee. Contrast-enhanced CT demonstrates a thick-walled, enhancing, fluid-filled, suprapatellar recess with adjacent inflammatory fat stranding.
c,d   Septic elbow in a child. Radiograph shows erosion of the distal humeral articular surface. Fat-suppressed postgadolinium MRI shows enhancement of the elbow joint and adjacent muscles.
e,f   Septic ankle joint and talar osteomyelitis in an immunocompromised patient. Radiograph shows lucency and superior erosion of the talar head and large anterior joint effusion. Fat-suppressed postgadolinium MRI shows two marginally enhancing fluid collections within the anterior ankle joint capsule, osteomyelitis of the talus, and an incidental bone infarct in the distal tibial metaphysis.

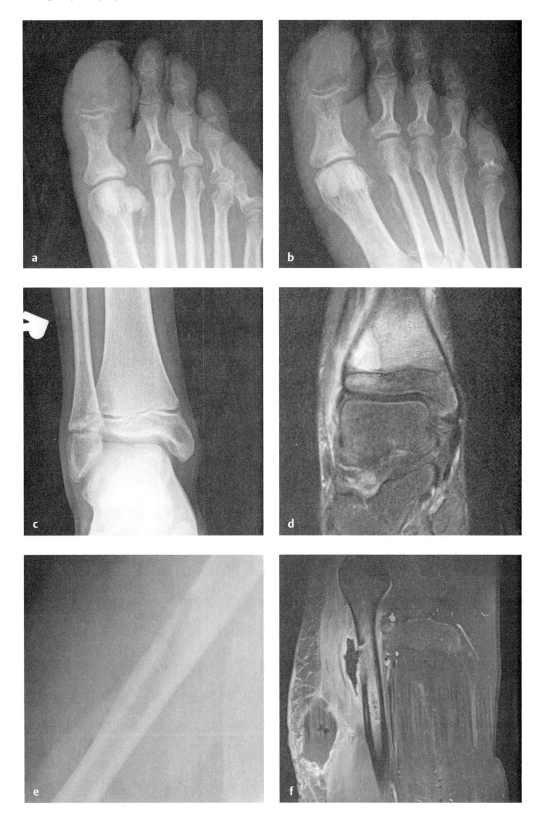

◆ Osteomyelitis

Bone infection can result from hematogenous dissemination, direct extension infection from cellulitis, or inoculation following instrumentation or open injury. While osteomyelitis can occur at any age, it is particularly common in children between 2 and 12, the elderly, and patients with impaired immune response, particularly diabetics. In children, osteomyelitis is usually due to hematogenous seeding, and it primarily affects the long bones. Osteomyelitis in adults is related to either local soft tissue infection or direct inoculation. When its origin is hematogenous, the spine is the most common site of involvement.

Pain, local soft tissue swelling, and erythema are typical. Fever and an elevated erythrocyte sedimentation rate may be seen, but the serum white blood cell count is frequently normal.

In the first 7–14 days of symptoms, radiographs may be normal or show only soft tissue swelling, poor subcutaneous definition, or joint effusion. Once osteomyelitis is established, more specific findings include periostitis, cortical destruction or permeation, and sclerosis. In contrast to plain radiographs, MRI is highly sensitive for early osteomyelitis and is generally preferred for the detection and characterization of soft tissue and intraosseous abscesses. Findings include replacement of the normal T1-hyperintense marrow signal, cortical destruction, abscess, or ulcer involving an abnormal portion of bone.

Treatment consists of systemic antibiotics for 4 to 6 weeks. Surgical intervention is reserved for patients requiring abscess drainage or débridement of necrotic bone (**Fig. 7.40**).

Fig. 7.40a–f
a,b Great toe osteomyelitis in a diabetic patient. Cortical destruction, fracture, and fragmentation with soft tissue swelling. Arterial calcifications are consistent with longstanding diabetes.
c,d Early distal tibial osteomyelitis in a child. Subtle lucency in the distal lateral tibial metaphysis on plain radiograph corresponds to marrow edema on coronal T2-weighted, fat-suppressed MRI.
e,f Humeral osteomyelitis in a diabetic patient. Well-defined intramedullary lucency in the humeral diaphysis with focal cortical defect at its proximal margin. Postgadolinium fat suppressed T1-weighted MRI shows intramedullary edema, cortical disruption, periosteal abscess, subcutaneous abscess, and extensive muscle edema.

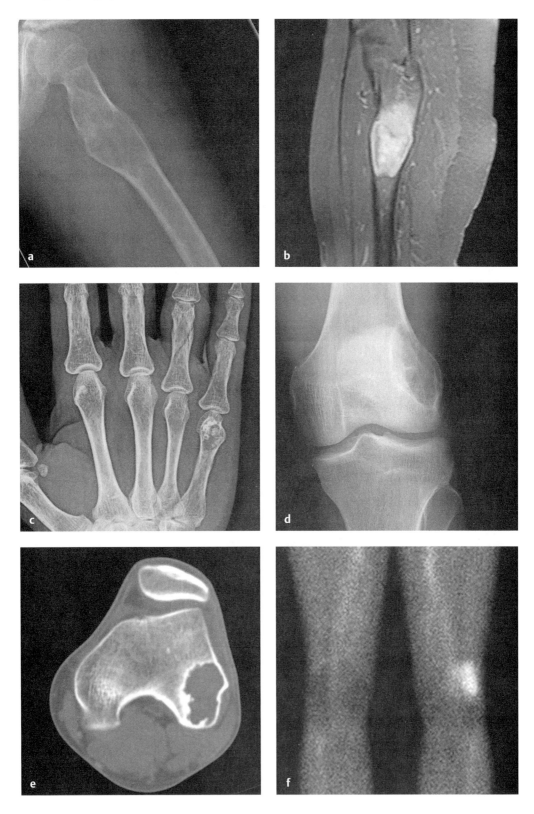

◆ Lucent Bone Lesions I

Incidental bone lesions are often encountered on plain radiographs obtained for trauma or nonspecific symptoms. Many are benign, and these tend to be painless, have sharply defined borders, and do not usually incite periosteal new bone formation. Metastases and osteomyelitis can sometimes appear benign and should also be considered. The common (and some uncommon) benign-appearing bone lesions can be remembered by the well-known mnemonic FEGNOMASHIC or its anagram FOGMACHINES:

- Fibrous dysplasia
- Enchondroma, eosinophilic granuloma
- Giant cell tumor
- Nonossifying fibroma
- Osteoblastoma
- Metastasis, myeloma
- Aneurysmal bone cyst
- Simple (solitary or unicameral) bone cyst
- Hyperparathyroidism (brown tumor)
- Infection
- Chondroblastoma/chondromyxoid fibroma

Fibrous dysplasia is a condition in which fibrous tissue replaces and expands medullary bone. It usually, but not necessarily, is limited to a single site. Its appearance on radiographs can vary from that of a well-defined lucent lesion to bizarrely deformed bone. Fibrous dysplasia tends to affect long bones such as the femur but can occur anywhere. It is usually asymptomatic but may be painful when associated with bone expansion or pathologic fracture.

Enchondroma is a common, painless, cartilaginous neoplasm found in the intramedullary cavity of the small bones of the hands and feet, the femur, the tibia, or the humerus. Radiographically, most tumors appear as small lytic lesions with sharp borders, no periosteal reaction, and rings or arcs of central chondroid calcifications. Most enchondromas are benign and, if asymptomatic, do not require specific treatment. Some can be the site of pathologic fracture due to local bone weakness, and the rare enchondroma can degenerate into low-grade chondrosarcoma. Pain without fracture or extension beyond the cortex of the parent bone suggests the possibility of malignant degeneration. Treatment, when indicated for pathologic fracture or biopsy, is curettage and bone graft.

Giant cell tumor (GCT) is a bone neoplasm with a peak incidence in the 20s and 30s that involves the metaphysis and epiphysis of a long bone, usually the distal femur or proximal tibia. Giant cell tumors are lucent, well-defined lesions and can have a similar appearance to metastases, aneurysmal bone cysts, and nonossifying fibromas.

Most GCTs are benign, but they may sometimes recur after curettage and bone grafting. Pulmonary metastases are seen in up to 2% of cases and are more likely to occur in patients with locally recurrent tumors (**Fig. 7.41**).

Fig. 7.41a–f
a,b Lucent bone lesions. Fibrous dysplasia. "Ground glass" slightly expansile lesion in proximal femur. Mildly heterogeneous enhancement on fat-saturated T1-weighted MRI.
c Enchondroma. Medullary lucent lesion with central chondroid calcification.
d–f Giant cell tumor. Distal femoral lesion with sharply defined, sclerotic borders. Increased uptake on technetium 99m radionuclide bone scan.

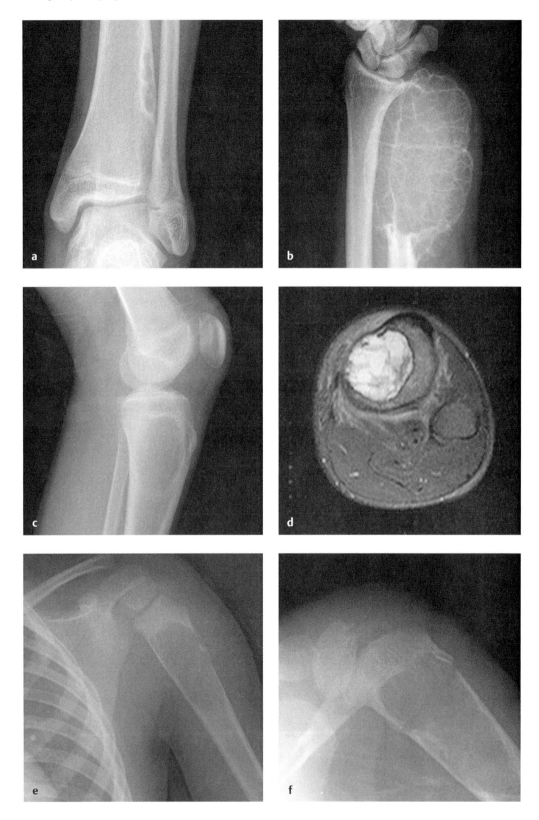

◆ Lucent Bone Lesions II

Nonossifying fibroma (NOF), also known as a fibrous cortical defect, is a benign, asymptomatic, cortical osseous lesion that occurs in the metaphysis of long bones in children and adolescents. NOFs are characterized by a thin sclerotic rim, may be multiple, and tend to resolve completely by adulthood. They are not associated with a soft tissue mass or periosteal reaction. Healed NOFs can appear as a cortical or subcortical area of hyperostosis. A large NOF, like any other lytic osseous lesion, can fracture.

Aneurysmal bone cyst (ABC) is a benign lesion containing blood-filled spaces traversed by connective tissue septa. It is found in children or adolescents who present with insidious bone pain that worsens over weeks to months. Aneurysmal bone cysts are eccentric, expansile, metaphyseal osteolytic lesions with sharply defined, sclerotic margins. They are usually located adjacent to the growth plate and can occur in any bone, but most commonly they involve the humerus, tibia, or pelvis. MRI shows blood-filled cysts with a rim of low T1 and T2 signal.

Although pathologically benign, ABCs may be locally aggressive, weakening the involved bone and compressing surrounding soft tissue. If an ABC involves the posterior elements of the spine, it can lead to spinal cord compression. Treatment options include intralesional curettage, en bloc excision, and selective arterial embolization. Bone grafting may be necessary, and recurrence is not uncommon.

A simple bone cyst (SBC), also known as a solitary or unicameral bone cyst, is a fluid-filled, benign lytic lesion of the proximal humeral and femoral diaphyses found in children and teenagers. In older patients, SBCs can be found in the calcaneus, talus, and ilium. Solitary bone cysts are sharply defined, lucent lesions, and their cyst contents have MRI and CT characteristics that correspond to simple fluid. Pathologic fractures complicate SBCs in about two-thirds of cases, and the cyst may contain a "fallen fragment," a finding that does not occur in lesions that can otherwise mimic SBC such as enchondroma, fibrous dysplasia, or bone abscess.

Small cysts can be observed. Cysts that have fractured may heal spontaneously. Larger cysts, particularly in active or athletic children, may be treated by curettage and bone grafting (**Fig. 7.42**).

Fig. 7.42a–f
a Nonossifying fibroma. Cortically based lucent lesion involving the distal tibia with bubbly appearance and sclerotic margins.
b Aneurysmal bone cyst. Expansile, osteolytic mass with lacelike expanded cortex and innumerable internal septations. The distal ulnar articular surface is distorted but intact.
c,d Sharply defined, metaphyseal lucent lesion that extends to but does not traverse the physeal plate. Fat-saturated, T1-weighted postgadolinium MRI shows fluid-fluid level characteristic of intracyst hemorrhage.
e,f Simple bone cyst. Sharply defined proximal humeral cyst with traversing pathologic fracture and small dependent bone fragment within the cyst.

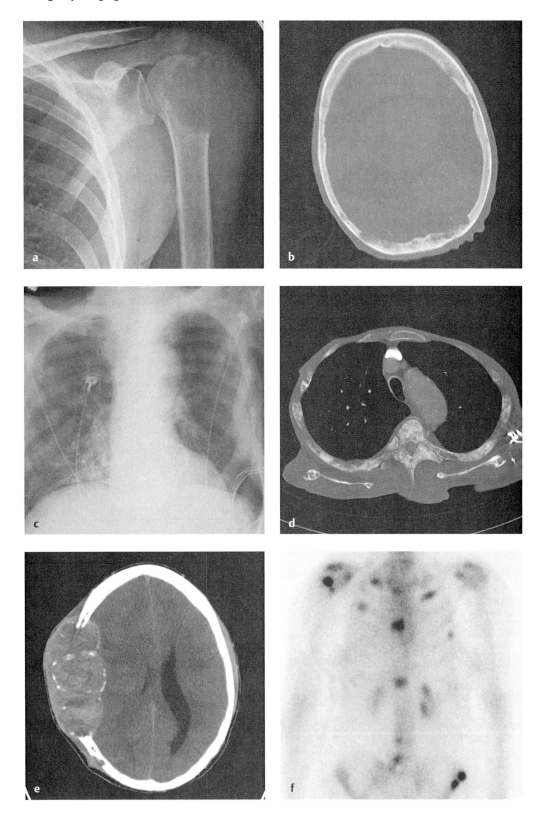

◆ Skeletal Metastasis

Skeletal metastases are most frequently seen in lung, breast, renal cell, and prostate carcinoma. While diagnosis is often straightforward in the setting of a known malignancy, metastases can mimic benign diseases or primary bone tumors. Although most osseous metastases are asymptomatic, metastatic disease may cause local bone pain, pathologic fracture, soft tissue deformities, or palpable masses.

Metastases preferentially involve the vertebrae, pelvis, proximal femur, proximal humerus, and skull. A combination of bone resorption and formation can produce lytic, sclerotic, or mixed lesions. Skeletal metastases can be diffuse, permeative, focal, or expansile.

Plain radiographs may not show a lytic lesion until significant bone mineral loss (30–50%) has taken place. CT is typically not employed for the evaluation of metastases except in areas such as the spine, where the multiplanar imaging capacity of CT better defines the extent of bony involvement and risk of pathologic fracture.

Treatment focuses on addressing the underlying malignancy and managing local pain. If metastatic tumor has compromised the structural integrity of a bone, surgical pinning or targeted radiotherapy may be required to prevent pathologic fracture (**Fig. 7.43**).

Fig. 7.43a–f
a   Lung carcinoma. Lytic metastasis involving the left humeral head.
b   Prostate carcinoma. Lytic calvarial metastases.
c,d   Prostate carcinoma. Sclerotic/blastic rib and vertebral metastases.
e   Renal cell carcinoma. Expansile calvarial metastases.
f   Breast carcinoma. Radionuclide bone scan showing vertebral, rib, pelvic, and humeral osseous metastases.

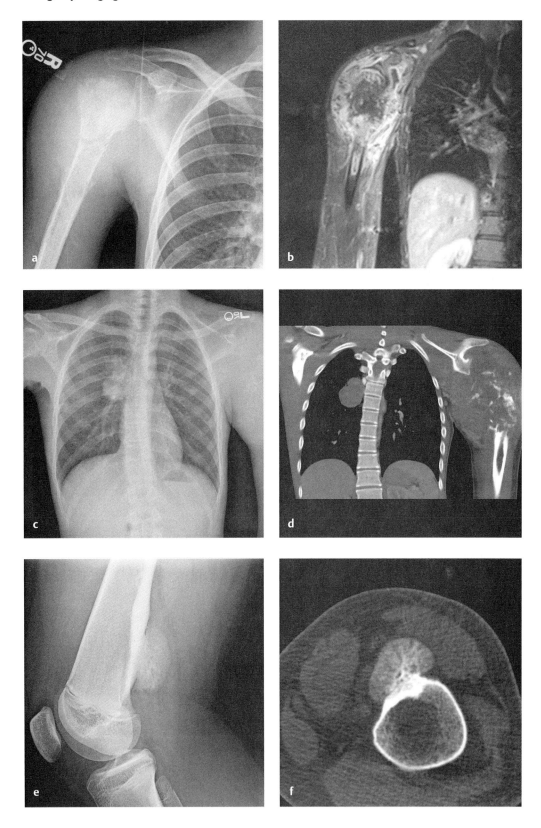

◆ Osteosarcoma and Parosteal Osteosarcoma

Osteosarcoma is the most common primary bone malignancy of adolescents and young adults, usually diagnosed before age 20. It involves the diametaphyseal junction of tubular bones, most commonly the distal femur, proximal tibia, and humerus. In older patients, secondary osteosarcoma may arise in an area of preexisting Paget disease of bone or within the radiation field of a previously treated malignancy. Osteosarcoma presents with dull, aching pain, more pronounced at night, and is sometimes accompanied by a soft tissue mass. Less commonly, minor trauma may result in a pathologic fracture through involved bone, or it may simply bring attention to a previously unnoticed soft tissue mass.

Osteosarcomas may be osteolytic, osteoblastic, or a combination of the two. Radiographs frequently show a mixed sclerotic and lytic lesion centered at the metaphysis, with a broad zone of transition and a moth-eaten appearance that indicates both cortical and medullary bone destruction. Intra- and peritumoral calcification is common and has several characteristic appearances: the "Codman triangle," marking elevation and calcification of the periosteum adjacent to an osteosarcoma, and the "sunburst" appearance of fine linear radial calcification within a tumor that has traversed the periosteum. CT and MRI are used to define the tumor margins for operative planning.

Osteosarcoma treatment consists of excision, ideally with limb-sparing surgery. Adjuvant chemotherapy is generally required to manage micrometastatic disease, which is often present at presentation.

Parosteal osteosarcoma is a low-grade osseous malignancy with ~ 95% survival after resection. Most are located along the dorsal aspect of the distal femur, with the remainder arising from the tibial or humeral metaphyses. They are usually diagnosed in adolescence and early adulthood, and patients often present with subacute limb pain. Arising from the outermost portion of the periosteum, parosteal osteosarcomas often have a large exophytic "cauliflower-like" osseous mass with adjacent dense cortical hyperostosis. Treatment is by surgical excision, usually without adjuvant chemotherapy or radiation therapy (**Fig. 7.44**).

Fig. 7.44a–f
a,b Pathologic fracture in osteosarcoma. Sclerotic and permeative bone changes involve the proximal humerus and are associated with a large soft tissue mass and surgical neck fracture. Calcified, elevated periosteum is visible at the distal aspect of the mass (Codman triangle). T1-weighted postgadolinium MRI shows the extent of soft tissue and marrow involvement.
c,d Osteosarcoma with pulmonary metastatic disease. The left proximal humerus is completely replaced by soft tissue and heterogeneous irregular areas of ossification. A 4-cm lobulated right upper lobe mass reflects a pulmonary metastasis.
e,f Parosteal osteosarcoma. Well-defined, oval, ossific mass that arises from the dorsal aspect of the distal femur. Dense hyperostosis of the adjacent dorsal femoral cortex.

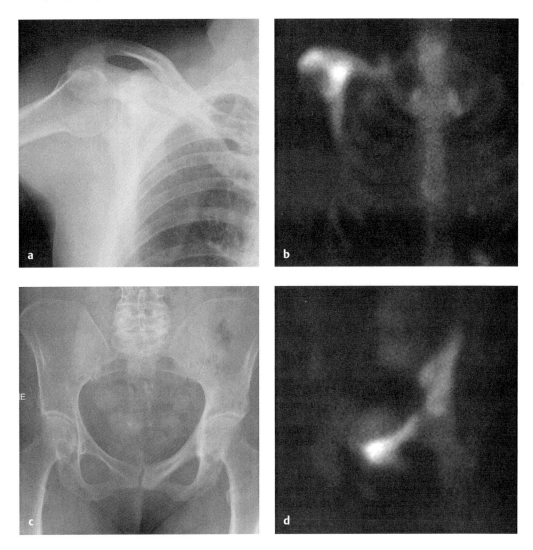

◆ Paget Disease of Bone

Paget disease of bone (osteitis deformans) is a chronic disorder characterized by exaggerated remodeling and hypertrophy. It is a relatively common disease of the elderly, with a slight male predilection. In this disease, osteoclastic overactivity results in structurally disorganized bone that is mechanically weaker than normal adult bone. Most patients are asymptomatic at diagnosis, but pain, tenderness, or excessive warmth due to hypervascularity may prompt medical attention. The pelvis, the skull, and the proximal portion of long bones are most frequently involved.

Paget disease of bone begins as an osteolytic or lucent bone lesion that evolves into an area of local bony enlargement with thickened trabeculae. Sclerosis is a late finding. Radionuclide bone scan shows intense technetium 99m uptake.

In long bones, osteolysis begins as epiphyseal demineralization that advances over time toward the middle of the bone, forming a wedge-shaped radiolucency. The border between normal and pagetic bone has been descried as the "blade of grass" or "flame" sign. In the skull, Paget disease begins as a well-defined lucency in the frontal and occipital bones, known as osteoporosis circumscripta. When Paget disease involves the vertebrae, it can appear as sclerotic thickening of the cortices, creating a "picture frame" on plain radiographs; this appearance should be distinguished from renal osteodystrophy, which involves only the superior and inferior vertebral endplates ("rugger jersey spine"). In the pelvis, Paget disease shows cortical thickening and sclerosis of the iliopectineal and ischiopubic lines or frank enlargement of a pubic ramus or ischium; it is typically asymmetric and more commonly seen on the right side.

The prognosis is generally good with early treatment. Medications such as calcitonin and alendronate are used to slow bone turnover. Morbidity from untreated Paget disease may be severe and is characterized by pain, pathologic fractures, and bone deformities (**Fig. 7.45**).

Fig. 7.45a–d
a,b Paget disease of the scapula. The right scapula is sclerotic with cortical thickening and marked enlargement of the acromion.
c,d Paget disease of the pelvis. The left superior pubic ramus and acetabulum are dense with cortical thickening and bone expansion, most conspicuous over the pubic ramus. In both cases, radionuclide bone scan shows increased focal uptake of technetium 99m.

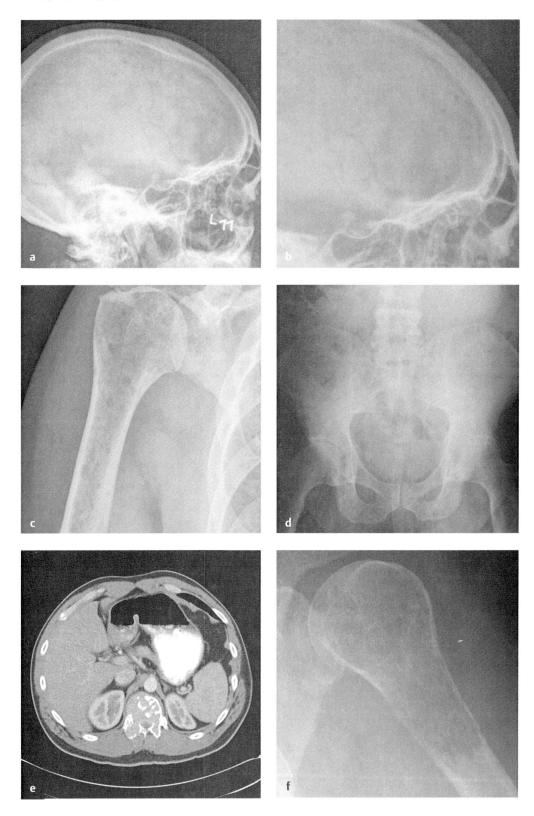

◆ Multiple Myeloma and Plasmacytoma

Multiple myeloma is a hematologic malignancy characterized by proliferation of marrow plasma cells and serum elevation of monoclonal paraprotein (M protein). It is a disease of older adults, with most patients in their 60s or 70s at the time of diagnosis. Bone pain, anemia, renal insufficiency, and hypercalcemia are common findings at presentation. The diagnosis is confirmed by laboratory detection of serum monoclonal immunoglobulin A (IgA) or immunoglobulin G (IgG). On plain radiographs, multiple myeloma is characterized by both generalized osteoporosis and innumerable small lucent, well-defined endosteal and cortical skeletal lesions.

A plasmacytoma, which can occur either in isolation or in association with systemic myeloma, is a homogenous, localized soft tissue mass, comprised of plasma cells. Plasmacytomas arise from bone marrow, often with osseous expansion, destruction, and soft tissue extension beyond the parent bone. Vertebral plasmacytomas can result in spinal cord compression.

Systemic remission is possible with chemotherapy, immunotherapy, and stem cell transplantation, with radiation and surgical care reserved for focal manifestations of the disease such as spinal cord compression or pathologic fracture (**Fig. 7.46**).

Fig. 7.46a–f
a–d Multiple myeloma involving the skull, humerus, spine, and pelvis. Innumerable, well-defined "punched-out" cortical osseous lesions.
e Vertebral plasmacytoma. The T12 vertebra is infiltrated and expanded by homogeneous soft tissue that extends into the spinal canal. Trabecular thickening reflects a combination of bone destruction and remodeling.
f Proximal humeral plasmacytoma involving the humeral head and proximal diaphysis. This is radiographically indistinguishable from metastatic disease.

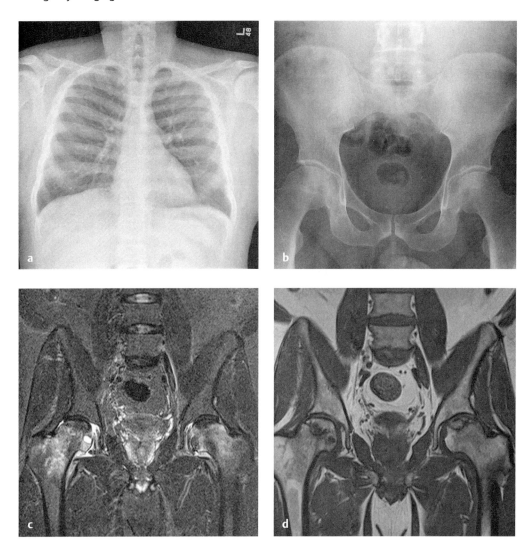

◆ Avascular Necrosis

Avascular necrosis (AVN), or osteonecrosis, consists of death of the cellular components of bone. Any process that interrupts blood flow to a portion of bone can result in AVN, including trauma, hemoglobinopathies, gout, corticosteroid therapy, alcoholism, pregnancy, collagen vascular disorders, lymphoproliferative disorders, and osteomyelitis. Because its vascular supply is often tenuous, the epiphysis is the most frequently involved part of an affected bone. Microinfarctions lead to edema, necrosis, and subchondral microfractures, which are further complicated by insufficient healing, abnormal joint remodeling, and dysfunction.

When symptomatic, patients will have localized bone pain. The femoral head is an especially vulnerable site, and AVN usually occurs at its anterolateral aspect, immediately below the weight-bearing articular surface. In nontraumatic hip AVN, subacute intermittent groin pain with restricted joint mobility is typical.

Hip radiographs may show subchondral lucency, or the "crescent sign." This finding, best seen on frog-leg lateral view, indicates imminent collapse of the articular surface. Other findings include subchondral sclerosis, cyst formation, flattening of the femoral head or other articular surface, and narrowing of the joint space.

MRI is more sensitive than radiographs for detection of early AVN. The most common appearance is that of a focal subchondral lesion in the anterosuperior femoral head with a fatty center and a low-T1-signal linear rim. Osteochondral fragmentation and secondary degenerative changes may also be seen.

Treatment involves reducing the physical load on the affected bone and promotion of revascularization. Depending on location, therapy may include anticoagulation, bisphosphonates, core compression, or total joint replacement (**Fig. 7.47**).

Fig. 7.47a–d
a Right humeral head AVN with subchondral sclerosis in a patient with sickle-cell disease.
b–d Bilateral femoral head avascular necrosis. Subchondral sclerosis involving both femoral heads with MRI showing corresponding marrow edema on fat-suppressed T2-weighted images and juxta-articular serpiginous low-signal changes on T1-weighted images, indicating condensed bone.

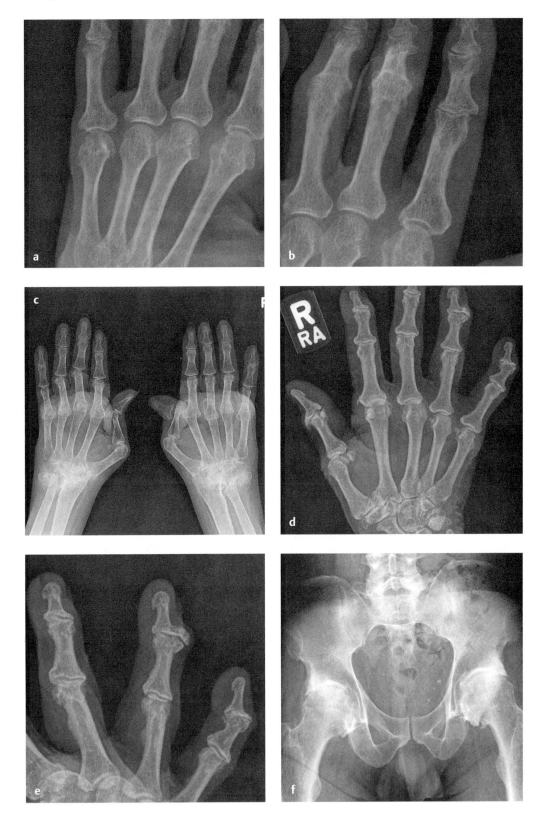

◆ Rheumatoid Arthritis and Osteoarthritis

Rheumatoid arthritis (RA) is a chronic systemic autoimmune disease two to three times more common in women than in men and with a peak incidence in the fourth and fifth decades. RA primarily involves the small joints of the hands, wrists, and feet. Its onset is insidious, beginning with malaise, arthralgias, weakness, and morning stiffness before progressing to frank joint inflammation and swelling. Fever and other constitutional symptoms may be present.

Soft tissue swelling, osteoporosis, uniform joint space narrowing, and marginal erosions are the imaging hallmarks of RA. In the hands and wrists, the disease is bilaterally symmetric with a predilection for the proximal interphalangeal (PIP) and metacarpophalangeal (MCP) joints. The distal interphalangeal (DIP) joints are characteristically spared. In advanced disease, joint space loss and subchondral cystic changes can resemble osteoarthritis. Joint laxity and subluxations are common and can lead to boutonnière and swan neck deformities of the fingers. The upper cervical spine can be affected with inflammatory pannus formation at the C1–C2 articulation with potential odontoid erosion and atlantoaxial subluxation.

Treatment is focused on slowing disease progression via a combination of cortico-steroids, NSAIDs, disease-modifying anti-rheumatoid drugs (DMARDs), and tumor necrosis factor (TNF) antagonists.

Osteoarthritis, or degenerative joint disease, is the most common arthropathy and results from either overt trauma or repetitive microtrauma. A hereditary form (primary osteoarthritis) may be seen in middle-aged women.

Signs and symptoms of osteoarthritis include joint pain, reduced range of motion, crepitus, and stiffness after periods of immobility. In contrast to RA, the DIP joints are characteristically involved, with relative sparing of the MCP joints. The PIP joint and the first CMC joint (also known as the basal joint) are also common locations. Heberden nodes, which represent palpable osteophytes at the DIP joint, are another characteristic finding of osteoarthritis and are more frequently seen in women than in men.

Diagnosis is based on clinical and radiographic findings, which include joint space narrowing, subchondral sclerosis, subchondral cyst formation, osteophytes, deformity, and malalignment. Joint space narrowing is the least specific of these findings, as it is seen in almost every other arthropathy.

Osteoarthritis is managed medically with acetaminophen, NSAIDs, and intra-articular corticosteroid injections (**Fig. 7.48**).

Fig. 7.48a–f
a–c (**a,b**) Rheumatoid arthritis. MCP and PIP joint space narrowing with marginal erosions of the distal fifth metacarpal and second proximal phalanx. Relative sparing of the DIP joints. (**c**) Advanced RA with severe and symmetric intercarpal, radioulnar, and radiocarpal joint destruction, subluxation of the proximal phalanges, and boutonnière deformities of all digits.
d–f Osteoarthritis. (**d**) Preferential DIP, PIP, and first CMC joint space narrowing and productive bone changes. (**e**) A large osteophyte at the ulnar aspect of the fourth DIP corresponds to a Heberden node. (**f**) Hip osteoarthritis with marked joint space narrowing, subchondral sclerosis, and subchondral cysts.

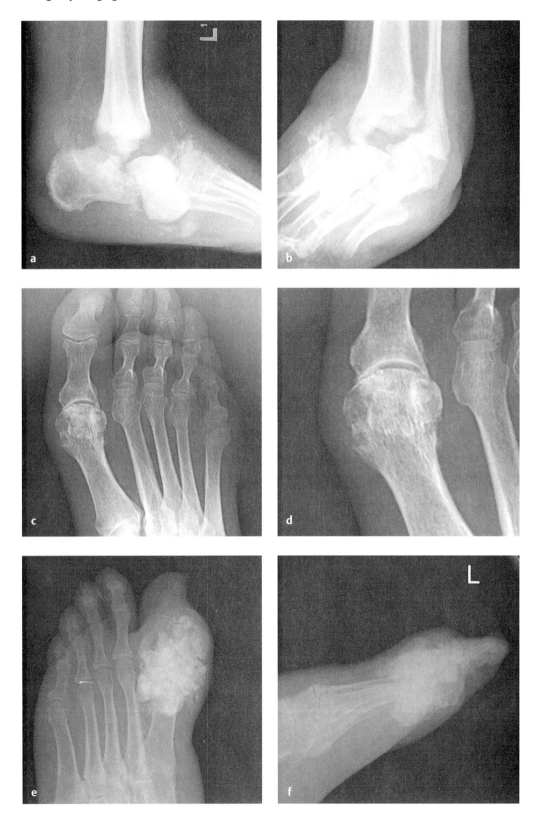

◆ Neuropathic Arthropathy and Gout

Neuropathic arthropathy is the progressive, destructive, and degenerative bone and joint disease of patients with diminished pain sensation and proprioception. It is the consequence of repeated microtrauma, hyperemia, and osteoclast activation. Most patients are diabetic; other causes include syphilis, leprosy, syringomyelia, and alcoholism. The involved joint may suggest the etiology; patients with neurosyphilis tend to have knee involvement, whereas neuropathic shoulder arthropathy is exclusively seen in cervical syringomyelia. Inflammatory arthritis with bilateral distributions can have a similar appearance but should be distinguishable based on history.

In neuropathic arthropathy, joint pain and deformity develop insidiously. The foot and ankle are most commonly affected in diabetic patients. In contrast to septic arthritis, the involved joint is swollen but painless, and patients do not have fever or elevated serum markers for inflammation. Neuropathic arthropathy can be classified into hypertrophic arthropathy, which is seen in younger patients, and atrophic arthropathy, which affects the elderly. Hypertrophic changes are common in upper motor neuron lesions, while atrophic changes are more characteristic of peripheral neuropathy.

Radiographic features include subchondral sclerosis, articular cartilage destruction, deformity, joint debris, and dislocation. These findings can be seen in severe degenerative joint disease from many causes, but in the patient with diminished sensation, they point to neuropathic arthropathy. In advanced disease, the affected joint is disorganized with gross deformity, debris, and osteophytosis. Treatment varies, depending on location and extent of joint involvement, but is usually either protected immobilization or arthrodesis. Joint replacement is generally contraindicated, because underlying bone quality is poor.

Gout, caused by monosodium urate monohydrate crystal deposition in and around a joint, results from underexcretion or overproduction of uric acid and is associated with high-fat and high-protein diets, alcohol overuse, and various metabolic, myeloproliferative, and renal diseases. Gout is primarily an asymmetric and polyarticular arthritis of the hands and feet. The first joint affected is usually the great toe metatarsophalangeal (MTP) articulation. Acute attacks are characterized by severe pain, swelling, warmth, erythema, and tenderness.

Radiographs may be normal or show eccentric periarticular erosions with sclerotic margins, preservation of the joint space, and normal periarticular mineralization. In long-standing disease, tophi (crystal-containing nodules) can develop in the fingers, toes, prepatellar bursa, olecranon, or helix of the ear. These can show bulky calcification.

Management is focused on ameliorating acute symptoms with anti-inflammatory medication and prophylactic pharmacotherapy to prevent future attacks depending on the etiology (**Fig. 7.49**).

Fig. 7.49a–f
a,b Neuropathic arthropathy in diabetes. The talus is inferolaterally dislocated with respect to the calcaneus. The distal tibial articular surface and the superior aspect of the calcaneus are grossly eroded. Extensive osseous debris, soft tissue swelling.
c,d Gout. Sharply defined, "punched-out" erosions of the medial first metatarsal head and lateral base of the first proximal phalanx. The adjacent joint space and mineralization are preserved.
e,f Tophaceous gout. Large conglomerate of soft tissue calcification surrounding the first metatarsal and proximal phalanx.

8
Pediatrics

◆ Approach and Analysis

A number of emergent conditions are unique to the pediatric and neonatal age groups, and these are addressed in this chapter. Conditions also seen in adults, such as intussusception and appendicitis, can be found in the corresponding chapters organized by anatomy.

Studies that do not utilize ionizing radiation are preferred in the pediatric age group. Because the lifetime risk of developing a radiation-induced cancer is greater with early exposure, it is prudent to avoid unnecessary X-ray and CT examinations in children and to minimize radiation dose in any necessary study that utilizes ionizing radiation. Fortunately, most practices and equipment manufacturers have protocols and techniques that reduce radiation dose to the minimum needed for accurate diagnosis. Ultrasound and MRI are preferred for cross-sectional imaging, especially in the diagnosis of pediatric abdominal pain and in the often-repeated evaluation of hydrocephalus in children with ventriculoperitoneal shunts.

In children with suspected appendicitis, ovarian torsion, testicular torsion, intussusception, or pyloric stenosis, ultrasound should be attempted prior to CT. Radiographs are the primary imaging modality for acute thoracic disease, ingested foreign bodies, and musculoskeletal injuries, and they can be helpful in evaluating abdominal pain by establishing the diagnosis of severe constipation as well as bowel obstruction. In the emergency setting, CT is generally reserved for significant traumatic injury and for acute abdominal pain that cannot be diagnosed by clinical and laboratory findings, plain radiography, and ultrasound.

◆ Imaging and Anatomy

Skeletal Survey for Nonaccidental Trauma

- Indications: Suspected child abuse.
  - AP/lateral skull
  - AP/lateral cervical and lumbar spine
  - AP/lateral thorax and abdomen
  - AP humeri, forearm, hand, femora, tibiae and fibulae, and feet

CT—Abdomen

- Indications: Appendicitis, acute abdomen.
- Technique: ~ 175 mA, 120 kV
- Oral contrast: Dilute Gastrografin (up to 1 liter depending on age and size)
- IV contrast: 1.5 mL/kg at 3 mL/sec, 90-second delay (symphysis to pubis)
- Images: 5-mm axial, 0.6-mm reconstruction, 3-mm coronal and sagittal reformation
- Approximate radiation dose: 400 mGy

Ultrasound—Generalized Abdominal Pain

Indications: Pain, mass, hernia.

Probe: Linear probe (9 MHz for infants, curved 6 MHz for older children)

Views:

- Liver—longitudinal and transverse
- Porta hepatis—main portal vein and common bile duct
- Pancreas/aorta/superior mesenteric artery—midline transverse
- Hepatorenal space (demonstrate lack of free fluid)
- Kidneys—longitudinal and transverse (measure length)
- Spleen—longitudinal and transverse (measure maximal length)
- Bladder—midline longitudinal and transverse (demonstrate lack of extravesical free fluid)
- Lymph nodes—mesenteric, right lower quadrant, and periaortic

Ultrasound—Suspected Appendicitis

Indications: Right lower quadrant pain.

Probe: Linear probe (12 MHz or 9 MHz depending on body habitus)

Views:

- Right psoas muscle—transverse including iliac artery and vein (± color Doppler
- Cecum and terminal ileum—longitudinal and transverse
- Region of appendix—transverse of region of appendix (± color Doppler)
- Bladder—midline longitudinal and transverse (show lack of extravesical free fluid)
- Right kidney—longitudinal and transverse

- Abnormal appendix:
  - Measure greatest diameter, color Doppler to show hyperemia
  - Hepatorenal space (demonstrate lack of free fluid)
- No appendicitis/appendix not seen:
  - Right kidney (exclude stone or hydronephrosis)
  - Gallbladder

- Ovaries (in girls) document volume and color flow
- Adnexal region if ovaries are not seen

Ultrasound—Suspected Intussusception

Indications: Abdominal pain.

Probe: 12 MHz linear probe (9 MHz may be used for evaluating the right kidney and hepatic flexure)

Views:

- Transverse images of colon—cecum, ascending, hepatic flexure, transverse, splenic flexure, and descending
- Mesenteric, right lower quadrant, and periaortic lymph nodes should be measured if identified
- Right kidney—longitudinal and transverse
- Hepatorenal space (demonstrate lack of free fluid)
- If an intussusception is identified, evaluate flow with color Doppler
- Identify any free or loculated peritoneal fluid

Ultrasound—Suspected Hypertrophic Pyloric Stenosis (HPS)

Indications: Projectile vomiting in young infant.

Probe: 12 MHz linear probe. Patient should be scanned supine and in right posterior oblique positions. It may be necessary to fill the stomach with a small amount of water if gastric air prevents visualization of the antrum

Views:

- Midline transverse images of pancreas/aorta/superior mesenteric artery
- Pylorus—image maximal canal length (normal is less than 17 mm), image maximal wall thickness from outer wall to mucosa (normal is less than 3 mm). Pyloric thickening should be fixed in HPS. If mobile, consider pylorospasm.

Ultrasound—Testicular or Appendix Testis Torsion

Indications: Scrotal pain.
Probe: Linear probe (12 MHz or higher)
Views:

- – Three transverse views of both testes on one image (upper, lower, mid)
- – Three longitudinal views of each testicle
- – Color and arterial flow Doppler both testes (longitudinal and transverse)
- – Epididymis (longitudinal and transverse ± color Doppler)
- – Document hydrocele if present
- – Measure testicular dimensions

Salter-Harris Classification of Pediatric Fractures

Salter-Harris classification of pediatric fractures is seen in **Fig. 8.1**.

◆ Clinical Presentations and Differential Diagnosis

Clinical Presentations and Appropriate Initial Studies

Cough and Dyspnea

- • Chest X-ray
  - – Bronchiolitis/reactive airway disease (young children)
  - – Pneumonia
  - – Congenital cardiac disease
  - – Tracheoesophageal fistula (newborns)

Vomiting in the Newborn

- • Abdominal plain radiograph
- • Ultrasound
  - – Duodenal or other small-bowel atresia
  - – Midgut volvulus/malrotation
  - – Pyloric stenosis

Abdominal Pain

- • Ultrasound
- • CT or MRI may be necessary if ultrasound not diagnostic
  - – Appendicitis
  - – Testicular or ovarian torsion
  - – Intussusception
  - – Colitis

Hip Pain

- • Pelvis plain radiograph
- • Ultrasound
- • MRI for evaluation of osteomyelitis and bone tumors
  - – Septic arthritis
  - – Toxic synovitis
  - – Osteomyelitis
  - – Eosinophilic granuloma
  - – Slipped capital femoral epiphysis
  - – Avascular necrosis
  - – Legg-Calvé-Perthes disease
  - – Juvenile rheumatoid arthritis
  - – Ewing sarcoma
  - – Osteoid osteoma

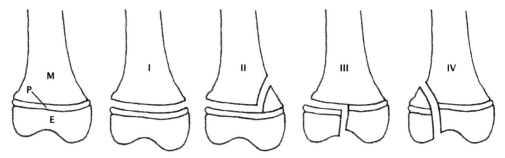

Fig. 8.1 The Salter-Harris classification of pediatric fractures describes five basic fractures that involve the physeal growth plate. Salter-Harris I fractures may be subtle and involve separation of the metaphysis (M) and epiphysis (E) through the physis (P). Salter-Harris II–IV fractures are growth plate fractures that extend to the metaphysis (II), the epiphysis (III), or both (IV). Type V fractures are impaction fractures at the growth plate.

Differential Diagnosis

Supratentorial Brain Tumors

- Astrocytoma
- Primitive neuroectodermal tumor (PNET)
- Choroid plexus papilloma (lateral ventricle)
- Pineal tumors

Infratentorial Brain Tumors

- Juvenile pilocytic astrocytoma
- Brainstem glioma (fibrillary astrocytoma)
- Medulloblastoma (fourth ventricle)
- Ependymoma (fourth ventricle)

Suprasellar/Parasellar Mass

- Craniopharyngioma
- Optic glioma
- Germinoma

Supraglottic Narrowing

- Croup
- Epiglottitis
- Retropharyngeal abscess

Pulmonary Mass

- Metastatic tumor (osteosarcoma, Wilms, neuroblastoma)
- "Round" pneumonia

Focal Pulmonary Opacity in Newborn

- Pulmonary sequestration
- Bronchogenic cyst
- Congenital cystic adenomatoid malformation

Lucent or Cystic Pulmonary Lesion in Newborn

- Congenital lobar emphysema
- Cystic adenomatoid malformation
- Diaphragmatic hernia

Mediastinal Mass

- Normal thymus (< 2 yrs)
- Lymphoma
- Germ cell tumor
- Bronchogenic or enteric cyst
- Adenopathy
- Neuroblastoma (posterior mediastinum)

Abdominal Mass

- Neuroblastoma
- Hepatoblastoma
- Wilms tumor
- Appendiceal abscess
- Rhabdomyosarcoma

Intestinal Obstruction in Newborn

- Duodenal atresia/stenosis/web
- Annular pancreas
- Jejunal atresia
- Meconium plug syndrome/meconium ileus
- Ileal or anal atresia
- Hirschsprung disease

Intestinal Obstruction in a Child

- Intussusception
- Incarcerated inguinal hernia
- Adhesions
- Appendicitis
- Malrotation/volvulus
- Meckel diverticulum

Right Lower Quadrant Mass in a Child

- Appendicitis
- Intussusception
- Duplication cyst

Aggressive Bone Lesion in a Child/Adolescent

- Osteosarcoma
- Ewing sarcoma
- Osteomyelitis
- Eosinophilic granuloma
- Neuroblastoma metastasis
- Leukemia/lymphoma

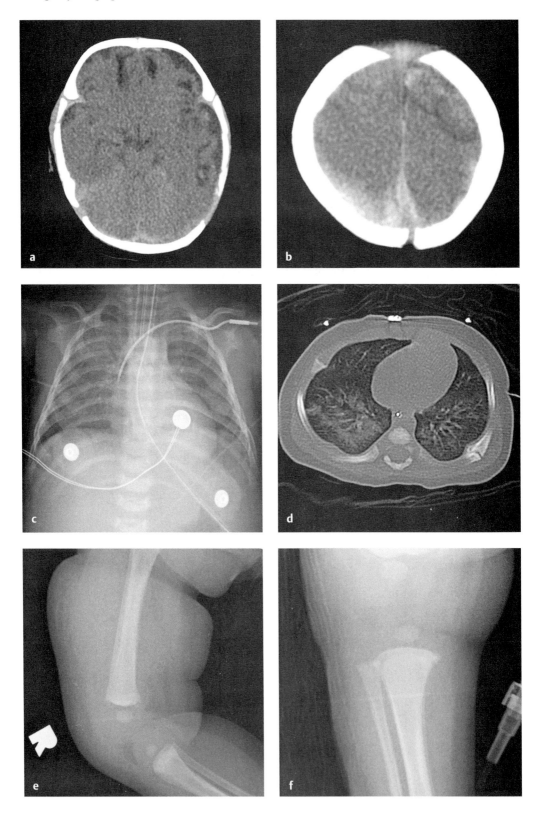

◆ Nonaccidental Trauma

Children who suffer nonaccidental trauma (NAT) are often brought to the emergency department with minor rather than catastrophic injuries. Emergency physicians and radiologists are therefore in a unique position to first identify NAT, and recognition of characteristic injury patterns can potentially avert future abuse or neglect. Common injuries include fractures, intracranial hemorrhage or contusion, and intra-abdominal injuries. Head injury is important to recognize, because it represents a frequent cause of death in abused children below the age of 3.

Suspicious injuries include any fracture in a preambulatory child, any injury incompatible with the clinical history, unusual delay in seeking medical attention, retinal hemorrhage, multiple fractures in the absence of any family history of osteogenesis imperfecta, and subdural hematomas of different ages. A skeletal survey should be performed in cases of suspected abuse to evaluate the location and extent of present and remote osseous injuries.

Certain fractures have been recognized as indicative of NAT: metaphyseal (bucket-handle or corner) fractures, posterior rib fractures, skull fractures, scapular fractures, and sternal fractures. Periosteal reactions and juxtaosseous soft tissue calcifications signify healing fractures and should be carefully documented for medicolegal purposes.

Head CT may identify skull fractures missed by skeletal survey as well as more significant brain injury. Nonparietal skull fractures, diastatic sutures, cross sutures, or depressed fractures should be considered suspicious. MRI can evaluate the brain parenchyma more sensitively and show subdural hematomas of varying ages, hypoxic-ischemic injury, cerebral contusions, and traumatic subarachnoid hemorrhages (**Fig. 8.2**).

Fig. 8.2a–f
a,b Head injury in NAT. Bilateral inferior frontal and anterior temporal cortical encephalomalacia consistent with remote injury; acute right parietal and left frontal vertex subdural hematomas.
c,d Bilateral posterior rib fractures. Healing fractures related to squeezing of the infant's thorax during a past episode of forceful shaking. Right lung consolidation versus contusion is likely a more acute injury.
e,f Metaphyseal corner fractures. Fractures of the distal femoral and proximal tibial metaphyses result from a whiplash movement of the arms when shaken.

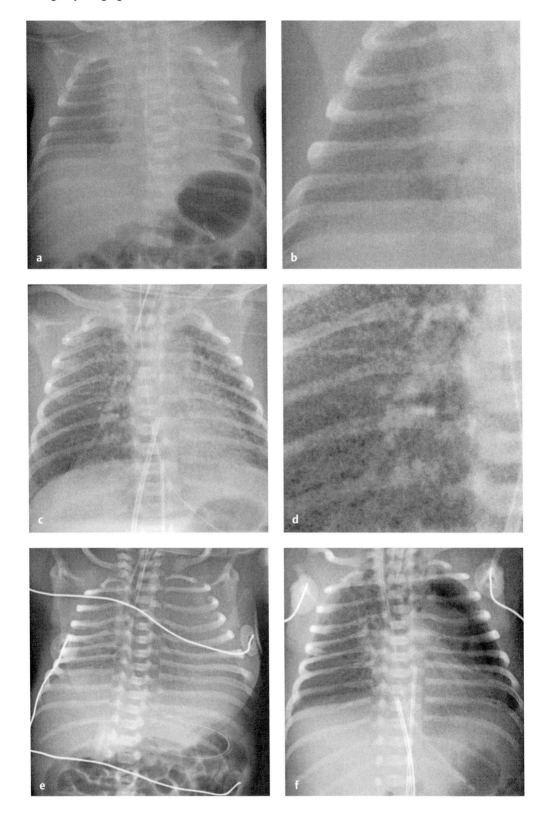

◆ Lung Disease of Prematurity

Lung disease of prematurity, also known as respiratory distress syndrome (RDS), is an acute lung disease seen in children born before the lungs produce adequate surfactant to maintain alveolar expansion. It is seen in neonates younger than 32 weeks gestational age or who weigh less than 1,200 grams. Symptoms, which are usually evident within hours of delivery, include tachypnea, expiratory grunting, nasal flaring, and substernal and intercostal retractions. In addition to prematurity, other risk factors include maternal gestational diabetes, prenatal asphyxia, and multiple gestations.

Radiographs show a bell-shaped thoracic contour. The lung parenchyma has a fine granular, or "ground glass," appearance, often with air bronchograms.

Complications of RDS are related to ventilation and barotrauma and include pulmonary interstitial emphysema, pneumothorax, and bronchopulmonary dysplasia.

Treatment consists of administration of artificial pulmonary surfactant and supportive ventilation and oxygen therapy. With the increased use of antenatal steroids to accelerate pulmonary maturity, the incidence and severity of hyaline membrane disease has been declining (**Fig. 8.3**).

Fig. 8.3a–f
a,b Lung disease of prematurity. Diffuse ground glass opacity involving all lung zones. Nasogastric tube.
c,d Pulmonary interstitial emphysema. Interval placement of endotracheal tube, umbilical arterial and umbilical venous catheters. The lungs now contain multiple linear lucencies corresponding to air that has dissected from the alveoli into the pulmonary interstitium.
e,f Pneumothorax complicating RDS. (**e**) Initial study showing bell-shaped thorax with diffuse ground glass opacity and endotracheal and nasogastric tubes. (**f**) Subsequent radiograph with left-sided pneumothorax and interval placement of umbilical arterial and venous catheters.

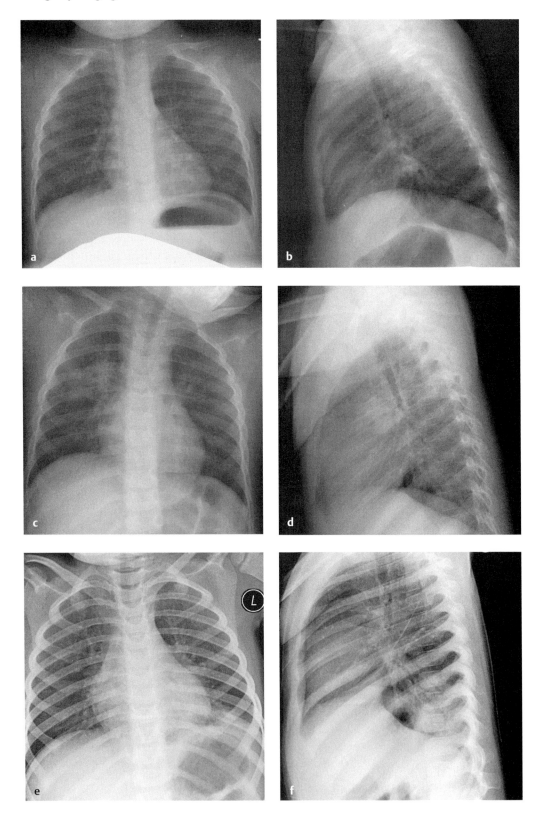

◆ Bronchiolitis and Acute Pediatric Pneumonia

Bronchiolitis, or bronchiolar inflammation, is the most common lower respiratory tract infection among children less than 2 years of age. It typically occurs in the late fall to early spring, and affected children have symptoms of congestion, cough, and rhinitis. Tachypnea, chest wall retractions, wheezing, and crackles may also be present.

Younger infants, ex-premature infants, and infants with congenital heart and lung disease are at higher risk of bronchiolitis and may show only nonspecific signs such as low-grade fever and decreased oral intake. Bronchiolitis is most commonly due to respiratory syncytial virus (RSV), but rhinovirus, influenza, parainfluenza, and adenovirus are other causes.

Although the American Academy of Pediatrics does not recommend routine imaging for children with a clinical picture of bronchiolitis, plain chest radiographs are sometimes obtained in the emergency department to exclude pneumonia. Radiographic findings, when present, may overlap with those of acute pneumonia and include peribronchial thickening, hyperinflation, atelectasis, and consolidation.

Management consists of supportive care with supplemental oxygen and antipyretics as needed. Some physicians advocate a trial of inhaled bronchodilator to assess for any clinical response. Antibiotics are not routinely indicated.

Acute focal pneumonia in children is usually caused by *Streptococcus pneumoniae* and appears on plain radiographs as a dense peripheral opacity, sometimes spherical and mass-like ("round" pneumonia). Any focal airspace opacity can be due to pneumonia and should be correlated with supporting clinical features: fever > 102°F, toxic appearance, and leukocytosis. In children, basilar pneumonias can mimic acute abdominal disease such as obstruction or appendicitis. Aspiration pneumonia can be seen in children with neurological conditions that reduce their ability to protect the airway. When aspiration occurs in the supine position, the upper lobes are often involved (**Fig. 8.4**).

Fig. 8.4a–f
a,b Bronchiolitis. Hyperinflation with mildly indistinct central vessels. No dense focal opacity.
c,d Right upper lobe pneumonia. Diffuse perihilar opacity visible on both PA and lateral radiographs.
e,f Left lower lobe pneumonia. Dense, mass-like, consolidation with air bronchograms that abuts the hemidiaphragm and is much more conspicuous on the lateral radiograph. Pediatric pneumonia in this location could present clinically as acute abdominal pain.

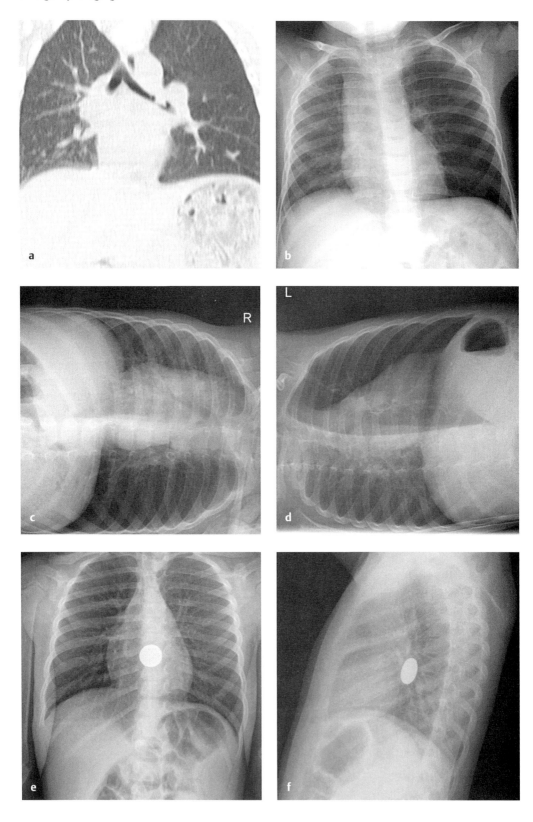

◆ Aspirated or Swallowed Foreign Body

Children, usually between age 1 and 3 years, may ingest or aspirate foreign bodies. Choking, gagging, coughing, unilateral wheezing, and respiratory distress are clinical signs. Large objects can lodge in the larynx or trachea and cause complete airway obstruction with subsequent asphyxia or anoxia. Smaller objects will pass beyond the carina and can result in less severe acute manifestations, but if aspirated material cannot be cleared from the tracheobronchial tree, chronic pulmonary infection or bronchiectasis may result.

Unless an aspirated foreign body is metallic, it is unlikely to be seen on a chest radiograph. Indirect signs of bronchial obstruction may be detected, however, and include air trapping, unilateral hyperinflation, lobar or segmental atelectasis, mediastinal shift, or pneumomediastinum. Most often an aspirated object passes into the right main bronchus, since it is more vertically oriented with respect to the carina and trachea. Unilateral hyperinflation that persists on decubitus positioning (with the hyperinflated side downward) is one sign. Postobstructive atelectasis and pneumonia may also be seen.

Primary management in the emergency department aims to relieve any airway obstruction or compromise. Bronchoscopy or endoscopy can permit retrieval of an impacted foreign body. Antibiotics are not indicated except in the case of delayed presentation and secondary pulmonary infection.

Many ingested foreign bodies that reach the stomach will eventually pass through the gastrointestinal tract without requiring endoscopic removal. Perforation or obstruction are risks, particularly with foreign bodies in the esophagus, with sharp objects, and in patients with developmental gastrointestinal anomalies or prior surgery. Emergent endoscopy is indicated for sharp objects or disk batteries lodged in the esophagus and in any patient who cannot manage secretions due to complete esophageal obstruction. Sharp-pointed objects, objects greater than 6 cm in length or greater than 2.5 cm in diameter, and magnets that are located in the stomach or duodenum should be removed promptly. In asymptomatic patients, coins in the esophagus can be observed for 48 hours. Disk or cylindrical batteries should be removed if they do not pass from the stomach for more than 48 hours (**Fig. 8.5**).

Fig. 8.5a–d
a,b Aspirated turkey burger. Rightward mediastinal shift that persists on left-side-down decubitus radiograph. CT shows foreign body in right mainstem bronchus.
c,d Swallowed coin. A round metallic object is located in the mid-esophagus.

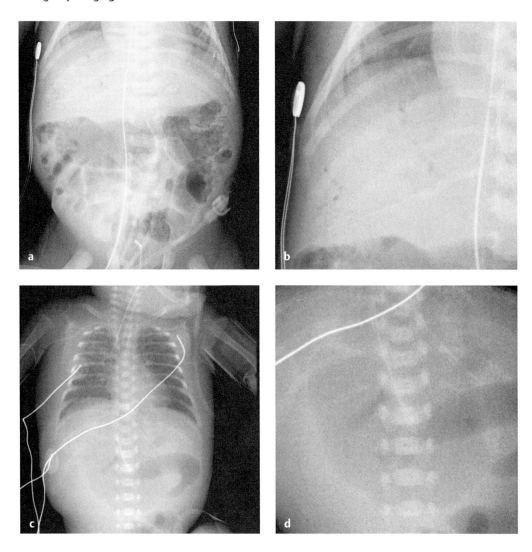

◆ Necrotizing Enterocolitis

Necrotizing enterocolitis (NEC)—mucosal or transmucosal ischemic necrosis of segments of the intestine—is commonly seen in premature and low-birth-weight infants. The condition reflects a combination of infection, ischemic injury, and incompletely developed immunity. NEC usually develops in the first 2–10 days of life, with an incidence inversely proportional to gestational age. Presentation is often nonspecific but includes feeding intolerance, vomiting, bile-stained vomitus, abdominal distention, and gross or occult blood in stool. Predisposing factors include prematurity, congenital heart disease, birth anoxia, and sepsis.

Abdominal radiographs may show ileus, bowel wall edema with thumbprinting, and loss of the normal polygonal gas shape within the dilated intestine. Pneumatosis intestinalis is considered pathognomonic, and portal venous gas and pneumoperitoneum indicate severe disease and perforation, respectively.

Medical management is pursued in most cases of NEC with bowel rest, placement of an orogastric tube, fluid resuscitation, and treatment with broad-spectrum antibiotics. Surgical intervention is reserved for patients with clinical and imaging evidence of perforation. Free intraperitoneal air is detected by identifying air on both sides of the bowel wall; nondependent free air is detected on decubitus radiograph or by identifying the falciform ligament outlined by air (**Fig. 8.6**).

Fig. 8.6a–d
a,b (**a**) Necrotizing enterocolitis. Intramural gas within the bowel causes portions of the left colon to appear granular or mottled. (**b**) Portal venous gas.
c,d Bowel perforation in newborn. Large oval lucency over upper abdomen with linear density overlying the spine that corresponds to the falciform ligament outlined by free intraperitoneal air.

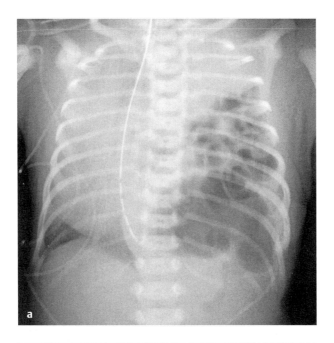

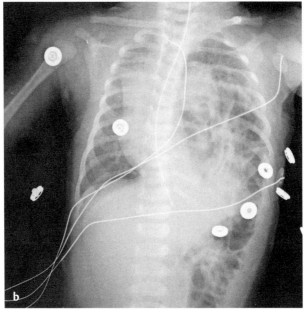

◆ Congenital Diaphragmatic Hernia

Congenital diaphragmatic hernia (CDH) is a consequence of incomplete diaphragmatic fusion, in which abdominal viscera herniate into the fetal thorax and prevents normal pulmonary development. Because of this, the clinical consequences of CDH are pulmonary hypoplasia and pulmonary hypertension. The affected hemithorax may contain a combination of stomach, intestine, liver, and spleen. CDH may occur in isolation or may be associated with chromosomal abnormalities in up to half of cases.

Bochdalek hernias are the most common variety of CDH and are almost exclusively seen on the left side. These result from posterolateral defects in the developing pleuroperitoneal folds. This hernia often presents in the neonatal period or the first year of life and is associated with a poorer outcome. Morgagni hernias are less common, present later, and are located more anteriorly and often on the right side. Small, fat-containing Bochdalek and Morgagni hernias are commonly incidentally detected in adults.

CDH is often diagnosed by prenatal ultrasound and is sometimes surgically repaired in utero. In some cases it may not be detected until after a child is born, and in that case CDH is a surgical emergency. If the defect is large enough, neonates may develop respiratory distress and cyanosis in the first hours of life. Clinical findings include decreased breath sounds and intrathoracic bowel sounds on the affected side.

Plain radiographs show intrathoracic bowel or viscera with contralateral mediastinal shift and compressive atelectasis or hypoplasia of the ipsilateral lung. A gasless abdomen may be seen if most bowel loops have herniated into the hemithorax. Ultrasound confirms the clinical radiographic diagnosis and can identify any herniated solid organs.

An antenatal diagnosis of CDH mandates delivery in a tertiary care hospital with access to neonatologists, pediatric surgeons, and extracorporeal membrane oxygenation (ECMO). Poorer prognosis is associated with larger diaphragmatic hernias, early gestational age at diagnosis, intrathoracic liver, and the presence of a small contralateral lung (**Fig. 8.7**).

Fig. 8.7a,b Congenital diaphragmatic hernia in two newborns. Air-filled bowel fills the inferior aspect of the left hemithoraces, with rightward mediastinal shift and compression of airless, hypoplastic left lungs. Relative paucity of intra-abdominal bowel loops.

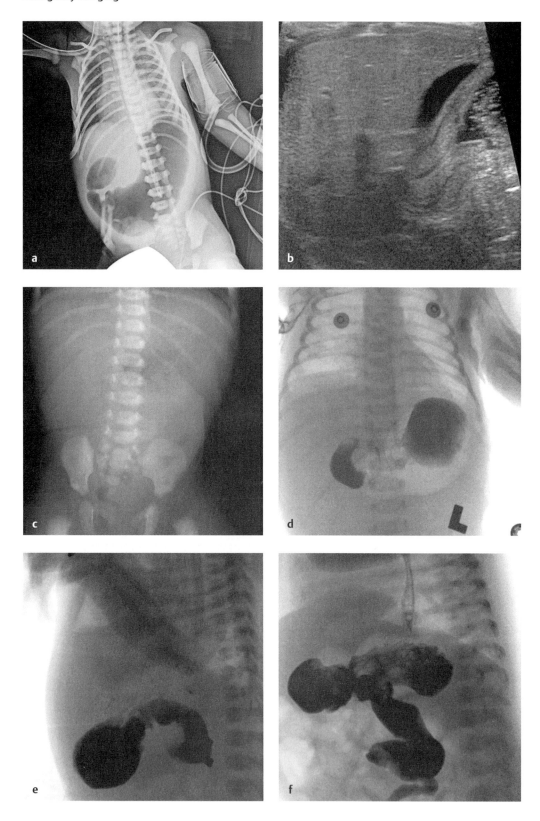

◆ Proximal Bowel Obstruction

Duodenal atresia, stenosis, or web are the most common causes of proximal bowel obstruction in the neonate. Clinical findings are abdominal distention, vomiting, and failure to pass meconium. In cases of complete atresia, the distal bowel will not contain gas. Because obstruction is usually distal to the pancreatic ampulla, vomiting in duodenal atresia is usually bilious. Associated congenital disorders are common and include Down syndrome and the VACTERL association (vertebral defects, anal atresia, cardiac defects, tracheoesophageal fistula, renal anomalies, and limb abnormalities).

Radiographs show a dilated stomach and small bowel proximal to the obstruction. The "double bubble" sign corresponds to isolated air-filled distended stomach and duodenal bulb separated by the normal pylorus. Ultrasonography may also reveal similar findings perinatally, but duodenal atresia is often not detectable until the mid to late second trimester. Incomplete duodenal obstruction may show gas in distal bowel loops and is seen with duodenal webs and stenosis. Annular pancreas or volvulus can present with a similar clinical and imaging picture.

Surgical correction is required, and the prognosis is excellent, especially in nonsyndromic cases.

Pyloric stenosis is idiopathic hypertrophy of the pylorus muscle, leading to gastric outlet obstruction. It is more common in males than in females and usually presents between 3 and 6 weeks of age with gradual development of nonbilious projectile vomiting. Occasionally the hypertrophied pylorus muscle can be palpated as an olive-sized mass in the upper right quadrant.

Abdominal radiographs in pyloric stenosis may show a dilated, gas-filled stomach. Ultrasound is diagnostic; the pyloric channel is thickened and elongated with a length exceeding 12 mm and muscle thickness greater than 3 mm.

Emergent management consists of bowel rest, volume resuscitation, and correction of any electrolyte abnormalities. Definitive treatment is surgical pyloromyotomy.

Midgut volvulus is due to failure of normal small-bowel fixation (malrotation) or to congenital fibrous bands that permit twisting of the proximal small bowel about its mesentery with potential bowel ischemia and necrosis. Most cases occur in the first week of life, presenting with bilious vomiting and abdominal distention.

Imaging diagnosis is by upper gastrointestinal examination. Complete duodenal or proximal jejunal obstruction will be evident, sometimes with "beaking" at the point of obstruction.

Management is surgical, with lysis of Ladd bands (if present) and detorsion of any twisted bowel. Complications include bowel necrosis and septicemia. Short gut syndrome and malabsorption may result if extensive bowel resection is necessary (**Fig. 8.8**).

Fig. 8.8a–f
a Double bubble sign in complete duodenal atresia. Markedly distended air-filled stomach and proximal duodenum. The remainder of the abdomen is entirely gasless.
b Pyloric stenosis. The pylorus is thickened and elongated measuring 18 mm in length and 6 mm in wall thickness.
c–f Midgut volvulus. (**c**) Air-filled, mildly distended stomach with paucity of distal bowel gas. (**d,e**) Contrast-filled distal duodenum tapers to a "beak." (**f**) Postrepair study shows passage of contrast to small bowel.

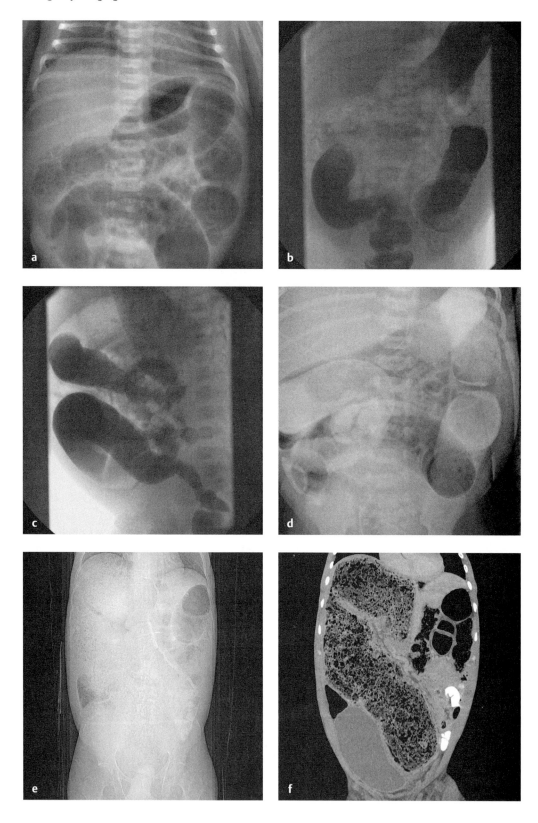

◆ Hirschsprung Disease

Hirschsprung disease, a common cause of neonatal colonic obstruction, is due to congenital absence of ganglion cells in the rectum and distal colon and is usually seen in full-term neonates who fail to pass meconium in the first 48 hours following birth. It is more common in males and is only rarely seen in premature infants. Although Hirschsprung disease is often an isolated abnormality, it can be associated with Down syndrome and multiple endocrine neoplasia type II.

Abdominal radiographs of the neonate with Hirschsprung disease show bowel obstruction: multiple dilated loops of large and small intestine with air-fluid levels. The affected colonic segment is typically small in caliber, with normal or dilated co-lon proximal to the transition, which usually occurs at the rectosigmoid junction. No gas or stool is seen in the rectum. Contrast enema may be helpful in diagnosis and evaluation of length of involvement, and imaging findings include a transition zone, abnormal or irregular contractions of the aganglionic segment, thickening or nodularity of the colonic mucosa, and delayed evacuation of contrast material. While a transition zone is considered highly suggestive of Hirschsprung disease, its absence does not rule out the diagnosis.

Treatment consists of removal of the poorly functioning aganglionic bowel and creation of an anastomosis from the proximal, unaffected colon to the distal rectum (**Fig. 8.9**).

Fig. 8.9a–f
a–d Hirschsprung disease in a newborn. (**a**) Radiograph shows distended bowel with mottled contents. (**b–d**) Contrast enema and subsequent radiograph with narrowed rectosigmoid and marked proximal colonic dilatation.
e,f Adult with Hirschsprung disease. Massively dilated, stool-filled colon.

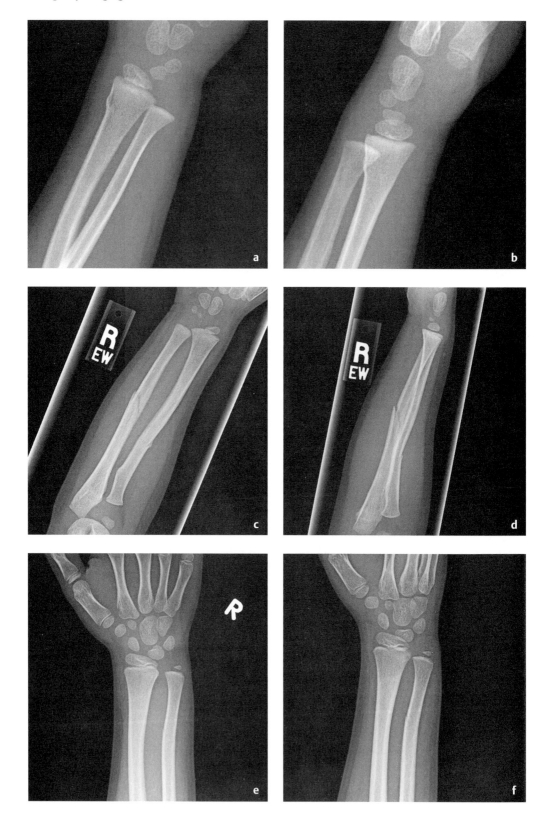

◆ Incomplete and Impacted Pediatric Fractures

Buckle or torus fractures of the forearm are extremely common in children after a fall on an outstretched hand. The mechanism is an axial loading force along the axis of the extremity that results in compression of the trabecular bone and bulging of the adjacent cortex without a distinct transverse fracture line. Subtle cortical buckling or angulation may be the only radiographic finding.

Treatment consists of immobilization and prompt orthopedic follow-up. These fractures have a good prognosis, and complications are quite rare.

Greenstick fractures are incomplete fractures of long bones of children that result from forces perpendicular to the axis of the bone. Young children have more compliant long bones that have a greater tendency to bow and bend under stress rather than fracture. Greenstick fractures consist of a complete fracture or cortical disruption of the bone opposite the impacted side while the ipsilateral cortex remains intact.

Treatment of a greenstick fracture consists of closed reduction and immobilization (**Fig. 8.10**).

Fig. 8.10a–f
a,b Buckle (torus) fracture. Skeletally immature; mild cortical buckling along the radial aspect of the radial metaphysis. No displacement or angulation.
c,d Greenstick fracture. Skeletally immature. Distal radial and ulnar bowing with apex volar angulation and with incomplete disruption of the volar cortices of both bones.
e,f Subtle greenstick fracture. Skeletally immature. The distal ulnar diaphysis is bowed toward the radius with subtle disruption of the radial aspect of the distal ulnar cortex.

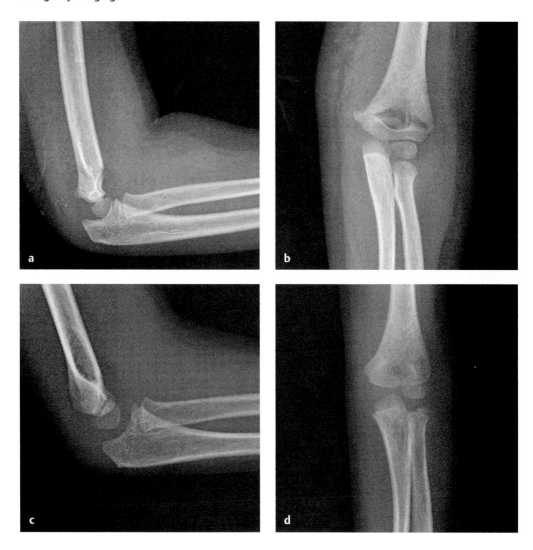

◆ Humeral Supracondylar Fracture

Humeral supracondylar fractures involve the distal humerus above the joint capsule, with highest incidence in children between the ages of 3 and 11. Supporting connective tissue about the elbow is fully developed by age 20, and ligamentous strains without associated fracture are more typical of adult injuries. Comminuted supracondylar fractures can be seen in osteopenic adults and the elderly, particularly women over 80.

AP and lateral radiographs are usually adequate for diagnosis, but oblique views may be helpful for fracture definition. Supracondylar fractures can be subtle and can be completely invisible in children, indicated only by the presence of an elbow effusion following trauma. On lateral radiographs, the anterior humeral fat pad should closely parallel the anterior humer-

al cortex. With elbow effusions, this fat pad is elevated and resembles a sail (sail sign). The posterior fat pad is normally hidden on the lateral view but becomes visible when dorsally displaced by an elbow effusion. In children, a line drawn along the anterior humeral cortex should intersect the middle third of the capitellum on the lateral view; with angulated supracondylar fractures, this relationship is disrupted.

Fractures can be described as undisplaced (type I), displaced with intact cortex (type II), or completely displaced (type III). Type I injuries are stable and can be managed with immobilization and analgesia. Type II and III injuries need orthopedic consultation for definitive management, which usually consists of open reduction and plate fixation (**Fig. 8.11**).

Fig. 8.11a–d
a,b Transverse supracondylar fracture with dorsal angulation. The anterior humeral line does not intersect the capitellum on the lateral view. Anterior and posterior fat pad signs are both present. The fracture is subtle on the lateral view but apparent on frontal view as a transverse lucency in the distal humeral metaphysis.
c,d Subtle supracondylar fracture. Large elbow effusion with anterior and posterior fat pad signs. Normal anterior humeral line–capitellar alignment.

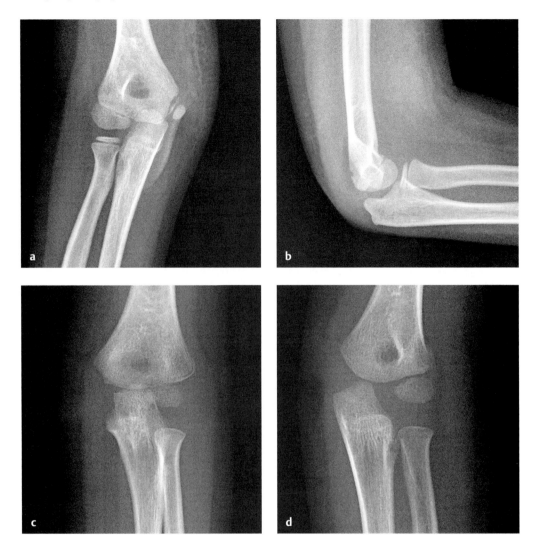

◆ Humeral Epicondyle Avulsion Fractures

Medial epicondylar fractures are the most common avulsion fractures at the elbow and are typically seen in children and adolescents who fall on an outstretched hand with the elbow extended. The epicondyle does not fuse to the distal humerus until approximately age 20, accounting for both acute avulsions as well as chronic injuries due to repeated valgus stress from ball throwing. Common in adolescent baseball players, "Little League elbow" is characterized by a widened medial epicondylar physeal plate and fragmentation. Comparison with the opposite normal elbow is helpful for detecting subtle injuries.

Patients present with localized pain over the epicondyle, increased with flexion of the elbow or pronation of the forearm. In transient dislocation, the avulsed epicondylar fragment can be entrapped within the elbow joint. The ulnar nerve may be directly injured or secondarily impaired by soft tissue edema.

Because a detached and entrapped fragment from the medial epicondyle can be mistaken for the normal trochlear ossification center, it is important to appreciate the normal order in which elbow epiphyseal ossification centers appear on radiographs. This begins at 6 months, is usually complete by 12 years, and is summarized by the mnemonic CRITOE: capitellum, radial head, internal (medial) epicondyle, trochlea, olecranon, external (lateral) epicondyle.

The trochlear ossification should never be visible unless the medial epicondyle is already ossified in its normal position. If an apparent trochlear ossification is the only medial fragment seen after trauma, an avulsed medial epicondyle should be diagnosed. Contralateral comparison views can be very useful in this setting.

Humeral epicondyle avulsion fractures that are nondisplaced or only minimally displaced (< 4 mm) can be managed nonoperatively with immobilization in a long-arm posterior splint. The elbow is flexed to 90° with the forearm in neutral or pronation.

Lateral epicondyle avulsion fractures are much less common than medial avulsions. The clinical mechanism is similar: a fall on an outstretched arm, with avulsion of the common extensor muscle origin rather then the flexor/pronator muscle attachment. Treatment is similar, with immobilization for nondisplaced or minimally displaced fractures and internal fixation for those with significant displacement (**Fig. 8.12**).

Fig. 8.12a–d
a,b Medial epicondyle avulsion fracture. The medial epicondylar ossification center is displaced 5 mm from the medial humerus. A linear bone flake is interposed between the ossification center and the medial distal humerus. Moderate associated elbow effusion, with anterior and posterior fat pad signs. All ossification centers except for the lateral epicondyle have appeared.
c,d Lateral epicondyle avulsion fracture. Subtle cortical separation at the lateral humeral epicondyle.

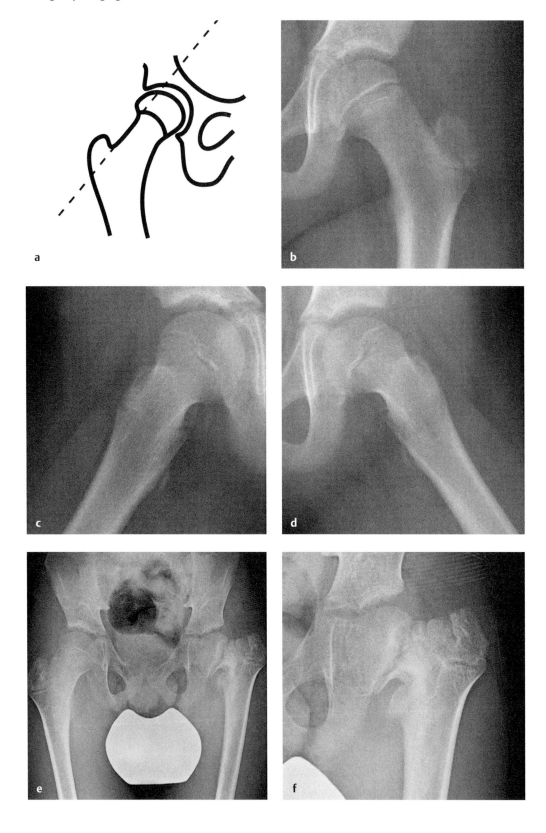

◆ Slipped Capital Femoral Epiphysis

Slipped capital femoral epiphysis (SCFE) is a Salter-Harris type I growth plate injury in which the femoral epiphysis slips posteriorly with respect to the metaphysis, with consequent hip or knee pain and impaired internal rotation. Likely related to repeated microtrauma in predisposed patients, it is often diagnosed in adolescence and is more common in overweight children.

Imaging investigation should include a frog-leg lateral view in addition to the standard AP hip radiograph. In the preslip phase, the physis may appear widened with adjacent metaphyseal demineralization. An acute SCFE occurs posteriorly, and to a lesser extent medially, and is best seen on the frog-leg view, where the offset epiphysis and metaphysis are better visualized. This can be described as "ice cream slipping off a cone." The height of the epiphysis may also be decreased as the femoral head rotates posteriorly with the slippage.

The patient should be made non-weight-bearing with urgent referral to a pediatric orthopedic surgeon for pinning. Early recognition and treatment is important because, left untreated, SCFE may progress to leg length discrepancy, avascular necrosis of the femoral head, or chondrolysis (**Fig. 8.13**).

Fig. 8.13a–f
a A line drawn along the superolateral edge of the femoral neck (Klein line) should normally intersect a portion of the epiphysis. In slipped femoral capital epiphysis, the Klein line will be lateral to the epiphysis.
b–d Acute SCFE. (**b**) AP view of the hip shows subtle blurring of physeal plate but near-anatomic alignment. (**c,d**) Frog-leg lateral view with comparison of right and left hips shows slight but definite medial displacement of the symptomatic left femoral head with respect to the neck.
e,f Chronic SCFE. Inferomedial slip of femoral head with sclerosis (indicating an element of avascular necrosis), proximal migration, and rotation of the femur.

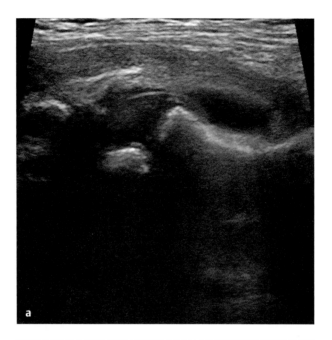

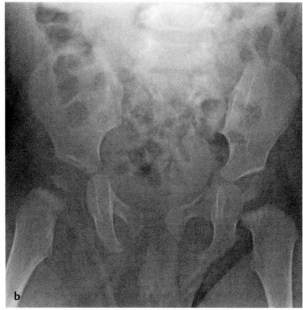

◆ Hip Effusion

A hip effusion indicates an inflammatory process or other abnormality within the joint. Children typically present with acute hip pain, joint stiffness, or limp—nonspecific symptoms that can be seen in several conditions, including septic arthritis, osteomyelitis, and transient synovitis, among others.

Septic arthritis or osteomyelitis require prompt diagnosis and treatment to prevent permanent joint damage. Fever, elevated white blood cell count, increased erythrocyte sedimentation rate, and elevated C-reactive protein indicate a likely infectious etiology and should prompt hip aspiration. Transient synovitis, which appears as pain or limp in a young, otherwise well child, is a diagnosis of exclusion. These patients may have blood tests that show mild inflammation but otherwise have a self-limited process.

Hip effusion can be seen on AP plain radiograph as widening of the teardrop distance, defined as the distance from the lateral margin of the pelvic teardrop to the most medial aspect of the femoral head. Unfortunately, this finding is not very sensitive, and ultrasound is preferred for identification of effusion in the child with hip pain with no history of trauma.

An effusion will appear as a hypoechoic collection ballooning out from the cortex of the femoral head when viewed along the long axis of the femoral metaphysis. Although ultrasound is particularly helpful in the diagnosis of hip effusion, it is unable to differentiate between a sterile and purulent effusion. Consequently, if there is a high suspicion of infection, an ultrasound-guided aspiration of joint fluid should be performed (**Fig. 8.14**).

Fig. 8.14a,b Hip effusion in a child with septic arthritis. The right femoral head is displaced laterally with respect to the acetabulum. Lentiform hypoechoic collection superficial to the proximal femoral metaphysis on ultrasound.

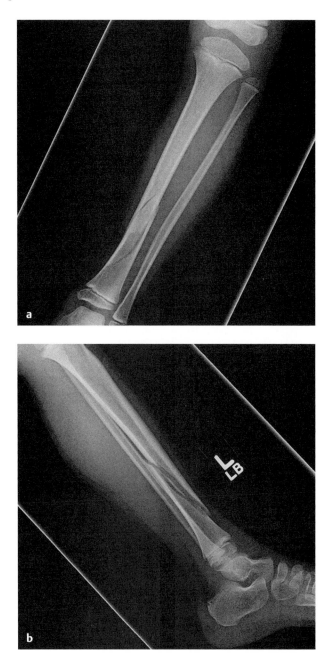

◆ Toddler Fracture

Toddler fractures are spiral fractures of the distal lower extremity seen in newly ambulating toddlers. Most are nondisplaced and occur in children under 3 years of age. These fractures result from external rotation of the foot relative to the knee with failure of newly developing bone. They are common and do not indicate child abuse.

AP, lateral, and mortise views of the ankle should be obtained to exclude concomitant ankle injury. Multiple views may be necessary, as the fracture may not be apparent on one or even two views. Frac-

tures may be subtle or invisible, and sclerosis and periosteal reaction may be the only radiographic signs of injury. Repeat images obtained 7 to 10 days after injury are sometimes helpful if there is strong clinical suspicion of fracture and initial radiographs are unrevealing.

Toddler fractures are generally treated with a long-leg cast for 2 to 3 weeks followed by a short-leg walking cast for an additional 2 to 3 weeks. Prognosis is excellent, with complications exceedingly rare (**Fig. 8.15**).

Fig. 8.15a,b Toddler fracture. Spiral fracture of the proximal tibial diaphysis with slight dorsal displacement of the distal fragment. The fibula is intact.

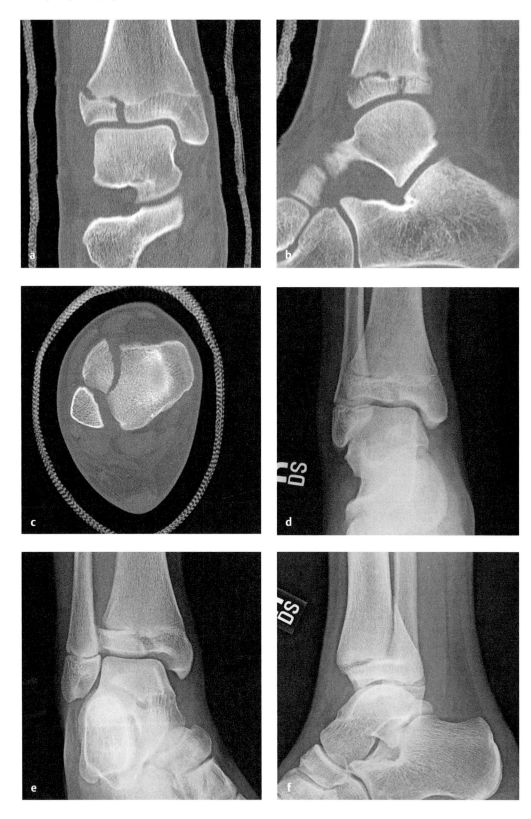

◆ Tillaux and Triplane Fracture

The Tillaux fracture is a Salter-Harris type III fracture in which the anterolateral aspect of the tibial epiphysis is avulsed by stress on the anterior tibiofibular ligament. It is common among older adolescents in whom the anterolateral growth plate has not yet completely fused, and it is usually caused by external rotation of the ankle.

Tillaux fractures are usually diagnosed with plain radiographs but often require CT for operative planning. The mortise view is most helpful for detection of the fracture because in this view the lateral tibia is not obstructed by the fibula and the talar dome may be visualized best. The Tillaux fracture is distinguished from the triplane fracture by the absence of a coronal component when evaluated on lateral view or CT.

A triplane fracture is a Salter-Harris type IV fracture of the distal tibial physis in coronal, sagittal, and transverse planes. Distal fibula fractures also frequently occur with this fracture. Triplane fractures occur in adolescence before complete closure of the distal tibial physis and consist of a sagittal fracture through the epiphysis, a transverse fracture through the physis, and an oblique or coronal fracture through the metaphysis. The characteristic pattern of a triplane fracture results from the asymmetric closure of the growth plate. The medial tibial physis closes first, followed by the lateral physis.

On AP view, the sagittal fracture may be seen as a vertically oriented lucency through the anterior epiphysis, usually at the midportion of the tibial plafond. The coronal fracture is best seen on lateral view and involves the posterior tibial metaphysis and a portion of attached epiphysis. The axial fracture is difficult to appreciate on radiograph but occurs through the physis.

Triplane fractures may occur as two-, three-, or four-part fractures depending on the number of fragments produced. Two-part fractures are the most common and consist of the lateral epiphysis attached to the posterior metaphyseal spike and the distal tibia with the anteromedial epiphysis. Three-part fractures consist of a large rectangular anterolateral fragment of the epiphysis, the epiphysis attached to a posterolateral spike of the tibial metaphysis, and the distal tibia attached to the remainder of the tibial metaphysis and a small portion of the anteromedial epiphysis. Four-part fractures include a fourth fragment that arises from the medial malleolus.

CT accurately characterizes these fractures for operative planning. Nondisplaced triplane fractures (less than 2 mm displacement) and extra-articular fractures may be managed with immobilization in a short-leg cast; all other fractures warrant operative fixation (**Fig. 8.16**).

Fig. 8.16a–f
a–c Tillaux fracture. The anterolateral physeal plate is widened with lateral displacement of an anterolateral epiphyseal fragment. The posterior physeal plate is fused, and there is no metaphyseal component.
d–f Two-part triplane fracture. The anterolateral physeal plate is widened with lateral displacement of an anterolateral epiphyseal fragment. The posterior aspect of the epiphyseal fragment is fused to a triangular portion of the metaphysis, separated from the distal tibia in the coronal plane.

Index

Note: Page numbers followed by f or t indicate figures or tables, respectively.

A

AAST. *See* American Association for the Surgery of Trauma
abdomen and pelvis checklist, 268
abdomen and pelvis imaging, 267–397.
    See also specific conditions of the abdomen and pelvis
– checklist, 268
abdominal abscess, 364f, 365
abdominal aortic aneurysm, 372f, 373
abdominal foreign bodies, 334f, 335
abdominal lymphoma, 366f, 367
abscesses
– abdominal, 364f, 366
– brain, 64f, 65
– buccal space, 134f, 135
– epidural, 184f, 185
– hepatic, 318f, 319
– lung, 240f, 241
– masticator space, 134f, 135
– odontogenic, 134f, 135
– orbital, 138f, 139
– peritonsillar, 120f, 121
– prevertebral, 122f, 123
– renal, 322f, 323
– retropharyngeal, 120f, 121
– submandibular, 134f, 135
– tubo-ovarian, 388f, 389
abuse. *See* nonaccidental trauma
acetabular fracture, 448f, 449
achalasia, 224f, 225
Achilles tendon rupture, 464f, 465
acromioclavicular separation, 412f, 413
acute pediatric pneumonia, 516f, 517
adenocarcinoma
– of the lung, 260f, 261
– of the pancreas, 300f, 301
adenoma, adrenal, 328f, 329
adrenal adenoma, 328f, 329
adrenal hemorrhage, 330f, 331
adrenal myelolipomas, 328f, 329
adrenal nodules and masses, 328f, 329
adverse reaction classification, 6t
American Association for the Surgery of Trauma
– grading for hepatic injury, 283t
– grading for renal injury, 285t
– grading for splenic injury, 281t
amyloid angiopathy, 46f, 47
anatomy
– abdomen and pelvis, 271

– chest, 206, 207f
anatomy, and imaging
– abdomen and pelvis, 268–271
– brain, 10, 11f, 12f–13f
– chest, 205–206
– head and neck, 86–87, 87f, 88f
– mandible, 106f
– pediatric, 507–509
anchors, orthopedic, 406f
aneurysmal bone cyst, 490f, 491
angiography, of the neck, after trauma, 84
angiography, images
– arteriovenous malformation, 50f
– nasopharyngeal masses, 114f
– spinal dural arteriovenous fistula, 196f
– subarachnoid hemorrhage, 48f
ankle fracture, 466f, 467
ankle fracture fixation, 404f
ankle, septic arthritis in, 484f, 485
ankylosing spondylitis, 190f, 191
anoxic injury, 54f, 55
anterior cruciate ligament (ACL) injury, 452f, 453
anterior shoulder dislocation, 414f, 415
anterior spinal compression fracture, 172f, 173
anterior-posterior compression pelvis fracture, 446f, 447
aortic dissection, 228f, 229
aortic injury, traumatic, 222f, 223
aortic rupture, nontraumatic, 228f, 229
apical petrositis. *See* petrous apicitis
appendicitis, 348f, 349
appendix testis, torsed, 392f, 393
arachnoid cyst, 18f, 19
arachnoid granulation, 18f, 19
arterial cerebral infarct, 58f, 59
arteriogram, CT
– imaging protocols
–– brain, 10
–– neck, 85–86
arteriovenous fistula, spinal dural, 196f, 197
arteriovenous malformation, 50f, 51
– pulmonary, 244f, 245
arthritis
– rheumatoid, 502f, 503
– septic, 484f, 485, 536f
arthropathy
– neuropathic, 504f, 505
– total hip, 406f

aspirated foreign body, 518f, 519
atlantoaxial rotatory subluxation, 158f, 159
atlantooccipital dislocation, 156f, 157
atrophy, posttraumatic, 42f, 43
avascular necrosis, 500f, 501

B

B-cell lymphoma, 366f, 367
bacterial meningitis, 70f, 71
Baker cyst, 460f, 461
Balthazar grading for acute pancreatitis, 296f, 297, 297t
Bankart lesion, 415
Bankart lesion, reverse, 416f, 417
base of thumb fractures, 438f, 439
basicervical fracture, 450f, 451
Bellevue Hospital Radiology Department practice policy, 4, 5–7
benign pneumatosis coli, 362f, 363
Bennett fracture, 438f, 439
bilateral interfacet dislocation, 167
bladder injury, 290f, 291
Bochdalek hernias, 522f, 523
body packing, 334f, 335
Boehler angle, 470f, 471
Boerhaave syndrome, 226f, 227
bone lesions, lucent, 488f, 489, 490f, 491
bone scan. *See* radionuclide bone scan, images
boutonniere deformity, 442f, 443
bowel ischemia and necrosis, acute, 344f, 345
boxer's fracture, 436f, 437
brain abscess, 64f, 65
brain imaging, 9–81. *See also specific conditions of the brain*
branchial cleft cyst, 132f, 133
breast carcinoma
– pulmonary metastasis, 264f, 265
– skeletal metastasis, 492f, 493
bronchial rupture, 220f, 221
bronchiectasis, 238f, 239
bronchiolar inflammation, 516f, 517
bronchiolitis, 516f, 517
bronchogenic carcinoma, 260f, 261
bucket-handle fracture, 447
buckle (torus) fracture, 528f, 529
Budd-Chiari syndrome, 308f, 309
bursitis, 482f, 483
burst fracture, 172f, 173
buttress plates, 405f

543

C

C1 burst (Jefferson) fracture, 158f, 159
C2 spondylolisthesis, traumatic, 162f, 163
calcaneal fracture, 470f, 471
calvarial fracture, 20f, 21
cancellous screws, 403f
cannulated screws, 403f
carcinomas
– breast
–– pulmonary metastasis, 264f, 265
–– skeletal metastasis, 492f, 493
– bronchogenic, 260f, 261
– cholangiocarcinoma, 314f, 315
– head and neck, metastatic, 130f, 131
– hepatocellular, 312f, 313
– lung, skeletal metastasis, 492f, 493
– ovarian, 380f, 381
– prostate, skeletal metastasis, 492f, 493
– renal cell, 326f, 327
– renal cell, skeletal metastasis, 492f, 493
– testicular, 396f, 397
carotid space, 86, 87f
catheters, 6, 6t
cavernous hemangiomas, 52f, 53
cavernous malformation, 52f, 53
cavum septum pellucidum, 18f, 19
cecal volvulus, 340f, 341
cellulitis, 480f, 481
cerclage wires, 405f
cerebral contusion, 32f, 33
cerebral edema, 16f, 17
cerebral herniation, 40f, 41
cerebral infarct
– arterial, 58f, 59
– ischemic, 56f, 57
– venous, 60f, 61
cerebral metastasis, 78f, 79
cerebral swelling, 38f, 39
cerebritis, 64f, 65
cervical adenitis, 126f, 127
cervical developmental cysts and masses, 132f, 133
cervical hyperflexion teardrop fracture, 168f, 169
cervical lymph node levels, 88f
cervical spine hyperextension injury, 170f, 171
cervical spine hyperflexion injury, 166f, 167, 168f, 169
cervical spine measurements, 151
cervical vascular injury, 110f, 111
Chance fracture, 174f, 175
chauffeur's fracture, 428f, 429
checklists
– abdomen and pelvis, 268
– chest, 205
– face/neck, nontraumatic, 84
– facial trauma, 83–84
– musculoskeletal, 400–402
– spine, 152
chest checklist, 205
chest imaging, 205–266. *See also specific conditions of the chest*
– checklist, 205
chest wall injuries, 212f, 213

choking injury, 110f, 111
cholangiocarcinoma, 314f, 315
cholecystitis, acute, 302f, 303
cholesteatoma, 146f, 147
choroidal fissure cyst, 18f, 19
cirrhosis, 306f, 307
clay shoveler fracture, 166f, 167
clinical presentation
– abdomen and pelvis imaging, 271–276
– brain imaging, 10, 14–15
– chest imaging, 206, 208–211
– head and neck imaging, 88–90
– musculoskeletal imaging, 408–409
– pediatric imaging, 509–510
– spine imaging, 153–154
CNS lymphoma, primary, 76f, 77
colitis
– ischemic, 346f, 347
– neutropenic, 354f, 355
– pseudomembranous, 354f, 355
– ulcerative, 358f, 359
Colles fracture, 428f, 429
colon carcinoma, liver metastasis, 316f, 317
compression plates, 404f
computed tomography (CT)
– contrast, 4, 5–7, 6t
– imaging protocols
–– abdomen and pelvis, 268–269
–– brain, 10
–– chest CT, 206
–– face CT (helical + contrast), 85
–– face CT (noncontrast helical), 85
–– head CT (noncontrast), 10
–– head CT (noncontrast helical), 10
–– neck CT (helical + contrast), 85
–– pediatric, 507
–– spine CT, 152
–– temporal bone CT, 86
– window and level, 3–4, 5f, 25f
congenital diaphragmatic hernia, 522f, 523
contrast-induced nephropathy, 7
contrast, CT, 4, 5–7, 6t
cortical plates, 404f
cortical screws, 403f, 404f
craniocervical junction injuries, 154f, 155
Crohn disease, 356f, 357
croup, 116f, 117
CT. *See* computed tomography (CT)
cystic fibrosis, 238f, 239
cysts
– aneurysmal bone, 490f, 491
– arachnoid, 18f, 19
– Baker, 460f, 461
– branchial cleft, 132f, 133
– choroidal fissure, 18f, 19
– dermoid, 132f, 133
– simple bone, 490f, 491
– thyroglossal, 132f, 133
cytotoxic edema, 16f, 17

D

dacryocystitis, 142f, 143
dancer's fracture, 478f, 479
Danis-Weber classification of fibular fracture, 467t
deep venous thrombosis, 230f, 231

degenerative joint disease. *See* osteoarthritis
demyelinating disease, 62f, 63
dens fracture, 162f, 163
dental disease, 134f, 135
Denver Modified Blunt Cerebrovascular Screening Criteria, 84
dermoid cyst, 132f, 133
diaphragm rupture, 278f, 279
diaphragmatic hernia, congenital, 522f, 523
differential diagnosis
– abdomen and pelvis imaging, 271–276
– brain imaging, 10, 14–15
– chest imaging, 206, 208–211
– head and neck imaging, 88–90
– musculoskeletal imaging, 408–409
– pediatric imaging, 509–511
– spine imaging, 153–154
diffuse axonal injury, 34f, 35
diffuse idiopathic skeletal hyperostosis, 180f
dinner fork deformity, 429
disk herniation, 188f, 189
diskitis, 182f, 183
dislocations
– anterior shoulder, 414f, 415
– atlantooccipital, 156f, 157
– bilateral interfacet, 169
– elbow, 420f, 421
– Essex-Lopresti fracture-dislocation, 422f, 423
– fracture-dislocation of the spine, 178f, 179
– Lisfranc fracture-dislocation, 476f, 477
– lunate, 432f, 433
– perilunate, 432f, 433
– posterior shoulder, 416f, 417
– spine fracture-dislocation, 176f, 177
– sternoclavicular, 212f, 213
– unilateral interfacet, 168f, 169
distal articular fracture, 434f, 435
distal radius fractures, 428f, 429
diverticulitis, 360f, 361
dorsal plate avulsion fracture, 444f, 445
double bubble sign, 524f, 525
drugs. *See* body packing
duodenal atresia, 524f, 525
duodenal perforation, 294f, 295
dynamic hip screws, 404f

E

ectopic pregnancy, ruptured, 390f, 391
edema
– cerebral, 16f, 17
– cytotoxic, 16f, 17
– interstitial, 16f, 17
– pulmonary, 248f, 249
– vasogenic, 16f, 17
Edwards classification, 164f, 165
Effendi/Levine classification, 164f, 165
Ehler-Danlos syndrome, 111
elbow bursitis, 482f, 483
elbow dislocation, 420f, 421
elbow, septic arthritis in, 484f, 485
emergency imaging, generally, 1–7
emphysema, 250f, 251
empyema, 242f, 243
encephalomalacia, 42f, 43

enchondroma, 488f, 489
enlarged perivascular space, 18f, 19
enterocolitis, necrotizing, 520f, 521
ependymoma, 202f, 203
epididymitis, 394f, 395
epididymo-orchitis, 394f, 395
epidural abscess, 184f, 185
epidural hematoma, 22f, 23
– spinal, 180f, 181
epiglottitis, 116f, 117
epiploic appendagitis, 350f, 351
Epstein-Barr virus (EBV) infection, 114f,
    115, 118f, 119
esophagogram, images
– achalasia, 224f
– Boerhaave syndrome, 226f
Essex-Lopresti fracture-dislocation, 422f,
    423
external fixators, 406f
external otitis, necrotizing, 144f, 145

F

face/neck checklist, nontraumatic, 84
facial trauma checklist, 83–84
fasciitis, necrotizing, 480f, 481
femoral neck fractures, 450f, 451
fibrous dysplasia, 488f, 489
fibular fracture, 462f, 463
finger deformities, 442f, 443
flail chest, 214f, 215
fleck sign, 476f, 477
flexion-distraction injury of the spine,
    174f, 175
flow rate, of catheters, 6, 6t
fluoroscopy, images
– hepatic abscess, 318f
Foix-Alajouanine, 197f
forearm fractures, 426f, 427
foreign bodies
– abdominal, 334f, 335
– aspirated/swallowed, 518f, 519
fracture
– acetabular, 448f, 449
– ankle, 466f, 467
– anterior spinal compression, 172f, 173
– anterior-posterior compression pelvis,
    446f, 447
– base of thumb, 438f, 439
– basicervical, 450f, 451
– Bennett, 438f, 439
– boxer's, 436f, 437
– bucket-handle, 447
– buckle (torus), 528f, 529
– burst, 172f, 173
– C1 burst (Jefferson), 160f, 161
– calcaneal, 470f, 471
– calvarial, 18f, 19
– cervical hyperflexion teardrop, 168f, 169
– Chance, 174f, 175
– chauffeur's, 428f, 429
– clay shoveler, 166f, 167
– Colles, 428f, 429
– dancer's, 478f, 479
– dens, 162f, 163
– distal articular, 434f, 435
– distal radius, 428f, 429
– dorsal plate avulsion, 444f, 445

– Essex-Lopresti fracture-dislocation,
    422f, 423
– femoral neck, 450f, 451
– fibular, 462f, 463
– forearm, 426f, 427
– fused-spine, 178f, 179
– Galeazzi, 426f, 427
– greenstick, 528f, 529
– hamate, 434f, 435
– hangman's, 164f, 165
– humeral epicondyle avulsion, 532f, 533
– humeral head, 418f, 419
– humeral supercondylar, 530f, 531
– Hutchison, 428f, 429
– intertrochanteric, 450f, 451
– Jefferson, 158f, 159
– Jones, 478f, 479
– laryngeal, 108f, 109
– Le Fort, 96f, 97, 97f
– Lisfranc fracture-dislocation, 476f, 477
– Maisonneuve, 462f, 463
– Malgaigne, 447
– malleolar, 466f, 467
– mandible, 106f, 107
– metacarpal neck, 436f, 437
– metaphyseal corner, 512f
– metatarsal, 478f, 479
– midface smash injury, 98f, 99
– Monteggia, 426f, 427
– nasal, 92f, 93
– naso-orbito-ethmoid, 92f, 93
– navicular, 474f, 475
– nightstick, 426f, 427
– nonscaphoid carpal, 434f, 435
– occipital condyle, 156f, 157
– odontoid (dens), 162f, 163
– orbital wall, 100f, 101
– osteochondral, 468f, 469
– patellar, 454f, 455
– pedicle, 164f, 165
– pelvis, 446f, 447
–– anterior-posterior compression, 446f,
    447
– pilon, 466f, 467
– pseudo-Jones, 478f, 479
– Rolando, 438f, 439
– scaphoid, 430f, 431
– scapular, 410f, 411
– Segond, 452f, 453
– skull, 20f, 21
– skull base, 18f, 19
– Smith, 428f, 429
– spinal compression, anterior, 172f, 173
– sternal, 212f, 213
– subcapital, 450f, 451
– subtalar, 472f, 473
– subtrochanteric, 450f, 451
– talar, 472f, 473
– temporal bone, 104f, 105
– tibial, 462f, 463
– tibial plateau, 458f, 459
– tibial spine avulsion, 452f, 453
– Tillaux, 540f, 541
– toddler, 538f, 539
– torus (buckle), 528f, 529
– triplane, 540f, 541
– triquetral, 434f, 435

– trochanter avulsion, 450f, 451
– ulnar olecranon, 424f, 425
– vertical shear pelvis, 446f, 447
– volar plate avulsion, 444f, 445
– zygomaticomaxillary complex, 94f, 95
fracture-dislocation of the spine, 176f,
    177
fused-spine fracture, 178f, 179

G

Galeazzi fracture, 426f, 427
gamekeeper's thumb, 440f, 441
garden spade deformity, 429
gastric lymphoma, 366f, 367
gastric outlet obstruction, 292f, 293
gastric ulcer, 292f, 293
giant cell tumor, 488f, 489
glioblastoma multiforme, 74f, 75
glioma, low-grade, 72f, 73
globe injury, 102f, 103
gout, 504f, 505
Goyrand fracture. *See* Smith fracture
Gradenigo syndrome, 149
grading, 2
grading, American Association for the
    Surgery of Trauma
– for hepatic injury, 283t
– for renal injury, 285t
– for splenic injury, 281t
grading, Balthazar, for acute pancreatitis,
    296f, 297, 297t
Graves myositis, 140f, 141
Graves orbitopathy, 140f, 141
greenstick fracture, 528f, 529

H

hamate fracture, 434f, 435
hardware, orthopedic, 402, 403f–408f
Hawkins classification of talus fractures,
    473t
head and neck imaging, 83–150. *See also*
    specific conditions of the head and neck
headless variable compression screws,
    403f
hematoma, subdural. *See* subdural
    hematoma
hemiarthroplasty, 406f–407f
hemorrhage
– adrenal, 330f, 331
– hypertensive, 44f, 45
– subarachnoid, 48f, 49
– subarachnoid, traumatic, 30f, 31
hemothorax, 216f, 217
hepatic abscess, 318f, 319
hepatic injury, 282f, 283
hepatic metastases, 316f, 317
hepatitis, 304f, 305
hepatocellular carcinoma, 312f, 313
hereditary hemorrhagic telangiectasia,
    64f, 65, 244f, 245
hernia
– Bochdalek, 522f, 523
– congenital diaphragmatic, 522f, 523
– incarcerated inguinal, 376f, 377
– Morgagni, 522f, 523
herpes simplex encephalitis, 66f, 67
Hill-Sachs lesion, 414f, 415

Hill-Sachs lesion, reverse, 416f, 417
hip effusion, 536f, 537
Hirschsprung disease, 526f, 527
HIV encephalitis, 62f, 63
Hodgkin lymphoma, 128f, 129, 254f, 255, 366f, 367
Houndsfield units (HU), 3, 3t
HU. *See* Houndsfield units (HU)
humeral epicondyle avulsion fracture, 532f, 533
humeral head fracture, 418f, 419
humeral supercondylar fracture, 530f, 531
Hutchison fracture, 428f, 429
hydrocephalus, 80f, 81
hygroma, subdural, 28f, 29
hypertensive hemorrhage, 44f, 45
hypoxic-ischemic injury, 54f, 55

I

imaging report, 1–2
immunodeficiency-associated lymphoproliferative disorder, 128f, 129
incarcerated inguinal hernia, 376f, 377
incidental findings, 2
inguinal hernia, incarcerated, 376f, 377
interference screws, 403f
interlocking nails, 406f
interstitial edema, 16f, 17
intertrochanteric fracture, 450f, 451
intramedullary nails, 406f
intussusception, 332f, 333
ischemic cerebral infarct, 56f, 57
ischemic colitis, 346f, 347

J

Jefferson fracture, 160f, 161
Jones fracture, 478f, 479
jugular vein thrombosis, 124f, 125
juvenile nasopharyngeal angiofibroma, 114f, 115

K

kidney. *See* renal
kidney injury. *See* renal injury
Kirschner wires (K-wires), 405f
Klatskin tumor, 314f
Klein line, 534f
knee bursitis, 482f, 483
knee prostheses, 408f
knee, ligamentous injuries of, 452f, 453
knee, septic arthritis in, 484f, 485

L

laryngeal fracture, 108f, 109
laryngotracheobronchitis. *See* croup
lateral compression pelvic fracture, 446f, 447
Le Fort fractures, 96f, 97, 97f
Lemierre syndrome, 124f, 125, 243
LeTournel acetabular fracture classification, 449t
ligamentous injuries of the knee, 452f, 453
lightbulb sign, 416f, 417
lingual thyroid, 132f, 133
Lisfranc fracture-dislocation, 476f, 477
Little League elbow, 532f, 533

liver. *See* hepatic
liver injury. *See* hepatic injury
liver masses, incidental, 310f, 311
low contact plates, 404f
low-grade glioma, 72f, 73
lucent bone lesions, 488f, 489, 490f, 491
lunate dislocation, 432f, 433
lung abscess, 240f, 241
lung cancer, 260f, 261
lung carcinoma, skeletal metastasis, 492f, 493
lung disease of prematurity, 514f, 515
luxatio erecta, 414f, 415
lymphangitic carcinomatosis, 264f, 265
lymphoma
– abdominal, 366f, 367
– B-cell, 366f, 367
– gastric, 366f, 367
– of the head and neck, 128f, 129
– Hodgkin, 128f, 129, 254f, 255, 366f, 367
– immunodeficiency-associated lymphoproliferative disorder, 128f, 129
– of the lungs, 254f, 255
– non-Hodgkin, 128f, 129
– primary CNS, 76f, 77
– T-cell, 254f, 255

M

magnetic resonance imaging (MRI)
– imaging protocols
–– spine MRI, 152–153
Maisonneuve fracture, 462f, 463
Malgaigne fracture, 447
malleolar fractures, 466f, 467
mallet finger, 442f, 443
mandible fracture, 106f, 107
Marfan syndrome, 111
Mason classification of radial head fracture, 423t
masticator space, 86, 87f
mastoiditis, 146f, 147
measurements, cervical spine, 151
measuring, 2
mediastinitis, 226f, 227
melanoma, adrenal metastasis, 328f, 329
meningioma, spinal, 200f, 201
meningitis, bacterial, 70f, 71
mesenteric adenitis, 352f, 353
metacarpal neck fractures, 436f, 437
metaphyseal corner fractures, 512f
metastasis
– adrenal, from melanoma, 328f, 329
– breast carcinoma
–– to the lung, 264f, 265
–– to the skeleton, 492f, 493
– cerebral, 78f, 79
– colon carcinoma, to the liver, 316f, 317
– hepatic, 316f, 317
– lung carcinoma, to the skeleton, 492f, 493
– ovarian carcinoma, to the lung, 264f, 265
– pancreatic carcinoma, to the liver, 316f, 317
– parotid carcinoma, to the lung, 264f, 265
– prostate carcinoma
–– to the liver, 316f, 317

–– to the skeleton, 492f, 493
– pulmonary, 264f, 265
– renal cell carcinoma, to the skeleton, 492f, 493
– spinal, 198f, 199
metatarsal fractures, 478f, 479
midface smash injury, 98f, 99
midgut volvulus, 524f, 525
millisieverts (mSv), 4, 4t
mononucleosis, 118f, 119
Monteggia fracture, 426f, 427
Morgagni hernias, 522f, 523
MRI. *See* magnetic resonance imaging (MRI)
mSv. *See* millisieverts (mSv)
multiple myeloma, 498f, 499
multiple sclerosis, 62f, 63
musculoskeletal imaging, 399–506. *See also specific conditions of the musculoskeletal system*
– checklists, 400–402
myelitis, 186f, 187
myelolipomas, adrenal, 328f, 329

N

nails, orthopedic, 406f
nasal fracture, 92f, 93
naso-orbito-ethmoid fracture, 92f, 93
nasopharyngeal masses, 114f, 115
National Emergency X-ray Utilization Study (NEXUS), 151
navicular fracture, 474f, 475
necrotizing enterocolitis, 520f, 521
necrotizing external otitis, 144f, 145
necrotizing fasciitis, 480f, 481
Neer classification system, 418f, 419
nephrolithiasis, 320f, 321
neurocysticercosis, 68f, 69
neuropathic arthropathy, 504f, 505
neutropenic colitis, 354f, 355
New York University Medical Center practice policy, 4, 5–7
NEXUS. *See* National Emergency X-ray Utilization Study (NEXUS)
nightstick fracture, 426f, 427
non-Hodgkin lymphoma, 128f, 129
nonaccidental trauma, 512f, 513
nonossifying fibroma, 490f, 491
nonscaphoid carpal fractures, 434f, 435

O

observing and reporting, 1
occipital condyle fractures, 156f, 157
odontogenic abscess, 134f, 135
odontoid (dens) fracture, 162f, 163
olecranon fracture, ulnar, 424f, 425
omental infarct, 350f, 351
orbital abscess, 138f, 139
orbital cellulitis, 138f, 139
orbital inflammatory disease, 140f, 141
orbital soft tissue injury, 102f, 103
orbital wall fractures, 100f, 101
orthopedic hardware, 402, 403f–408f
Osler-Weber-Rendu syndrome, 64f, 65
osteoarthritis, 502f, 503
osteochondral fracture, 468f, 469
osteomyelitis, 486f, 487
– vertebral, 182f, 183

osteonecrosis, 500f, 501
osteosarcoma, 494f, 495
otitis media, 146f, 147
otitis, necrotizing external, 144f, 145
ovarian carcinoma, 380f, 381
– pulmonary metastasis, 264f, 265
– staging, 381t
ovarian cysts, 378f, 379
ovarian cysts, ruptured, 384f, 385
ovarian teratoma, 382f, 383
ovarian torsion, 386f, 387

P

Paget disease of bone, 496f, 497
pancoast tumor, 262f, 263
pancreatic adenocarcinoma, 300f, 301
pancreatic carcinoma, liver metastasis,
   316f, 317
pancreatic injury, 286f, 287
pancreatic masses, 300f, 301
pancreatic necrosis, 298f, 299
pancreatitis
– acute, 296f, 297
– chronic, 298f, 299
parapharyngeal space, 86, 87f
parotid carcinoma, pulmonary
   metastasis, 264f, 265
parotid space, 86, 87f
patellar fracture, 454f, 455
patellar tendon rupture, 456f, 457
pediatric imaging, 507–541. *See also
   specific conditions affecting pediatric
   populations*
Pellegrini-Stieda disease, 452f, 453
pelvis and abdomen imaging, 267–397.
   *See also specific conditions of the pelvis
   and abdomen*
pelvis fracture, anterior-posterior
   compression, 446f, 447
pericardial effusion, 246f, 247
perilunate dislocation, 432f, 433
peritoneal carcinomatosis, 368f, 369
peritonsillar abscess, 120f, 121
perivascular space, enlarged, 18f, 19
petrous apicitis, 148f, 149
petrous temporal bone fracture, 20f, 21
pharyngeal mucosal space, 86, 87f
pilon fracture, 466f, 467
plasmacytoma, 498f, 499
plates, orthopedic, 404f–405f
pneumatosis coli, benign, 362f, 363
pneumocephalus, 36f, 37
pneumomediastinum, 252f, 253
pneumonia
– acute pediatric, 516f, 517
– aspiration, 232f, 233
– broncho-, 232f, 233
– influenza, 234f, 235
– interstitial, 234f, 235
– lobar, 232f, 233
– pneumocystis, 234f, 235
pneumothorax, 214f, 215
portal venous hypertension, 306f, 307
– postsinusoidal, 308f, 309
posterior cruciate ligament (PCL) injury,
   453
posterior shoulder dislocation, 416f, 417

postsinusoidal portal venous
   hypertension, 308f, 309
posttraumatic atrophy, 42f, 43
prevertebral abscess, 122f, 123
prevertebral space, 86, 87f
prostate carcinoma
– liver metastasis, 316f, 317
– skeletal metastasis, 492f, 493
prostheses, orthopedic, 407f–408f
proximal bowel obstruction, 524f, 525
pseudo-Jones fracture, 478f, 479
pseudomembranous colitis, 354f, 355
pulmonary arteriovenous malformation,
   244f, 245
pulmonary contusion, 218f, 219
pulmonary edema, 248f, 249
pulmonary embolism, 230f, 231
– septic, 240f, 241
pulmonary laceration, 218f, 219
pulmonary metastases, 264f, 265
pyelonephritis, 322f, 323
pyloric stenosis, 524f, 525

Q

quadriceps tendon rupture, 456f, 457

R

radial head fracture, 422f, 423
radiation doses, 4, 4t
radiation exposure, 507
radiculitis, 186f, 187
radiography
– imaging protocols
–– cervical spine, 152
–– chest, 205–206
–– lumbar spine, 152
–– pediatric, 507
–– thoracic spine, 150
radiology, learning, 2–3
radionuclide bone scan, images
– breast carcinoma, skeletal metastasis,
   492f
– giant cell tumor, 488f
– lucent bone lesions, 488f
– Paget disease of bone, 496f
– skeletal metastases, 492f
reconstruction plates, 404f
renal abscess, 322f, 323
renal calculi. *See* nephrolithiasis
renal cell carcinoma, 326f, 327
– skeletal metastasis, 492f, 493
renal colic. *See* nephrolithiasis
renal cyst, 326f, 327
renal infarct, 324f, 325
renal injury, 284f, 285
renal masses, 326f, 327
Rendu-Osler-Weber syndrome, 244f, 245
respiratory distress syndrome. *See* lung
   disease of prematurity
retroperitoneal hematoma, 374f, 375
retropharyngeal abscess, 120f, 121
retropharyngeal space, 86, 87f
reverse Bankart lesion, 416f, 417
reverse Barton fracture. *See* Smith
   fracture
reverse Colles fracture. *See* Smith fracture
reverse Hill-Sachs lesion, 416f, 417

rheumatoid arthritis, 502f, 503
Rolando fracture, 438f, 439

S

Salter-Harris classification of pediatric
   fractures, 509, 509f
sarcoidosis, 258f, 259
satisfaction of search, 399
scaphoid fracture, 430f, 431
scapholunate dissociation, 430f, 431
scapular fracture, 410f, 411
schwannoma, spinal, 200f, 201
sclerosing mesenteritis, 370f, 371
screws, orthopedic, 403f–404f
Segond fracture, 452f, 453
septic arthritis, 484f, 485, 536f
septic jugular thrombophlebitis, 124f,
   125
septic pulmonary embolism, 240f, 241
shock bowel, 288f, 289
shoulder dislocation
– anterior, 414f, 415
– posterior, 416f, 417
shoulder prostheses, 407f
sialadenitis, 136f, 137
sialodochitis, 136f, 137
sialolithiasis, 136f, 137
sigmoid volvulus, 342f, 343
simple bone cyst, 490f, 491
sinus obstruction and inflammation,
   112f, 113
sinusitis, 112f, 113
skeletal metastases, 492f, 493
skier's thumb, 440f, 441
skull base fracture
– anterior, 20f, 21
– posterior, 20f, 21
skull fracture, 20f, 21
slipped capital femoral epiphysis, 534f,
   535
small-bowel injury, 288f, 289
small-bowel obstruction, 336f, 337, 338f,
   339
Smith fracture, 428f, 429
spinal compression fracture, anterior,
   172f, 173
spinal cord infarct, 194f, 195
spinal dural arteriovenous fistula, 196f, 197
spinal epidural hematoma, 180f, 181
spinal meningioma, 200f, 201
spinal metastatic disease, 198f, 199
spinal schwannoma, 200f, 201
spine checklist, 152
spine hyperextension injury, cervical,
   170f, 171
spine hyperflexion injury, cervical, 166f,
   167, 168f, 169
spine, flexion-distraction injury of, 174f,
   175
spine, fracture-dislocation of, 176f, 177
spine imaging, 151–204. *See also specific
   conditions of the spine*
– checklist, 152
spine measurements, cervical, 151
splenic injury, 280f, 281
spondylolisthesis, 192f, 193, 193t
– traumatic C2, 164f, 165

spondylolysis, 192f, 193
sternal fracture, 212f, 213
sternoclavicular dislocation, 212f, 213
subarachnoid hemorrhage, 48f, 49
– traumatic, 30f, 31
subcapital fracture, 450f, 451
subdural hematoma
– acute, 24f, 25
– chronic, 26f, 27
– subacute, 26f, 27
subdural hygroma, 28f, 29
sublingual space, 86, 87f
submandibular space, 86, 87f
subtalar fracture, 472f, 473
subtrochanteric fracture, 450f, 451
suture anchors, 406f
swallowed foreign body, 518f, 519
swan neck deformity, 442f, 443

T

T-cell lymphoma, 254f, 255
talar fracture, 472f, 473
temporal bone fracture, 104f, 105
temporal bone imaging, 85
tendon rupture
– Achilles, 464f, 465
– patellar, 456f, 457
– quadriceps, 456f, 457
tension band wires, 405f
terrible triad, 420f, 421
testicular carcinoma, 396f, 397
testicular torsion, 392f, 393

three-dimensional reconstruction, images
– bowel ischemia and necrosis, acute, 344f
– fracture-dislocation of the spine, 176f, 177
– Le Fort fractures, 96f, 97f
– mandible fracture, 106f
– midface smash injury, 98f
– pelvic fractures, 446f, 447
– zygomaticomaxillary complex fracture, 94f
thymoma, 256f, 257
thyroglossal duct cyst, 132f, 133
tibial fractures, 462f, 463
tibial plateau fracture, 458f, 459
tibial spine avulsion fracture, 452f, 453
Tillaux fracture, 540f, 541
tissue densities, on CT, 3t
toddler fracture, 538f, 539
tonsillitis, 118f, 119
torsed appendix testis, 392f, 393
tracheobronchial rupture, 220f, 221
triplane fracture, 540f, 541
triquetral fracture, 434f, 435
trochanter avulsion fractures, 450f, 451
tuberculosis, 236f, 237
tubo-ovarian abscess, 388f, 389

U

ulcerative colitis, 358f, 359
ulnar olecranon fracture, 424f, 425

ultrasound
– imaging protocols
–– abdomen and pelvis, 269–270
–– pediatric, 508–509
unilateral interfacet dislocation, 168f, 169
urethral injury, 290f, 291

V

vascular injury, cervical, 110f, 111
vasogenic edema, 16f, 17
venogram, CT
– imaging protocols
–– brain imaging, 10
venous cerebral infarct, 60f, 61
venous sinus thrombosis, 60f, 61
vertebral osteomyelitis, 182f, 183
vertical shear pelvis fracture, 446f, 447
volar plate avulsion fracture, 444f, 445
voxels, 3

W

white matter disease, 62f, 63
window, CT, 3–4, 5f
wires, orthopedic, 405f

X

x-ray. *See* radiography; radiography, images

Z

zygomaticomaxillary complex fracture, 94f, 95